CARDIAC PACING

A Concise Guide to Clinical Practice

PHILIP VARRIALE, M.D.
Chief of Cardiology and
Attending Physician in Charge
Cardiac Pacemaker Division
Cabrini Medical Center
Attending Physician in Cardiology
St. Vincent's Hospital Medical Center
Associate Clinical Professor of Medicine
New York Medical College
New York

and

EMIL A. NACLERIO, M.D.
Attending Thoracic Surgeon and
Attending Surgeon in Charge
Cardiac Pacemaker Division
Cabrini Medical Center
Consultant in Thoracic Surgery
Harlem Hospital Center of Columbia University
Clinical Professor of Surgery
New York Medical College
New York

CARDIAC PACING

A Concise Guide to Clinical Practice

Lea & Febiger 1979 • *Philadelphia*

Library of Congress Cataloging in Publication Data

Varriale, Philip, 1934–
   Cardiac pacing.

   Bibliography.
   Includes index.
   1. Pacemakers, Artificial (Heart)   I.   Naclerio, Emil A., joint author.   II.   Title. [DNLM:
1.   Cardiac pacing, Artificial.   2.   Pacemaker, Artificial. WG168.3 C267]
RC684.P3V37   1979   617'.412   79–16691
ISBN 0–8121–0668–7

Published in Great Britain by Henry Kimpton Publishers, London

PRINTED IN THE UNITED STATES OF AMERICA

Print No.   3   2   1

To all pioneering cardiologists, surgeons, and

biomedical engineers who have made significant

contributions to the field of cardiac pacing

Preface

Steady and at times spectacular advances in the development of new and more reliable pacemaker power sources, circuits, and electrodes have led to the introduction of a wide variety of sophisticated and specialized pacemaker devices. Concomitant rapid expansion has occurred in the indications for cardiac pacing, techniques for pacing, hemodynamic benefits, and longevity of the implantable pacemaker system.

Recent pacemaker statistics attest to the pervasive import of electrical pacing and its widespread application to patient management as an incisive therapeutic modality. Approximately 400,000 people throughout the world are living with a pacemaker, and of these, over 150,000 live in the United States. The United States has the highest rate of new pacemaker implants in the world—approximately 60,000 each year.

This book is a compilation of the science, major developments, and current clinical applications of cardiac pacing. It describes the present state of the art and is intended for the needs of those who require a useful, authoritative and fundamental reference source. This book is designed to be comprehensive, concise, but not extensively detailed. It is a teaching document created by clinicians and teachers and written to present the wide scope of cardiac pacing to resident house officers, internists, surgeons, nurses, and bioengineers.

The editors have gathered together talented contributors who are prominent, active, and expert in the technology and practice of cardiac pacing. The underlying theme of this book underscores the fundamental electrophysiologic concepts of pacing, the role of pacing in the management of patients with cardiac dysrhythmias, and the methods and techniques that ensure the integrity and long-term success of the implantable pacemaker system.

Clinical principles and guidelines are stressed; established facts are emphasized and controversial issues are minimized. The reader seeking quick references to varied pacemaker concepts, problems, and solutions will find valuable source material with a minimum of difficulty. Selected current references presenting original and authoritative research and clinical experiences in cardiac pacing are included at the conclusion of each chapter.

To make the discussions of the various subjects complete in themselves, a certain amount of repetition has been unavoidable—and desirable. It is hoped that this has been held to a minimum.

The editors are particularly fortunate for the cooperation received in the preparation of this book. To the contributors who have so generously given of their time, the editors are most gratefully indebted.

The editors are grateful to Dr. Angelo Taranta, Director of Medicine, and Dr. Raymond D. LaRaja, Director of Surgery, at the Cabrini Medical Center of New York for their valuable assistance and encouragement in the preparation of this book. Our gratitude is extended to Dennis Hepp, Medtronic engineer, and Richard O. Martin, Ph. D., Intermedics engineer, for their advice relative to bioengineering concepts and to Maureen Wynne for her tedious efforts in typing the manuscripts.

We also acknowledge the kindness and support of Sr. Josephine Tsuei, M.S.C., President, and Mr. John Reilly, Executive Vice President, of Cabrini Medical Center of New York.

To our publishers, Lea & Febiger, we are indebted for their moral support and sympathetic understanding; to Mr. Ken Bussy, Executive Editor, for his constant help and valuable suggestions; to Miss Isabelle Clouser, copy editor, for her painstaking care and diligent review of the manuscript, and to Mr. Thomas Colaiezzi and Mr. Samuel Rondinelli, other staff members who made early publication of this book possible.

Finally, to our wives—Eileen Varriale and Gloria Naclerio—and to our children—Donna, Philip, and David Varriale and Emil Jr. and Ronald Naclerio—we wish to express our sincerest gratitude for their patience, understanding, and cooperation during the preparation of this book.

New York, N.Y.   PHILIP VARRIALE, M.D.
EMIL A. NACLERIO, M.D.

Contributors

WILLIAM C. BOAKE, M.D., Professor of Medicine, Section of Cardiology, Department of Medicine, University of Wisconsin Clinical Science Center; Consultant Cardiologist, William S. Middleton Veterans Administration Medical Center, Madison, Wisconsin.

ROBERT R. BROWNLEE, M.S.E.E., Senior Research Associate, Department of Electrical Engineering, The Pennsylvania State University, State College, Pennsylvania; Adjunct Associate Professor of Surgery, University of Texas Medical Branch, Galveston, Texas.

CHARLES L. BYRD, M.D., Clinical Assistant Professor of Surgery, University of Miami School of Medicine; Clinical Assistant of Surgery, University of Miami Medical School; Associate Attending, Department of Thoracic and Cardiovascular Surgery, Mount Sinai Medical Center of Greater Miami, Miami Beach, Florida.

WILLIAM M. CHARDACK, M.D., Associate Professor of Surgery, State University of New York at Buffalo School of Medicine; Thoracic Surgeon, Veterans Administration Medical Center, Buffalo, New York.

KHALID R. CHAUDRY, M.D., Research Associate in Cardiology, Lankenau Hospital, Philadelphia, Pennsylvania.

ANTHONY N. DAMATO, M.D., Chairman, Department of Medicine, Chief of Cardiology, U.S. Public Health Service Hospital, Staten Island, New York.

LEONARD S. DREIFUS, M.D., Professor of Physiology and Medicine, Jefferson Medical College of the Thomas Jefferson University; Head, Division of Cardiovascular Disease, The Lankenau Hospital, Philadelphia, Pennsylvania.

KENNETH W. EXWORTHY, M.S.E.E., Senior Engineer and Manager of EMC Department, Physiological Research Laboratory, A Division of Medtronic, Inc., Minneapolis, Minnesota.

PETER R. FOSTER, M.D., Assistant Professor of Medicine, Indiana University School of Medicine; Associate Director Coronary Care Unit, Wishard Memorial Hospital; Research Associate, Krannert Institute of Cardiology, Indianapolis, Indiana.

SEYMOUR FURMAN, M.D., Professor of Surgery, Albert Einstein College of Medicine of Yeshiva University; Attending Physician, Department of Surgery, Cardiothoracic Division, Montefiore Hospital and Medical Center, Bronx, New York.

JOSEPH ANTHONY C. GOMES, M.D., Assistant Chief of Cardiology, Cardiopulmonary Laboratory, U.S. Public Health Service Hospital, Staten Island, New York.

WILSON GREATBATCH, M.D., Adjunct Professor of Physical Sciences, Houghton College, Houghton; Chairman of the Board, Wilson Greatbatch Ltd., Clarence, New York.

GEORGE M. KRONCKE, M.D., Associate Professor of Surgery, Division of Cardiovascular and Thoracic Surgery, University of Wisconsin Clinical Science Center; Chief of Cardiovascular Surgery, William S. Middleton Veterans Administration Medical Center, Madison, Wisconsin.

RAYMOND P. KWA, M.D., Fellow in Cardiology, Cabrini Medical Center, New York, New York.

GERALD M. LEMOLE, M.D., Clinical Assistant Professor of Surgery, University of Pennsylvania College of Medicine; Chief of Surgery, Deborah Heart and Lung Center, Browns Mills, New Jersey.

JAMES J. MORRIS, Jr., M.D., Professor of Medicine, Division of Cardiology, Duke Medical Center, Durham, North Carolina.

DRYDEN MORSE, M.D., Assistant Professor, Thoracic Surgery, Temple University, Philadelphia, Pennsylvania; Director of Pacemaker Clinic, Deborah Heart and Lung Center, Browns Mills, New Jersey.

GEORGE H. MYERS, Ph.D., Technical Director, Pacemaker Center, Beth Israel Medical Center, Newark, New Jersey.

EMIL A. NACLERIO, M.D., Clinical Professor of Surgery, New York Medical College; Attending Thoracic Surgeon and Attending Surgeon in Charge, Cardiac Pacemaker Division, Cabrini Medical Center; Consultant in Thoracic Surgery, Harlem Hospital Center of Columbia University, New York, New York.

JOSEF NIZNIK, M.D., Fellow in Cardiology, Cabrini Medical Center, New York, New York.

SATOSHI OGAWA, M.D., Head, Noninvasive Laboratories, Department of Internal Medicine, Cardiopulmonary Division, Keio University School of Medicine, Tokyo, Japan.

ROBERT A. O'ROURKE, M.D., Professor of Medicine, Chief, Division of Cardiology, The University of Texas Health Science Center at San Antonio, San Antonio, Texas.

VICTOR PARSONNET, M.D., Clinical Professor of Surgery, New Jersey College of Medicine and Dentistry at Newark; Director of Surgery, Newark Beth Israel Medical Center, Newark, New Jersey.

DAVID CHAS. SCHECHTER, M.D., Clinical Associate Professor (Cardiovascular and Thoracic Surgery), New York Medical College; Member of the Surgery Staffs, St. Vincent's Hospital and Medial Center, Doctors Hospital, New York, New York.

ESTHER SHILLING, R.N., Pacemaker Clinician, Newark Beth Israel Medical Center, Newark, New Jersey.

NICHOLAS P.D. SMYTH, M.D., Associate Clinical Professor of Surgery, The George Washington University School of Medicine; Department of Surgery, Washington Hospital Center, D.C. General Hospital, Washington, D.C.; Prince Georges Hospital, Cheverly, Maryland.

THEODORE STERN, Vice-President, Neurometrics, Inc., Philadelphia, Pennsylvania.

G. FRANK O. TYERS, M.D., Professor and Chief, Division of Cardiovascular and Thoracic Surgery, The University of British Columbia, Vancouver, British Columbia, Canada.

PHILIP VARRIALE, M.D., Associate Clinical Professor of Medicine, New York Medical College; Chief of Cardiology and Attending Physician in Charge, Cardiac Pacemaker Division, Cabrini Medical Center; Attending Physician in Cardiology, St. Vincent's Hospital Medical Center, New York, New York.

RICHARD A. WALSH, M.D., Assistant Professor of Medicine, Division of Cardiology, The University of Texas Health Science Center; Co-Director, Cardiac Catheterization Laboratories, The University of Texas Health Science Center and Veterans Administration Hospital, San Antonio, Texas.

G. DOYNE WILLIAMS, M.D., Professor of Surgery, University of Arkansas, School of Medicine; Chief, Section of Cardiovascular Surgery, University Medical Center, Little Rock, Arkansas.

DENNISON YOUNG, M.D., Professor of Pediatric Cardiology, Albert Einstein College of Medicine of Yeshiva University; Director of Pediatric Cardiology, Montefiore Hospital and Medical Center, New York, New York.

ALLAN ZINBERG, Vice-President, Cardiac Data Corporation, Inc., Bloomfield, Connecticut.

DOUGLAS ZIPES, M.D., Professor of Medicine, Director of Cardiovascular Research, Division of Cardiology, Indiana University School of Medicine; Senior Research Associate, Krannert Institute of Cardiology; University Hospital; Wishard Memorial Hospital; Veterans Administration Hospital, Indianapolis, Indiana.

Contents

1

Cardiac Pacing in Perspective

DAVID CHAS. SCHECHTER

There is, in truth, no such thing as a method of discovery. It may come to one man after immense systematic analysis, to another by analogy, to a third as a sudden thought or vision, to yet another even as a dream, and in a hundred other ways. There is a method (or methods) of scientific demonstration, but that is a different thing from discovery. It is demonstration that is the basis of science.

—Professor Charles Singer, 1960

A purist might, with some justification, date the advent of cardiac pacing to 50 years ago, when Hyman designed an apparatus (later named "artificial pacemaker" by him) for the specific purpose of delivering electrical impulses at a physiologic rate to the heart in standstill. Doing so and then chronicling subsequent happenings in temporal order would, however, provide too simplistic and narrow an introduction to the background of what has become the dominant preoccupation of cardiac electrotherapy.

Cardiac pacing did not culminate from a natural and orderly procession of research enterprises aimed primarily at treating heart block. These came about, in fact, almost as an afterthought, whereas pacing eventuated from the conjunction of somewhat superficially interrelated clinical trials with electricity and laboratory inquiries on the

anatomic and physiologic bases of cardiac activity. For the sake of historical propriety, therefore, it is advisable to examine the evolution of cardiac pacing methodology and technology in broader perspective than that alluded to above, especially owing to latter-day diversification of pacing beyond the curtilage of the management of Morgagni-Adams-Stokes syndrome.

Parts of the narrative which follows will illustrate that, as is true of history in general, and maybe of medical history in particular, seldom can a distinguishable causality pattern be traced in the unfolding of major contributions to progress. The ledger shows that for every advance born by dint of prescience, persuasiveness, ratiocination, above-average working facilities, or just plain hard labor there has been a multitude of missed opportunities, mistaken notions, obdurate opposition, or steps backtracked

1

from hindsight. This aspect is emphasized with respect to cardiac electrostimulation because many descriptions of the effects of electricity on the heart derived not from studious laboratory investigations but rather from serendipitous clinical circumstances that antedated experimental testing. Paradoxically, further clinical employment frequently was delayed until laboratory testimony could be procured. Little wonder, then, that the recital of sundry "recent" techniques and instruments against the backdrop of eighteenth and nineteenth century ideas and efforts sometimes imparts a sense of déjà vu.

Virtually all headway in science may be credited to the concepts and undertakings of numerous persons, but such indebtedness to the collective need not detract from legitimately singling out certain people for special recognition. Its objective would be a due acknowledgment of outstanding endeavor rather than obsession with claims to priority. In that regard, remote events and personages are safer to catalog than current ones without running the risk of unintentionally causing offense.

EARLY EXPERIMENTS ON ANIMAL HEARTS

We who take for granted that cardiac activity can be subjected to all sorts of manipulation by electricity may find it hard to understand why, during much of the eighteenth century, there was doubt whether that agency really had any direct effect on heart muscle. However, the arguments which focused on this aspect should be contemplated in the light of the great polemics that lasted many score years concerning whether the fundamental biologic property of generation and transmission of cardiac impulse was neurogenic or myogenic. Inasmuch as "vital spirits" or "electrical fluid" was thought to be inchoate to nerve, proponents of the neurogenic theory generally had the upper hand.

Until generators of static electricity were

produced, it was widely held that the electrical force either was deadly (viz., lightning), or near-deadly (viz., the torpedo-fish). The Leyden jar and analogous contrivances bestowed on electricity a posologic dimension which enabled ruling the intensity of its actions. One of the earliest observations made soon after the clinical beginnings of electrotherapy in the mid-eighteenth century was that mild doses of electricity caused the heart to beat slightly faster. As Wesley, that zealot electrotherapist, put it in 1759,

> ". . . electricity communicates Activity and Motion to Fluids in general, and particularly accelerates the Motion of the Blood in an human Body. This is quickened three or four Pulses in half a Minute, by a Person only standing on Glass, and being electrified."

That the exposed heart of small animals was capable of being stimulated mechanically had been known even before Aristotle's biology treatises. Curiously, pre-Galvanian experimentation with static electricity on the heart fell far short of that made on skeletal muscles, and research on the resuscitative powers of electricity implied that these were mediated to the heart by a systemic or neural mechanism rather than by any influence on the myocardium itself.

And yet, clues that heart muscle was inherently electroresponsive were not lacking. In 1760, when von Haller touched the heart of one frog with the leg of another frog sparks were received on the crural nerve.

> ". . . we were pleased to observe that the heart rhythms became more frequent and stronger. . . . We believe we may conclude . . . that nothing causes stronger irritation than electrical matter. It seems that it has the power to strengthen the movements of the heart, and this confirms the belief of the philosophers, who attribute a more rapid pulse to electrified subjects."

Along similar lines Shebbeare projected franklinic stimuli to the exposed arrested heart of an eel and made it beat again. Galvani apposed a live torpedo to the bare heart of dead frogs: spasmodic contortions, but not rhythmic movements, were elicited. Von Humboldt sent discharges from a Leyden jar to the isolated heart of a carp, changing its rate at will.

Accounts such as these verified that there was genuine potentiality of the quiescent heart to be goaded into motion by electricity. However, owing to the diversity of experimental subjects, methods of inducing cardiac stoppage, electrical apparatus, current strengths, and routes of administration, the factors or conditions most conducive to prompt and lasting cardiac revival were elusive.

Various physiologists asserted that the responsiveness of the stopped heart to electrostimulation was partly contingent upon myocardial integrity, which in turn was affected by the dose of current. Fontana in 1776 showed that potent, but sublethal, electric shocks themselves petrified the heart and made it nonreactive to further electrostimulation. He theorized that this irreversible state of rigor was due to cellular damage by the current. Valli mused about the possibility of a true *restituo ad integrum* of the heart "once that muscular exhaustion sets in because of prolonged anemia." Galvani denied that electricity had a sustained influence on cardiac activity after death of the organism. Volta was skeptical that the results of experiments on lower animal *ex vivo* hearts devoid of blood flow and nervous connections could be validly extrapolated to humans.

If the delivery of electricity to the chest wall or to the heart itself might so hurt the myocardium as to render it unresponsive, perhaps a safer way to conduct cardiac electrostimulation would be via the nerves to the heart. Fowler, who was one of the few scientists to believe this to be possible, contended that he had restarted a stilled frog heart by exciting the pneumogastric and cervical nerves. Fontana contravened that view.

"Let the chest of an animal with cold blood be opened (this experiment is subject to less uncertainty in these animals than in those with warm blood, on whom however the effect is the same), and let the nerves to the heart be stimulated, in any way whatever; it will not on this account quicken its contractions if it is in motion, nor will it recover its motions if at rest, although it is still in a state of contracting on the least stimulus thus offered to its fibers. . . .

"It is my opinion, then, a matter demonstrated by the fullest evidence, that no motion of the heart can in any case be brought about by the medium of the nerves, although the heart is, of all the muscular organs, the most susceptible to the affections of the mind."

EXPERIMENTS ON EXPOSED HUMAN HEARTS

Among the countless organizations spawned during the Age of Enlightenment were the humane societies dedicated to the cause of resuscitation. Besides social reformers, philosophers, and naturalists, their membership counted many physicians who availed themselves of any occasion to try electricity for reviving apparently dead persons.

The first successful human electroresuscitation took place in 1774. In that incident, as well as in subsequent ones, the electric shocks were aimed haphazardly at the chest. Therefore, the question whether the heart responded through a direct or reflex effect was not answered. From tests made in 1798 on the bodies of guillotined individuals, Bichat supported Fontana's assertion that the myocardium was susceptible to electrical stimulation without the intermediary of nerves.

Making do with the lone human cadaver that he was authorized to experiment on, Nysten found in regard to direct cardiac galvanization that (1) the left ventricle lost its contractile ability shortly after death, and always before that of other muscular structures; (2) in contrast, the right ventricle was still capable of being impelled nearly one hour after death; (3) both atria stayed excitable well after other muscles had ceased to be; (4) the contractile faculty of the right atrial appendage was preserved for a much more extended time than any other part of the heart; and (5) a segment of the superior vena cava adjoining the right atrium was sensitive to galvanic stimulation almost as much and almost as long as the auricle proper.

More of this kind of experimentation on human corpses borrowed from gibbets was undertaken by perfervid electrologists, such as Aldini. Although helpful in the sense of laying to rest any doubts about electrical restoration of obtunded cardiac motion, it did not clarify how the heart in different milieus behaved to electricity of varying magnitude, frequency, and energy. The truly meaningful work on this facet was launched around the mid-nineteenth century in conjunction with strivings to rein anesthesia-provoked fatalities. Added impetus sprang from new disclosures about neural regulation of cardiac action, as well as from refinements in methodology for graphic enregisteration of the pulse.

Electrical research on cadavers spanned less than a decade, being objected to on moral and juridical grounds. Direct access to the heart in living humans was unfeasible in those days, having to await the development of endotracheal anesthesia and safe pericardiotomy. Accordingly, von Ziemssen's article in 1882 was as spectacular as it was instructive.

Von Ziemssen seized a unique opportunity of testing the action of electricity on the exposed beating heart of a nonoperated person. His subject was a woman with a large defect of the anterior chest wall consequent to resection of a tumor. Her heart, covered by just a thin sheet of skin, was visible and palpable. Stimulating electrodes were fastened to various regions of the heart and thorax, and both central and peripheral responses were monitored. Distinct changes in cardiac tempo were produced by electrical discharges administered at varying strengths and with deliberately spaced regular interruptions.

One of the most telling deductions from von Ziemssen's data was that the normal heart could be compelled to assume an artificial cadence by virtue of an electrical staccato which was faster than the innate cardiac rate. Likewise informative and in keeping with what had been demonstrated recently in isolated amphibian hearts was the presence at the atrioventricular groove of a sharply localized patch of tissue which exhibited extraordinary sensitivity to the current. The response declined abruptly a mere centimeter or two outside that zone.

DIRECT CARDIAC ELECTROSTIMULATION WITHOUT THORACOTOMY

It is understandable that, of the endocardial and myocardial methods of direct stimulation, the former would long have been viewed as impracticable because of interference from blood clotting. However, why percutaneous needle stimulation of heart muscle was not essayed sooner is unclear.

Krimer in 1828 made two attempts to revive the heart in standstill by electric "acupuncture," but both failed owing to irreversible myocardial damage. This, plus publication of the report in a minor journal, relegated the technique to obscurity.

With the rising frequency of operating room misadventures following the inauguration of chloroform anesthesia, resuscitation ceased being an uncommon exercise directed chiefly to victims of drowning or gas asphyxiation and became a mandate in hospital practice. In 1851, a report given before the French Academy of Sciences advocated deployment of electroresuscitation apparatus in medical institutions. That same august gathering heard the identical recommendation reiterated two years later—an indication of the inattention or scant enthusiasm received by the first report!

The majority of experts who were canvassed on the most efficacious maneuvers for instituting speedy electroresuscitation favored discharges through moistened sponge electrodes pressed against the thorax. Electropuncture was cited also, but needle insertion was into the scalp, back, mouth, anus—anywhere, it seems, but into the heart!

Before the Royal Medical and Chirurgical Society of London, Althaus in 1864 showed on two dogs that cardiac electropuncture could reverse arrest of the heart induced by chloroform. Emboldened by successes from several dozen trials on sundry animals, Steiner employed electropuncture on a patient.

"An illustration of these investigations is furnished by a case of chloroformization which occurred during the year 1870 in Professor Billroth's clinic. A young woman in whom chloroform narcosis was attempted promptly developed progressive syncope. All resuscitative measures were unsuccessful, including galvanism directed to the heart. Finally a feeble current through an inserted needle proved effective. The excitability of the heart soon was reestablished."

Steiner's lengthy article supplied explicit directions *in extenso* for accurate percutaneous placement of intracardiac needle electrodes. Two years later an editorial in the *British Medical Journal* bestowed oblique endorsement of cardiac electropuncture, without once mentioning Steiner's name or paper.

There must have been considerable trepidation about impaling the heart with needles because the literature is devoid of other than scattered, mostly infructuous, instances when this procedure was done. As an alternative Smith in 1904 suggested laying bare the pericardium over the left ventricle and directly applying a blunt or sharp electrode over it instead of into the heart per se. A suprapericardial technique akin to Smith's was described exactly 50 years later by Chandler, Rosenbaum, and Hansen.

The endovascular pathway for electrostimulation was an offshoot of research on cardiac hemodynamics. In 1898 Chaveau catheterized the left ventricular outflow tract of horses with a metal cylinder in-

sinuated via the carotid artery. Inside the catheter was a delicate electromagnetic switch actuated by the play of the aortic valve cusps functioning as a make-and-break circuit. Minuscule currents sufficed to instigate marked cardiac acceleration, which phenomenon denoted the accentuated sensitivity of the endocardium in comparison with that of other layers.

Floresco described another ingenious cannulation technique, as well as "clip-on" electrodes for the heart exterior. He introduced hollow glass pipes coated with paraffin through the external jugular vein into the right ventricle. One variant of the tubes had a small side arm corresponding to the level of the atrium. Copper or platinum coils, insulated save at their tips, were then threaded down the probes until they abutted again at either atrial or ventricular endocardium. The heart rate could be speeded by extremely weak induction currents to those sides just as readily as stimuli conveyed to the interior of the left ventricle. However, pileup of coagulum on the naked wire ends was a vexatious limiting factor.

Whereas von Ziemssen had studied how electrostimulation of diverse areas on the epicardium affected cardiac performance, Marmorstein 45 years later did similar research from the standpoint of the inner topography of the heart. Like his predecessors he used a rigid sound, but sealed its tip to avert clotting on the electrode. He sedulously explored all heart chambers with a view to charting individual excitation thresholds of selected endocardial stations. Then he measured the influence on endocameral and systemic manometry of these liminal electric stimuli to each endocardial locale in turn.

Besides encompassing a quantitative assay of endocardial electrostimulation effects, Marmorstein's data furnished supplementary proof that the sinoatrial node was the natural pacesetter of the heart and that excitation of certain strata of the ventricular septum resulted in bradycardia or in frank atrioventricular dissociation.

REPETITIVE, EQUIPHASIC STIMULI

As mentioned before, the cardinal effect of electricity on the circulatory system was found to be a tonic one. But while solo electrical shocks of adequate force could be shown to quicken normoactive hearts or to reanimate arrested hearts with still-responsive myocardium, the same stimuli produced just transient velocity increments in dilatory hearts.

Various physiologists reasoned that maintenance of the artificially imposed speed probably would pivot on either one or both of two desideratums. The first was that impulses should be repetitive, in the guise of successive isochronal discharges at predetermined rates. The second was that, for maximum efficiency, stimulation should be targeted at the sinoatrial node rather than indiscriminately to any region of the heart or even to the entire heart.

The former desideratum was easier to satisfy inasmuch as it was not novel conceptually and many instruments already were at hand to accomplish it. The superiority of interrupted stimuli over continual unbroken ones or random barrages had been vouched for since the primal investigations on cardiac resuscitation. Even some rudimentary voltaic files were equipped with make-and-break components, and most of the electrophysiologic gadgetry of the nineteenth century had provisions for firing discontinuous, equispaced stimuli when desired.

Many investigators tested interrupted currents on obtunded animal hearts. However, the few of them who envisioned a clinical future for the technique believed that discharges should be sent to the heart through the medium of the cervical sympathetic nerves. MacWilliam and later Robinovich were among the minority who preconized rhythmic stimuli given transthoracically. The following passages are culled from MacWilliam's prolix literary offerings:

". . . Galvanic and faradic currents, too weak to induce fibrillar contractions in a heart of depressed excitability, have a comparatively trivial influence in exciting or accelerating its beat. We want a much more effective and speedy mode of exciting rhythmic contraction, and one that will have a direct and powerful influence in calling forth a series of beats in the depressed or inhibited heart, while at the same time free from the danger of throwing the ventricles into delirium. Such a mode of excitation seems to be available in the form of a periodic series of single induction shocks sent through the heart at approximately the normal rate of cardiac action. A single induction shock readily causes a beat in an inhibited heart, and a regular series of induction shocks (for example, sixty or seventy per minute) gives a regular series of heartbeats at the same rate. Never on any occasion have I seen fibrillar contraction excited by such a mode of stimulation. . . .

". . . it is evident that, in addition to the improvement in the blood-pressure resulting from direct excitation of the heart by a series of induction shocks, there is also a beneficial effect exercised upon the contractile mechanism of the inhibited heart. The depressing influence exerted through the vagus nerve upon the rhythm and contraction force are in large measure counteracted by direct excitation of the organ. In order that such excitation should be as effective as possible it is probably best to send the stimulating shocks through the whole heart, so that the auricles may come directly under their influence as well as the ventricles. In order to do this in man one electrode should be applied in front over the area of cardiac impulse, and the other over the region of the fourth dorsal vertebra behind, so that the induction shocks may traverse the organ. The electrodes should be of considerable extent (for example, large sponge electrodes), and they and the skin should be well moistened with salt solution. The shocks employed should be strong, sufficient to excite powerful contraction in the voluntary muscles.

"Such a method, it seems to me, is the only rational and effective one for stimulating by direct means the action of a heart which has been suddenly enfeebled or arrested in diastole by causes of a temporary and transient character."

SINOATRIAL NODE STIMULATION

Nobody disputed the desirability of electrically bombarding the sinoatrial node to combat bradysphygmia incidental to global cardiac depression unaccompanied by regionally deranged intracardiac conduction. It seemed only logical for the heart to be governed through operation of its natural pacesetter. Another premise was that the ultrasensitivity of the node would lower current requirements and permit protracted sessions of electrostimulation without supervention of premature myocardial "fatigue" from a rise in the excitation threshold.

The practicality of sinoatrial node stimulation was appraised originally by experiments in which the rhythm and rate of either exposed *in situ* or excised animal hearts were modified by thermal changes in the substance of the node. As has been discussed, Marmorstein in 1927 achieved electrical excitation of the node by means of a rigid glass cannula passed through the internal jugular vein. A couple of years later, Hyman initiated trials of cardiac resuscitation by electropuncture of the right atrium, his rationale being that a controlled ectopic focus might be geared to dominate cardiac activity during an interval of functional depression of the subject's sinoatrial node.

Hyman coined the name "artificial cardiac pacemaker" for the apparatus which he constructed to impart physiologically-stimulated impulses directly to atrial muscle. His blueprints called for the following:

> ". . . (1) a small source of electric current, i.e., a common flashlight battery; (2) an interrupter mechanism; (3) a timing device; (4) a method of regulating the duration of the injected current; and, (5) a suitable insulated needle to carry the current only to the right atrial area of the heart. The instrument would, of course, be easily portable, and small enough to fit into a doctor's bag."

Of all of this pacemaker's attractive features the most original and utilitarian probably was the "bipolar" needle electrode. Its fabrication concluded in the spring of 1931, it was utilized clinically 43 times, with successful outcome in 14.

The notion of reanimating the prostrated heart and ruling its cadence by sinoatrial stimulation made a comeback during the infancy of open heart surgery. In 1949 Bigelow, Callaghan, and Hopps performed experiments with ingenious "single-point"

and "two-point" focal electrodes inserted pervenously or placed directly against the location of the node. Their good results were not duplicated when the catheters were employed on a few desperately ill patients. Unfortunately, also, they confined their efforts to sinoatrial node stimulation. Had they perchance advanced the catheters just 4 or 5 centimeters into the right ventricle, it is likely that the pervenous cardiac pacing era would have dawned 10 years sooner.

Thoracotomy obviously was the ideal avenue for ensuring placement of an electrode precisely over the sinoatrial node. But, since odds were against the chest being conveniently open in the majority of candidates for this type of cardiac pacing, alternatives were sought. Though unequalled for celerity, transthoracic needling was shunned because of the inordinate number of complications carried in its wake.

It was hoped that the "noninvasive" and fairly fast technique of transesophageal cardiac electrostimulation would be adaptable to regional spurring of the sinoatrial node, but that likewise proved to be unsuitable. In Shafiroff and Linder's series in 1957 the voltages necessary for transesophageal cardiac rhythm control entrained chest pain and diaphragmatic flutter.

SYNCHRONOUS PACING

In the history of cardiac electrostimulation no bradydysrhythmia shared the limelight with Morgagni-Adams-Stokes disease until one decade ago, when entities such as "sick sinus syndrome" were unmasked and rendered amenable to electrical management. In the main, therefore, atrioventricular dissociation was the solitary conduction disturbance to be contended with.

Of various imaginable ways to electrically surmount atrioventricular dissociation, the chances of sinoatrial node excitation being successful might be expected to be practically nil, unless the ostensible complete heart block either was intermittent or not truly total, so that impulses could still traverse the node. That Hyman saw fit to use his atrial-stimulator on patients with Morgagni-Adams-Stokes disease and nevertheless reaped good results is mystifying.

Also in the realm of conceivable ways to combat complete heart block was electrical arousal of a sluggish atrioventricular bundle itself. In 1909 Erlanger and Blackman had created chronic, complete heart block in dogs by squeezing the bundle with a screw clamp and then converting the vise into a stimulating electrode. However, besides yielding erratic responses, the method plainly presented insuperable problems with regard to clinical applicability.

Logic dictated that the most desirable manner of compensating for a vitiated sector of the cardiac intrinsic innervation mechanism would be an arrangement for mimicking normal function of the faulty segment while retaining participation of uninvolved portions of the intrinsic system. In keeping with this idea were ventures to morphologically replace the role of the atrioventricular neuromuscular complex by tissue grafts containing the sinoatrial node, but all of them were to no avail. The next sensible step was to detour the blocked atrioventricular post without relinquishing the natural antegrade path of the activation and conduction processes. This alluring stratagem was, in short, to somehow sidestep the His bundle while cuing ventricular systole to intercepted and aggrandized sinoatrial node signals.

Intended originally for study of ventricular fusion beats, the archetypal circuitry was framed in 1942 by Butterworth and Poindexter. Impulses sensed by small leads on the right atrium were amplified several thousandfold, delayed, and then transferred to ventricular electrodes. Hellerstein,

Shaw, and Liebow's "extracorporeal electronic bypass of the A-V node," fabricated in 1950 and proposed for treating complete heart blocks had the same key elements except that the pickup and transmitting limbs were endocardial.

Other investigators improvised ingenious portative models of atrial-triggered ventricular stimulators. Regrettably, that family of pacers was long beset by annoyances emanating from exorbitant current consumption and the detail of a combination double detector and relay electrode to separate parts of the heart.

ASYNCHRONOUS PACING

The modern era of rational cardiac electrotherapy had its inception in the context of resuscitation enterprises with ventricular defibrillators. The principal impetus came, however, from demonstrations in 1952 that the Morgagni-Adams-Stokes syndrome was susceptible of being held in check by electrical maneuvers. This epochal contribution was made by Zoll, Belgard, Zarsky, and their colleagues. The only valid precedent rivaling it was Hyman's unpublished application of his percutaneous atrial electropuncture device in a few instances of the syndrome.

During the course of clinical and laboratory studies on resuscitation through reversal of dysrhythmias by electroshocks (subsequently denominated "cardioversion" by Lown), Zoll grew disenchanted with the transesophageal and transthoracic needle routes. He eschewed them in favor of electrodes clasped either onto or into the skin of the precordium when he ascertained that protracted rhythmic stimulation could be safely realized in this manner. The efficacy of the method in Morgagni-Adams-Stokes disease was confirmed when a patient whose ventricular asystole was abolished by a transthoracic electric discharge exhibited recrudescence of standstill unless repeated electrostimulation was continued.

This and additional cases attested to the practicality of long-term cardiac pacing, and to the absence of significant bodily jeopardies from unselective stimulation of the whole heart in the presence of atrioventricular dissociation.

The strongest corroboration of protracted artificial pacing stemmed from experiences during the genesis of open heart surgery, when complete heart block joined the unhappy list of iatrogenic diseases. The first patients whose cardiac activity was sustained for a few days by electronic machines had incurred intractable block in connection with operations on heart valves. In the majority of subsequent patients block sometimes eventuated after repair of complex congenital cardiopathies.

Unlike ordinary Morgagni-Adams-Stokes disease featuring remissions between intervals of ventricular indolence, complete heart block from accidental wounding of the atrioventricular bundle at surgery tended to linger indeterminately or irrevocably. Also, transthoracic stimulation with skin electrodes was likely to be painful and to provoke cutaneous burns or spasms of the pectoral musculature. These considerations guided the reexploration of techniques of direct myocardial stimulation for prolonged periods through indwelling ventricular electrodes.

The association of Lillehei and Bakken, with their respective teams, set the stage in 1956 for the manufacture of a carriable external pulse generator and for popularization of cardiac pacing by right ventricular stimulation via intramural wire electrodes placed under direct vision or introduced transthoracically. Coincidentally, mindful of how facile it was to stop and restart the heart electrically, surgeons resorted with confidence to deliberately induced cardiac arrest during some operative procedures.

The needle electrodes used at the outset for epicardial or intramural anchorage looked like darts. They had a predilection for becoming dislodged or broken and lacked foolproof insulation. Furthermore, scar tissue encased their tips rather quickly. Of the constellation of contrivances invented for abrogating such handicaps the best was the twin-spiked "platform" bipolar lead of Hunter, Roth, Bernardez, and Noble which eliminated the need for a dispersive electrode.

Ventricular stimulation through transthoracically inserted needle electrode was, owing to its latent dangers, justifiable only for emergencies. For durations beyond mere hours the specter of sepsis or cardiorrhexis loomed ever larger over it. Accordingly, right ventricular endocameral catheterization for pacing was reassessed so as to obviate the foreseeable hazards.

In 1958, Furman, Robinson, and Schwedel had recourse to that route for pacing uninterruptedly during 96 days the heart of an elderly man. A monopolar endocavitary catheter and an indifferent electrode buried subcutaneously into the chest wall were linked by a long cable to an electronic console wheeled on a small table. Espousal of their method was promoted when soon after bipolar catheters were developed by Battye and Weale and by Parsonnet, Zucker, Bilbert, and Asa.

INTRACORPOREAL ARTIFICIAL PACERS

The development of self-contained intracorporeal ("internal," "inlaying," "indwelling," "imbeddable," or "implantable") artificial pacemakers constitutes one of the most abiding triumphs of bioengineering. It was greatly aided by coeval inventions engendered by the nascent Space Age—miniature batteries, transistors, inert plastics, computers, stress-resistant alloys.

In 1958 Senning and Elmqvist installed in a patient (who happened to be an engineer) a permanent cardiac pacemaker assembly consisting of intramyocardial electrodes connected to an accumulator imbedded in the epigastrium. The unit was charged at intervals by induction from the exterior. A few months later, a radiofrequency receiver and transmitter designed in 1948 by Mauro for stimulation of biologic tissue was employed clinically by Glenn and his colleagues. The following year, Chardack implanted the first prototype of Greatbach's series of wholly battery-driven pulse generators that did not require charging from the outside. Kindred instruments were made and used by Kantrowitz's and Zoll's teams. A totally implantable atrial-triggered ventricular pacer designed by Keller was used by Nathan, Center, and Wu in 1962.

All of the aforementioned pacer emplacements were performed with epicardial or myocardial wires. In 1961, having to cope with the dilemma of a patient too sick to withstand thoracotomy, Abelson, Samet, Rand, and Monaca resorted to interim external pacing through an endocardial catheter until clinical amelioration permitted formal surgery for permanent myocardial electrode insertion. The great merits of this dual approach established it as the procedure of choice for most cases of persistent bradycardia refractory to medication.

The absolute need for thoracotomy was done away with after Lagergren and Johansson in 1962 obtained dependable performance from an intracorporeal pervenous pacemaker system. This singular achievement brought to a close the Golden Decade of the fledgling specialty of cardiac pacing.

OTHER THEMES AND VARIATIONS

The alliance between physicians and engineers which paved the way for implantable pacers has endured and flourished, ushering in a veritable boom in medical electronics. A mutuality of interests, serviced by creative talents, has yielded a cornucopia of versatile equipment and methods. These have been rewarded by ever-improving safety and reliability in clinical practice. And yet a host of frustrations still abounds, as do challenges galore.

An issue that has never ceased taunting pacemaker specialists is how best to harness cardiac autochthonous signals for the purpose of initiating appropriate pacer impulses as needed. Atrial-synchronized atrial stimulation certainly seems a logical solution, were it not for difficulties plaguing circuitry requirements and battery drain. Moreover, the system would not be applicable for the escalating population of people with sick sinus syndrome.

As early as 1953, well before the clinical trials with "fixed-rate" pacers, Dammann and his group engineered a makeshift apparatus which automatically detected spontaneous electrical signals from the ventricle and delivered stimuli after a preset pause had elapsed. This version of cardiac self-activation was the progenitor of the class of pacers called "demand," "standby," "ventricular-inhibited," "R-stop," or "ventricular-triggered."

Demand pacing with an external stimulator was used in 1956 by Leathem, Cook, and Davies. Usage of intracorporeal demand pacers was begun in 1963 by Zacouto and by Castellanos, Lemberg, and Berkovits, becoming in due time the choice mode of pacing. The latter group also acquainted the profession with the intriguing principle of "bifocal" or sequential atrioventricular demand pacing.

The disquieting factor of brief battery longevity led to concerted hunts for durable power sources with fewer impediments. The tantalizing prospect of tapping biologic energy from body fluids or tissues was scrutinized in the 1960's by Enger and Kennedy, by Myers, Parsonnet, and Zucker, by Satinsky, and by others. Unfortunately, the electromotive force of most biologic piles, with amplifiers and transformers notwithstanding, fell short of expectations.

Nuclear-fueled generators designed by Hursen and Kolenik, Lafferty, and Gerrard in 1969, and such as first used clinically by Piwnica and Laurens that same year, have not enjoyed wide application partly because of stringent government restrictions concerning radioisotope paraphernalia. Conversely, in ascendant vogue are solid-state lithium-powered pacers, originated by Greatbach, Schaldach, and other researchers.

The relatively low but nevertheless significant incidence of irksome endocardial catheter displacements has inspired the fashioning of a host of hooks, flanges, spurs, buttons, and prongs to catheter tips, the better to grapple trabeculae carneae. Either in situations of recurrent catheter dislodgment or out of personal preference for primary electrode placement, the epicardial route occasionally is substituted for the endocardial. The "sutureless" corkscrew-shaped lead devised by Hunter has been used with notable success by Naclerio and Varriale, who have also developed a convenient threshold tester probe for discerning on each individual heart the site of maximal sensitivity to electrical stimulation.

Ferrer's description of the sick sinus syndrome and Damato's dissertations on His electrography have been major incentives in opening new horizons for pacing. As the indications for pacing have expanded beyond that of complete heart block, so too have exquisitely sophisticated programmable features of instruments enabled adaptation of a multitude of variables, aside from rate and output intensity, to specific clinical exigencies. Currently, some 50 different pulse generators are marketed.

The pool of persons bearing artificial cardiac pacemakers has become so vast that special clinics have been organized in larger medical centers for periodic checks. Patients unwilling or unable to attend follow-up clinics have the option of submitting to analysis of pacer performance by transtelephonic monitoring of electrocardiograms.

Finally, since a sphere of human endeavor often is mirrored in what is spoken or written about it, the status of cardiac pacing may be gauged from those vantage points. A cursory survey of cardiology and bioengineering meetings over the last three years reveals pacing to be the topic of at least 10% of papers. Every month, numerous lectures, colloquia, workshops, or courses on pacing are announced on notice boards or in the medical press. The first European Symposium on Cardiac Pacing took place in London in 1978 with an overflow audience, and the VIth International Symposium on Cardiac Pacing scheduled for Montreal in 1979 promises to match record attendances as in the past.

During the last 25 years nearly 5000 articles pertaining to some subject about pacing have appeared in print. PACE, the only journal devoted exclusively to pacing and clinical electrophysiology, and the brainchild of Furman, Barold, Irnich, Parsonnet, and Thalen, made its debut in 1978. On average, one text has been published yearly since Siddons and Sowton in 1963 wrote the first book dealing entirely with cardiac pacing. The latest, this comprehensive literary rendition of Varriale and Naclerio's, reflects the fine tradition of excellence set forth by its predecessors.

SELECTED READINGS

Escher, D.J.W.: Historical aspects of pacing. In Cardiac Pacing. Edited by P. Samet. New York & London, Grune & Stratton, 1973, pp. 1–5.

Lagergren, H.: How it happened: My recollection of early pacing. PACE, 1:140, 1978.

Parsonnet, V.: Permanent pacing of the heart: 1952–1976. Am. J. Cardiol., 39:250, 1977.

Parsonnet, V.: Permanent transvenous pacing in 1962. PACE, 1:256, 1978.

Schechter, D.C., Lillehei, C.W., and Soffer, A.: History of sphygmology and heart block. Dis. Chest., 55:535, 1969.

Schechter, D.C., Lillehei, C.W., and Soffer, A.: Electrotherapy in noncardiac disorders. Bull. N.Y. Acad. Med., 46:932, 1970.

Schechter, D.C., Lillehei, C.W., and Soffer, A.: Origins of electrotherapy. N.Y. State J. Med., 71:997, 1114. 1971.

Schechter, D.C., Lillehei, C.W., and Soffer, A.: Early experience with resuscitation by means of electricity. Surgery, *69*:360, 1971.

Schechter, D.C., Lillehei, C.W., and Soffer, A.: Background of clinical cardiac electrostimulation. N.Y. State J. Med., *71*:2575, 2794, 1971; *72*:270, 395, 605, 953, 1166, 1972.

Schechter, D.C., Lillehei, C.W., and Soffer, D.A.: Electrical treatment of electrocution. PACE, *1*:114, 1978.

Schechter, D.C., Lillehei, C.W., and Soffer, D.A.: Experimental replication of heart block. PACE, *1*:269, 1978.

Zoll, P.M.: Historical development of cardiac pacemakers. Progr. Cardiov. Dis., *14*:421, 1972.

2

Organization of a Cardiac Pacing Service

VICTOR PARSONNET
GEORGE H. MYERS

Since the earliest days of permanent pacing of the heart responsibility for implantation of a pacemaker has alternated between surgeon and cardiologist. At first it rested with the surgeon, for only he was qualified to open the chest, then with the cardiologist, for only he had been trained in catheterization techniques, and now with the advent of more simply inserted myocardial electrodes it has returned once again to the surgeon. With the growing number of indications for pacemaker implantation, and with increased training (or partial training) of graduating residents, almost every hospital of 100 beds or more seems to have someone on the staff who can implant a pacemaker, whether or not such widespread use of pacemakers is desirable.[1] This increased use of pacemakers suggests that guidelines for organization of a pacemaker service be established, along with criteria for surgical privileges and encouragement of peer review, just as there are for any other established specialty service within the hospital. This chapter describes a pacemaker service that has been developed at the Newark Beth Israel Medical Center (NBIMC), its follow-up service, and organization.

IN-HOSPITAL SERVICES

CASE LOAD. In order to maintain both knowledge of the expanding field of cardiac pacing and technical proficiency we have recommended that a pacemaker service be limited to hospitals where the operating physician and the support team can perform 25 or more new pacemaker implantations each year.[1] This means that almost an equal number of pulse generator replacements are also performed.[2] The operations must be performed with a reasonably low complication and mortality rate. In the case of transvenous pacing, for example, the electrode dislodgment rate should be less than 5%, and operative mortality rates should be less than 1 to 2% with any technique.

STAFFING. It has been our policy that transvenous pacemakers must be implanted by a team of at least two physicians, one an

13

expert in catheterization and the other a surgeon. Of the six "pacemaker" physicians at our institution, three have "grown up" with pacemakers, and the others have been trained in our fellowship and residency programs. The credentials committee requires documentation of a physician's training and capability to implant pacemakers, and each practitioner's clinical privileges are carefully and specifically delineated, such as whether the physician may implant temporary or permanent pacemakers, or both. Adequate training for pacemaker implantation requires that any new applicant for privileges must have participated in an active program at a recognized center, where the physician has performed at least 20 new implants and an equal number of replacements and inserted at least 25 temporary pacemakers. Certificates or statements attesting to this training must be provided.

The nursing personnel have been specially trained by the physicians on the pacemaker service in basic electrocardiography, electrophysiology, pacemaker techniques, and complications. Nurses are *not* rotated from any other operating service, but are assigned permanently to the pacemaker facility. At the NBIMC, since pacemakers are implanted in the catheterization laboratory, this requirement is easily met. Paramedical personnel, such as bioengineering technicians, are essential for maintaining the necessary equipment for threshold and sensing analysis and for assuring that all aspects of electrical hazard control and equipment maintenance are attended to. There are three bioengineering technicians in the catheterization laboratory, and they assist in all pacemaker surgery. The bioengineering staff of the hospital is responsible for periodically inspecting the room and the equipment for electrical safety and appropriate grounding. (The ICHD report has recommended that if a bioengineering technician is not available on the hospital staff, appropriate consultative arrangements should be made.[2])

SPECIAL PROCEDURE ROOM. At our hospital pacemakers are implanted in the catheterization laboratory. The room is appropriately equipped, and it meets the clean environment specifications of an operating room. It is so located as to obviate the need for transporting support staff and sterile supplies from other areas of the hospital and to provide for immediate backup replacement in the event of equipment breakdown or contamination of materials during a procedure. Furthermore, the room is equipped with storage areas for spare electrodes and leads, pacemakers, monitors, and other essential devices.

For either myocardial or transvenous electrodes, threshold tests must be performed. For this reason the catheterization laboratory is equipped with a pacing system analyzer (PSA) now available from many pacemaker companies, although in most cases we still prefer to make direct measurements of the pacing parameters. Therefore the catheterization laboratory is equipped with oscilloscopes, digital counters, external pacemakers, and monitors, as well as with an image intensifying fluoroscope, television viewing system, electrocardiograph, standard surgical instruments, suture materials, intravenous fluids, and emergency equipment for management of cardiac catastrophes. This includes airways, emergency drugs, a DC defibrillator-cardioverter, mechanical hand ventilator, endotracheal tubes, and a source of oxygen supply.

RECORD KEEPING. For any pacing technique records must be maintained. In addition to the standard vital statistics, we provide the following information: a description of the primary cardiac rhythm disturbance, including the indication for pacemaker implantation, the date of implantation, the model and serial number of the pulse generator and electrodes, pacing thresholds, output of the pulse generator, and amplitude of the R wave. This information is readily available to our follow-up clinic. Now that programmable pacemakers are so widely used, we also record the way in which the pulse generator was programmed, accomplished by means of the computer which periodically prints a corrected updated report on the most recent programmed status of each unit. This report is posted outside the catheterization laboratory and in the Emergency Room and Coronary Care Unit.

A CLINICAL SERVICE. We have found that with our workload of 300 to 360 operations a year, and with 6 physicians on the staff who are actively interested in pacemaker implantation, it has become practical to set up a separate pacemaker service. Although this means double service responsibilities for all of the physicians, these responsibilities are kept light enough so that they are not unmanageable. In addition to the physicians there are two engineers, one nurse coordinator, and one administrator assigned to the service.

The responsibilities of the service include training of nurses, technicians, students, and house officers and rotation through the follow-up clinic, as well as nighttime and weekend coverage of the pacemaker center. All must attend a monthly conference at which the recent pacemaker procedures, complications, and mortalities are discussed and problem cases are presented.

An important advantage of such a service is the availability of peer review. Previously, the quality of pacemaker work had not been supervised adequately because pacemaker implantation did not seem to be attached to any of the major services of medicine, surgery, or cardiology.

IN-HOSPITAL FOLLOW-UP. After a patient has had a pacemaker implanted, some degree of postoperative surveillance is necessary. The patient is sent to the recovery room until the effects of anesthesia and sedation have subsided. Thereafter some patients are monitored for 24 to 48 hours, particularly those who are pacemaker-dependent and in whom failure of the pacing system may have serious consequences. Part of the record-keeping system includes identification of patients who are dependent upon the pacemaker. We believe that other patients do not require continuous postoperative monitoring, but they do require a certain number of basic tests before discharge.

There is daily evaluation of pacemaker function, either by electrocardiographic or oscilloscopic monitoring. Postoperative overpenetrated PA and lateral chest radiographs are taken to ensure that the electrode is properly positioned and to serve as a baseline for future evaluation. A complete test of pacemaker function is carried out to initiate the follow-up program.

For primary implants the length of stay in the hospital varies, depending upon the severity of the patient's overall medical status. Following transvenous implantation most patients are well enough to be discharged within three or four days. Only a day or two of postoperative hospitalization is required following pacemaker replacement, and monitoring is usually unnecessary.

The patient is provided with a set of written instructions regarding activity and follow-up programs. These instructions include information about suitable physical and social activities, the frequency and nature of postoperative visits, an appointment for the first clinic visit, and a procedure for obtaining medical care in emergency situations. The patient is also given an identification card to carry with him at all times, which indicates the date of implantation, type of pulse generator and electrode used, and the name, address, and phone number of the responsible physician.

FOLLOW-UP CLINIC

Pacemaker follow-up clinics have been in operation in this country and in Europe for over ten years.[3,4] In some of these, including the one at our institution, full waveform analysis coupled with telephone monitoring is done. Other methods range from simple

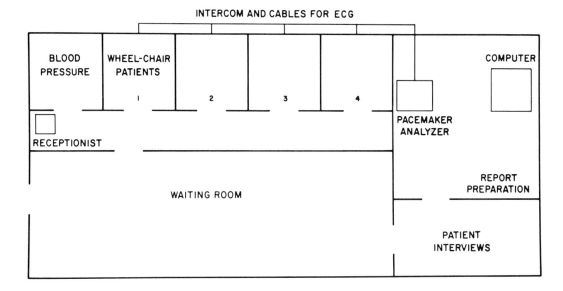

Fig. 2–1.   Floor plan of clinic showing examining areas, computer room, and intercom system.

interviews and ECG to full waveform analysis and vectorcardiography. Some services are performed privately by proprietary organizations which follow the patient for the physician or for the hospital.

In our system, pulse generators have been replaced electively, based upon clinic findings in 88% of cases since 1971. The average life of the pulse generator has been equivalent to that reported elsewhere;[5] emergency replacements have been avoided, but not at the expense of removing the pacemakers too early. All data indicate that the system is effective.

PATIENT EVALUATION AND PROCEDURE AREAS. At each clinic visit the pulse amplitude, width, and interval are measured, an electrocardiogram is taken, and a photograph of the pacemaker artifact is made. All readings are compared with previous findings. If the cardiac activity is not in competition with the pacemaker, and if this patient has a noncompetitive pacemaker, external overdrive (EOD) is also used to test the sensing circuit. EOD also permits measurement of the pacemaker refractory period and observation of the unpaced electrocardiogram. Special tests which are

occasionally performed include magnet rate differences (for Medcor pacers), special threshold tests (Vitatron), chest radiographs, and 24-hour dynamic monitoriing.

The purpose of the clinic is to examine the pacemaker, not to provide the patient with a routine check-up, because every patient sees his personal physician. If a nonpacemaker problem is disclosed at a clinic visit, the patient is advised to see his own physician. Emergencies, of course, are treated immediately. The final judgment concerning action to be taken as a result of the clinic examination rests with the physician attending the clinic, who always sees the entire past record and the results of the tests just taken at the clinic and interviews the patient.

In the clinic four examining rooms are connected by cables to a central station for an ECG and by an intercom for verbal communications (Fig. 2–1). All data are taken by technicians in the central station, using a Gutmann* pacemaker analyzer and Hewlett-Packard electrocardiographic recorder. The analyzer displays the pulse

---

* L.P.M., U.G. Gutmann, Eurasburg, W. Germany.

interval, width, and amplitude digitally, and the values are recorded by a Hewlett-Packard printer in order to minimize the possibility of transcription errors and to provide a permanent record. A Polaroid photograph is also taken of the pacemaker waveform. All numerical data are entered into the computer via a keyboard terminal, which then prints a report comparing the present data with all previous readings taken on that pacemaker. The physician at the clinic receives a copy of the report and the electrocardiogram and waveform photograph. The report is constructed so that the physician can see a summary of the findings of all of the previous visits, as well as all the written comments entered by previous examiners. Figure 2–2 shows a typical report ready to be presented to the physician.

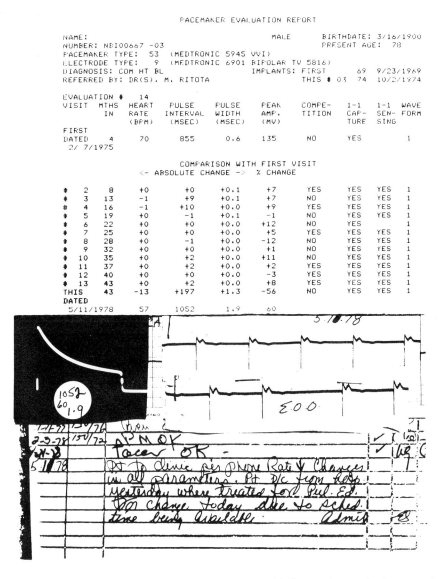

Fig. 2–2. Typical clinic report, with computer printout assembled onto sheet with electrocardiogram, waveform photograph, and comments from previous clinics.

STAFFING. The clinic is staffed by a clinic supervisor, two nurses (one of whom is the equivalent of a nurse practitioner), an attending physician and resident, two electronics technicians, a computer operator, a clerk, and four technicians (some of whom may be volunteers). The supervisor is responsible for the overall operation of the clinic. A nurse takes blood pressures, performs external overdrive tests (with physician supervision), and reprograms the pacemakers when necessary. The clerk assigns patients to the examining rooms and makes sure that all of the records are in proper order.

The electronic equipment for measuring the various parameters is operated by the electronics technicians, while the pacemaker technicians attach electrodes to the patients in the examining rooms. The computer operator inserts data into the computer and sees that the reports are properly prepared. A technician assembles the computer printout, waveform photograph, and ECG strip into a final report. (Since the clinic is held only once a week, most of the staff are not full-time but are borrowed from other functions, some of which are not related to the clinic. The departments lending these people are reimbursed for the time that their staff spends at the clinic, but even with this reimbursement the expenses for the clinic are much lower than they would be if it were necessary to use full-time staff for all of the functions.)

DETAILS OF PROCEDURE. A typical path of a patient through the clinic, illustrated in Figure 2–3, is as follows:

1. The patient reports at a reception desk, has his blood pressure taken, and then waits in the reception room until an examining room is free.

2. The patient is called, placed on the examining table, and ECG electrodes and cables are attached by the technician assigned to that room. The pacemaker area is exposed for examination and for external overdrive (EOD).

3. Data are taken by the technicians at the central station, who are in communication with the examining room by intercom. If EOD or reprogramming is necessary,

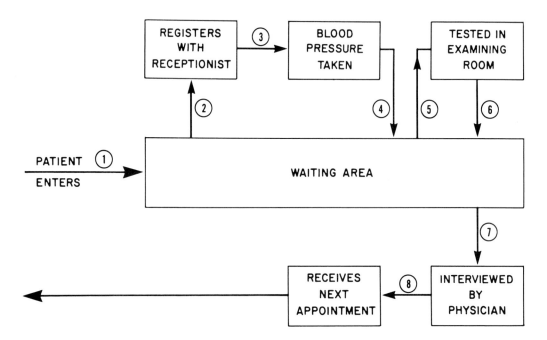

Fig. 2–3. Patient flow in clinic.

then either the resident or the nurse is called to perform these functions. If the pacemaker had been reprogrammed previously, it is always restored to its original setting before the examination and then returned to its therapeutically selected setting. All changes are documented.

4. The patient returns to the reception room until the report is prepared and he is called to see the physician.

5. Depending on the findings at the clinic and the interview with the physician, a decision is made as to whether to continue with the present schedule, to admit the patient to the hospital, to institute telephone monitoring, or to change the interval between visits.

6. If the patient is to be monitored by telephone, he is given a telephone monitor and is taught by a technician how to use it.

7. The patient is then given an appointment for his next visit by a clerk. Patients are given appointments for a particular hour and are called for examination according to the time of their appointments, not according to the time they arrive at the clinic. It has been found that calling patients according to the time of their appointments reduces the number of people waiting, since otherwise many people tend to come early to be the first one examined, and also reduces waiting time for the patient without affecting clinic operation.

If changes in a pacemaker are noted which are suspicious, but are not definitive enough to warrant changing a pacemaker, then the patient is usually followed more closely. This can be done either by starting to monitor him by telephone before monitoring would start on the regular schedule or by having him return to the clinic earlier than would usually be scheduled.

CLINIC SCHEDULES. Since schedules for routine monitoring are set by third-party payers (the schedules depend on the type of pacemaker), deviation from these schedules must have the reasons adequately documented.

TABLE 2–1

Follow-up Schedule for Pacemaker Clinics and Telephone Monitoring at Newark Beth Israel Medical Center

Clinics, all pacemakers	
First year:	Every four months
Succeeding years:	Every three months
Telephone Monitoring	
Mercury cells: Once a week after two years	
Lithium and nuclear cells: once a month after two years	

Patients come to the clinic every four months during the first year and every three months thereafter. They are monitored by telephone at various intervals, depending on the type of pacemaker. For the older mercury-zinc battery pacers, telephone monitoring starts at 18 months and at weekly intervals thereafter (except for the week of the clinic evaluation). For lithium- and nuclear-powered units, the starting time and intervals differ. Table 2–1 shows our present schedule.

The first recorded clinic visit is four months after discharge. Measurements taken earlier change considerably in the first few months, especially those for amplitude and waveform of unipolar units. Variations in interval have also been noted over this period and are probably caused by changes in the battery when current is initially drawn from it. Four months have proved to be a satisfactory "settling in" period.

COMPUTER FACILITY. The computer performs many other functions in addition to preparing the routine reports shown in Figure 2–2. At the end of each clinic it produces typewritten letters in which the results of the clinic examination are summarized automatically for the referring physician. The computer also is used for billing, inventory, maintaining schedules and delinquency lists, and for storing files of all types of pacemakers and leads used. Auxiliary functions include data retrieval for research purposes, calculation of beat-to-beat intervals (an additional method of confirming pacemaker failure), and providing calling lists for the telephone monitoring system. A new system for telephone monitoring is now being introduced in which the computer automatically determines whether a measured interval is within limits or not, and maintains, in the computer memory, all pertinent records concerning telephone measurements.

The computer is also of key importance in tying together a regional network of nine pacemaker clinics at different hospitals in New Jersey. These hospitals all have essentially the same type of pacemaker clinic, with its own computer terminal. When a clinic is run at one of these institutions, it has access to the central computer by means of telephone lines. Since the computer has time-sharing capability, other nonclinic programs can be run simultaneously at Newark Beth Israel Medical Center. Because of memory limitations in the present computer, only one clinic at a time can be operated.

TELEPHONE MONITORING. The clinic is held only once a week. During the rest of the week the full-time staff of the clinic are required for two principal functions: operating the telephone monitoring system and testing inpatients and emergency cases. All "telephone patients" have pulse generator rate monitored. In addition, approximately 60% of the patients also have their ECGs recorded by phone. About 100 telephone calls are made each day for telephone monitoring purposes. Making these calls, analyzing the results (including reading ECGs), and follow-up requires a staff of four technicians, a nurse, and the on call services of a resident or attending physician.

When suspicious findings are noted on telephone monitoring, the patient is usually asked to come into the hospital on a non-clinic day for the full range of clinic tests. A special examining room has been set up for this purpose, and a nurse and technician are always available. The examining room is equipped with a stretcher and its own monitoring equipment, which is also available as backup for general clinic use if there should be an equipment failure. The examining room equipment can also be used in an emergency by any affiliated hospitals in the regional network. Off-hour emergencies are handled by a telephone answering machine: the recorded message directs patients to an on-call physician. In case of nonemergency but still pressing situations, a message can be recorded on the tape, and the patient is called at the start of the next working day.

ADMINISTRATION. The pacemaker clinic has been separately incorporated as a not-for-profit corporation called the Pacemaker Center, Inc. Figure 2–4 is an organization chart showing the administrative structure of the Center. The president and the executive director of the hospital are ex-officio members of the board of directors. The nine active members include four from the hospital board, four from the professional staff of the Center, and one patient. Under the board are a president (one of the medical staff), an administrative director, and a technical director.

COSTS. Although the staff is concerned primarily with patient care, because the hospital provides most of the administrative functions, some personnel are needed for billing, which is done entirely by Center personnel. The full-time nonprofessional staff of the Center is responsible for the telephone monitoring program, and its size is appropriate to carry on this function. As mentioned, some staff personnel are "borrowed" for special functions from other hospital departments during clinics and for certain peak load hours. Use of part-time people is an efficient and cost-effective way of running the Center, but to use such part-time people requires that a clinic be held only once a week. Thus, the automa-

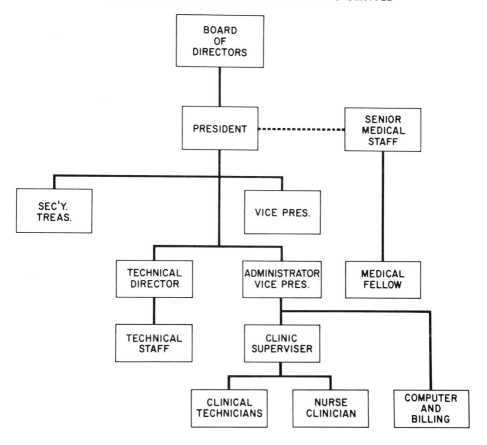

Fig. 2–4. Organization of the Pacemaker Center.

tion and efficiency of this clinic are actually dictated by the economics of the system and the availability of staff. If the clinic were held daily with fewer patients each day, the cost per patient would be considerably increased.

MISCELLANEOUS ACTIVITIES. The Pacemaker Center is in a unique position to gather research data on pacemakers and their clinical application because of its large patient load, computerized record keeping, and full-time professional staff. For a number of years the Center has participated in the FDA Pacemaker Registry, which maintains records on pacemakers and their failure modes based on data collected at the Newark Beth Israel Medical Center, the University of Southern California, and Montefiore Hospital and Medical Center.[6]

Together, the three organizations implant 2% of all pacemakers in the United States.

A computerized record-keeping system permits rapid retrieval of desired information, as well as periodic statistical reports. In many cases, the FDA project has detected problems in pacemakers before the manufacturers were aware of them. The project is also a source of unbiased life data on the types of pacemakers implanted in the centers. Since there is practically no problem with "loss to follow-up," the records are remarkably complete. In addition, the Pacemaker Center at Newark maintains many statistics on its patients and presents the results in the regular scientific literature.

Because of the necessity of maintaining an efficient operation, the Center also devotes time to studying ways of improving its activities. Much effort goes into developing new computer programs and new ways of improving diagnostic techniques. A computer program has recently been developed for automatically indicating from telephone monitoring data when a patient should be brought into the hospital for a detailed check on his pacemaker, and a completely automated system for data acquisition is now being planned.

RESULTS OF THE CLINIC PROGRAM. An analysis of six years of clinic experience is shown in Figure 2–5. In that time, 12% of all replacements were on an emergency basis. Most pacemakers were replaced for battery failure, but a large number were replaced for component and wire problems and miscellaneous other reasons. Because we might expect that problems other than battery might be missed by the waveform analysis system and phone monitoring, it is

interesting to note that most of the *nonbattery* failures were also detected in the clinic and the pacemakers were removed electively. Approximately 5% of all units were removed because of wire problems (about half of these were caught in the clinic).

The average age of pacers removed for battery exhaustion is shown in Figure 2–6. This age has climbed from a low of 20 months in 1971 to 35.9 months in 1976. Complementary data is shown in Figure 2–7, which records the percentage of units greater than 24 months old in 1975 and 1976. At the end of 1976, about 40% of all pacers implanted were more than two years old. As lithium pacemakers replace mercury-zinc units, one would expect that both of these curves would continue to increase. These curves indicate longevities that are comparable to those reported by manufacturers and thus indicate that pulse generators are not being replaced too soon.

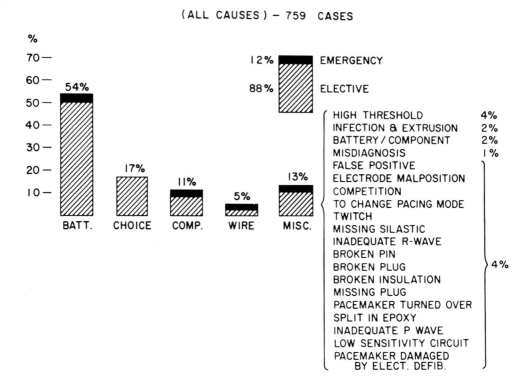

Fig. 2–5.   Pulse generator replacements for all causes from 1971 to 1976.

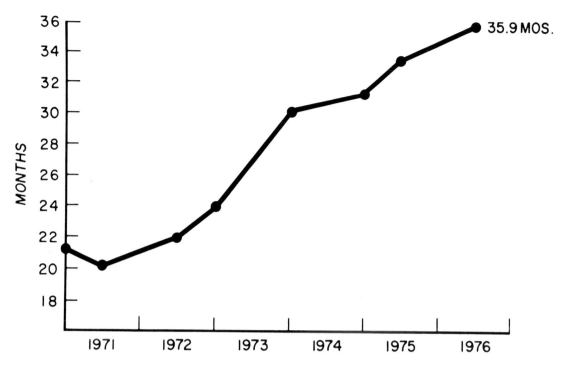

Fig. 2–6. Average age of pacers removed for battery exhaustion through 1976. This age has been steadily increasing.

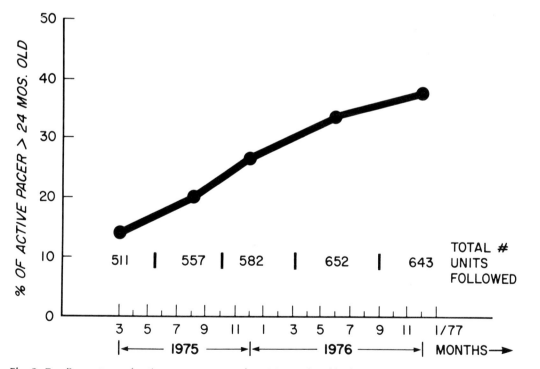

Fig. 2–7. Percentage of active pacers greater than 24 months old. This percentage has been increasing as a result of improvements in pacemaker technology.

TABLE 2-2

Reasons for Pulse Generator Replacement in 1976

80 CASES*		
Battery failure	58	(72.5%)
Component failure	9	(11%)
Broken wire	6	(7.5%)
High threshold	2	
Broken insulation	1	
Misinterpreted signs	2	(9%)
Accidental reprogramming	1	
Misdiagnosis	1	

(9%) bracket notes:
1 rate change not confirmed by tests
1 phone rate change not confirmed in clinic
Broken wire thought to be component failure

OTHER REASONS—23 CASES
13—Cases from elsewhere
4—Patient or physician choice
1—Extrusion
1—Early high threshold
1—Electrode malposition
1—Poor sensing-small R wave
1—Poor atrial sensing-small P wave
1—Pacer damaged by electrical defibrillation

* The 80 cases of particular interest are those caused by pulse generator failure or operator error.

Clearly, if all units were replaced too early, there would be few emergency replacements, but the interests of the patient would not be protected.

Table 2–2 summarizes the experience for 1976, when 103 pulse generators were replaced, and shows the reasons for replacement. Thirteen pulse generators originally implanted at other institutions were not followed by us and therefore are not included in the study. An additional four were removed electively at the request of the patient or the physician, and six were removed for a variety of uncommon reasons not related to the device. Of the remaining 80 cases, 72 were detected (90%)—63 first on the telephone, and 9 first at the clinic; this is about the same proportion as would be expected from the relative frequency of the two types of contact with the patient.

Battery exhaustion remained the most common cause for replacement (72.5%),

but component failure rose to 11%, and broken wires accounted for 7.5%, a persistent problem that has not begun to disappear. Other causes for pacemaker removal shown in the table accounted for approximately 10%.

To analyze the relative value of the measurements made in the clinic, the 72 cases of detected failures were studied in depth (Table 2–3). Change in interval was the most frequently detected alteration, but on retrospective analysis of the computer reports a preliminary change of amplitude was noticed in 25%. A variety of other signs were also detected, but these were relatively less frequent.

The 8 cases that were not detected are also shown in Table 2–3. In five of these the wire broke. This table also shows the earliest signs as they should have been detected in the 72 detected cases. In the retrospective analysis, the sign most fre-

TABLE 2–3

First Signs of Failure (1976)

	80 CASES DETECTED	
SIGNS	ACTUALLY DETECTED	RETROSPECTIVE ANALYSIS
Interval (I)	62 (86.1%)	48 (66.6%)
Amplitude (A)	3 (3.6%)	15 (20.8%)
Int.+Ampl. (I+A)	2 (2.7%)	2 (2.7%)
Bad pacing (B_p)	1 (1.4%)	1 (1.4%)
Sensing failure (S)	1 (1.4%)	0 —
Duration (D)	0 —	1 (1.4%)
I+D+A	0 —	1 (1.4%)
I+S	1 (1.4%)	1 (1.4%)
I+D	1 (1.4%)	2 (2.7%)
I+B_p	1 (1.4%)	1 (1.4%)
Total	72	72

8 CASES NOT DETECTED
1—Sudden zero output—no warning signs
5—Broken wire-zero output (1 other was detected by A change)
2—High threshold-sudden bad pacing

quently missed was drop in amplitude. Change in interval should be discernible in 94% of cases, and in 76% of cases it was the first sign. Change in amplitude should be seen in 71% of the cases, and in 25% as the first sign. Pulse duration should change in 60% of cases, but is rarely seen as a first sign. Pulse duration should change in 60% of cases, but is rarely seen as a first indication (5.5%). In no instance in 1976 was a change in wave shape or refractory period useful in detecting impending pacemaker failure, although two such instances were seen in 1977. The increase in pulse generator longevity reflects the combined effectiveness of a pacemaker clinic analysis and the growing reliability of the new pulse generators.

An analysis of reasons for replacement of pulse generators using the cumulative survival curve reveals that within a three-year period, about 30% of pacemakers must be replaced for reasons other than battery failure.[7] This fact calls attention to the persistence of nonbattery problems, particularly fractured wires and random component failures, clearly a directive to the manufacturer to continue the work of improving pacemaker design.

As batteries last longer, the percentage of failures caused by components and broken wires will continue to increase, even though the absolute numbers of such failures may become less. With older pacemakers, which lasted two years, the only component and wire failures that could be observed were those occurring early in the life of the unit. As battery life increases, we can expect to see more failures from these other sources, which are age-dependent. For example, metal fatigue will have more time to operate on the leads. Small moisture seepage might produce negligible effects in two or three years, but might cause failures after 10 years.

For many years the patients have maintained a Pacemaker Club for the purpose of helping each other, supporting potential pacemaker patients, and raising money for research. There are monthly executive and educational meetings and an annual party to which special guest speakers are invited. The activities of the club are supported and encouraged by the staff of the Pacemaker Service and Foundation, but the functions of the Club are in every other way independent of the hospital and professional staff.

PERSPECTIVE. The above analysis of the tangible results of our present follow-up system illustrates that it is possible to detect signs of about 90% of pacemaker failures before they occur, even in some situations in which sudden failure is to be expected without evident preliminary findings. We have shown that it is possible to detect almost all cases of battery exhaustion and perhaps 95% of all problems having to do with failure of the pulse generator. Other non-device problems (such as impending skin erosion) are usually detected and discussed in the follow-up clinic.

Although it is no longer necessary to argue for the merits of some sort of follow-up routine, it is important to show the many ways that a complete system may be of benefit to the patient and physician. The method provides highly accurate and sophisticated care at reasonable cost and is tremendously efficient for the physician. In this regard, one must picture the comfort and security to patient and physician alike with the knowledge that a replacement operation may be scheduled at a convenient time for both and an emergency operation avoided, the latter often requiring the additional preliminary insertion of a temporary pacing system.

The complexity of new pacemaker models in the multiplicity of real (and false or misinterpreted) signs of failure makes it almost obligatory to employ a follow-up clinic. Pacemaker programmability and the extension of pacemaker life, potentially 10 to 20 years in models implanted today, almost demand a systematic follow-up system, if not to program the pacer, then at least to have an organized long-lasting record-keeping system. (Many pacemaker patients will now outlive their physicians.) Computers that are capable of doing total waveform analysis and storing data indefinitely are now in use at several centers, and much of the work that we are doing now will eventually be accomplished by much smaller, more compact, cheaper, project-dedicated, and office-based microprocessors. Follow-up care, now complicated by technical detail, will become simpler and more easily available.

Some alternative systems of follow-up are feasible in specific situations, but are clearly less satisfactory. Elective pulse generator replacement is now uncalled for, because pacemaker life is potentially so long that a reasonable time for replacement cannot be selected. For example, lithium and nuclear pulse generators already show better than 95% survival in three years.[8] Telephone analysis by itself, although at times the only feasible system for a bedridden or geographically remote patient, as well as proprietary third-party methods, lacks some desirable features that are provided by a more thorough system, particularly the opportunity of examining the patient and providing personal counsel.

REFERENCES

1. Dodinot, B., et al.: Professional qualifications for pacemaker implantation. Panel Discussion. PACE, *1*:381, 1978.
2. Parsonnet, V., Furman, S., and Smyth, N.P.D.: Implantable cardiac pacemakers: Status report and resource Guideline. Pacemaker Study Group (ICHD). Circ., 50-A21–35 (#4), October 1974.
3. Siddons, H., and Sowton, E.: Cardiac Pacemakers. Charles C Thomas, Publisher, Springfield, Illinois, 1967, pp. 120–131.

4. Watanabe, Y.: Cardiac Pacing. Amsterdam, Excerpta Medica, 1971, pp. 231–317.
5. Bilitch, M.: Performance of cardiac pacemaker pulse generators. PACE, *1* (1):157, 1971.
6. Parsonnet, V., et al.: Pulse Generator Longevity as Determined by a Multi-Center Registry. Proc. of Int. Sympos. Troubles du Rythme et Electro-stimulation. Toulouse, France, Societé de La Nouvelle Imprimerie Fournie, 1977, p. 321.
7. Association for Advancement of Medical Instrumentation: Pacemaker Standard, August 1975, p. 116.
8. Bilitch, M.: op cit.

3

The Implantable Pacing System

WILLIAM M. CHARDACK
WILSON GREATBATCH

The first successful long-term correction of heart block in man by an implantable self-contained pacemaker was reported in 1960.[1] Since then important developments have taken place. In the clinical area, the indications for permanent pacing of the heart have been extended to brady- and tachyarrhythmias other than block. Technical advances have been made in the design and manufacture of all the components of the implantable pacing system. Sophisticated electronic instrumentation is now available. Its function is programmed from the intrinsic electrical activity of the heart and also permits the noninvasive adjustment by the physician of a number of functional parameters of the implanted device (Table 3–1).

The first pulse generators were the product of the transistor age and contained but eight discrete electronic components exclusive of the power source (Fig. 3–1). Today's pulse generators are the product of the era of the integrated circuit or a combination of such electronic "chips" (Figs. 3–13, 3–15) and numerous unmounted discrete components in a so-called hybrid circuit. They incorporate the equivalent of hundreds of discrete electronic elements in a highly complex structure of extremely small size that can be hermetically sealed.

The implantable pacing system consists of the pulse generator (power source and electronic circuitry) providing an appropriate electrical stimulus (usually biphasic, 4 to 5 volts, and of a duration of 0.5 to 1.0 milliseconds) and the electrode lead conducting the stimulus to cardiac tissue. The term *lead* applies to the insulated electrical conductor, and the terminal electrical contact point on cardiac tissue is designated as the *electrode*. Typical systems are schematically shown in Figure 3–2 and listed in Table 3–1.

ELECTRODE LEADS

The electrode lead system may be of a bipolar configuration, both negative and positive terminals being in or on the heart (Fig. 3–2A), or as is more common today,

TABLE 3–1

Fully Implantable Pacemaker Systems

1. *Electrode Leads*
   Endocardiac   Unipolar or bipolar
   Myo(epi-) cardial   Ventricular or atrial
2. *Pulse Generators*
   A. *Asynchronous* (fixed rate)
      (Emission of stimuli is independent of intrinsic cardiac activity.)
      1. Stimulation rate and output amplitude are fixed.
      2. Stimulation rate and output amplitude are noninvasively adjustable (programmable).
      3. Stimulus may be applied to ventricle or atrium or both (AV sequential) (VOO, AOO, DOO).
   B. *Synchronous* (Emission of stimuli is programmed from cardiac electrical activity.)
      1. From atrium (P-wave, synchronous) (VAT)
      2. From QRS
         a. QRS-suppressed ventricular demand pulse generator (VVI).
         b. QRS-triggered (standby) pulse generator (VVT).
            (Stimulus falls into absolute refractory during NSR.)
         c. AV bifocal, suppressed by QRS (DVI). (Stimulates atrium and/or ventricle.)
      3. Output parameters (rate, amplitude, pulse duration, etc.) Any of the above pulse generators may be noninvasively adjustable (programmable).

The capital letters in this table refer to the pulse generator terminology code developed by the Inter-Society Commission for Heart Disease (ICHD): V, ventricle; A, atrium; D, double chamber (both); I, inhibited; T, triggered; O, not applicable. The first letter refers to chamber paced, the second to chamber sensed, and the third to mode of response.

After Parsonnet, V., et al.: Implantable cardiac pacemakers: Status report and resource guideline. Circulation, 50:A21–A35, 1974.

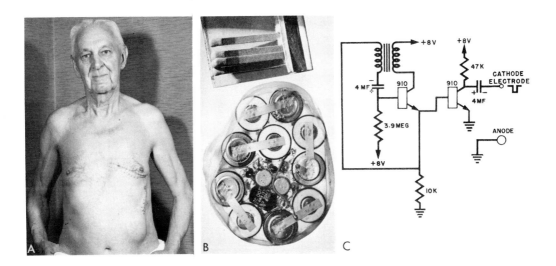

Fig. 3–1. A, First patient treated successfully in 1960.[1] He was 77 years old, had sustained a skull fracture after innumerable Stokes-Adams attacks, and lived several years after receiving his pacemaker. (From Chardack, W. M., Gage, A. A., and Federico, A. J.: In Davis-Christopher Textbook of Surgery, 11th ed. Edited by D. C. Sabiston, Jr. Philadelphia, W. B. Saunders Company, 1977.) B, Pacemaker similar to one used in patient in A. Note ten cells in series yielding a 14-volt pulse (high by current standards). Long-term stimulation requirements were, of course, unknown and unforeseeable at that time. (Reprinted by permission from the New York State Journal of Medicine copyright by the Medical Society of the State of New York. From Schechter, D. C.: Background of clinical cardiac stimulation. N.Y. State J. Med., 72:1183, 1971–1972.) C, Transistorized blocking oscillator used in pulse generator and for earlier experimental work. (From Chardack, W. M., Gage, A. A., and Greatbatch, W.: A transistorized, self-contained, implantable pacemaker for long-term correction of complete heart block. Surgery, 48:643, 1960. A similar circuit was also used in earlier experimental work reported by Greatbatch, W., and Chardack, W. M.: A transistorized implantable pacemaker. Proc. New England Research & Engineering Meeting. NEREM 1:8, 1959.)

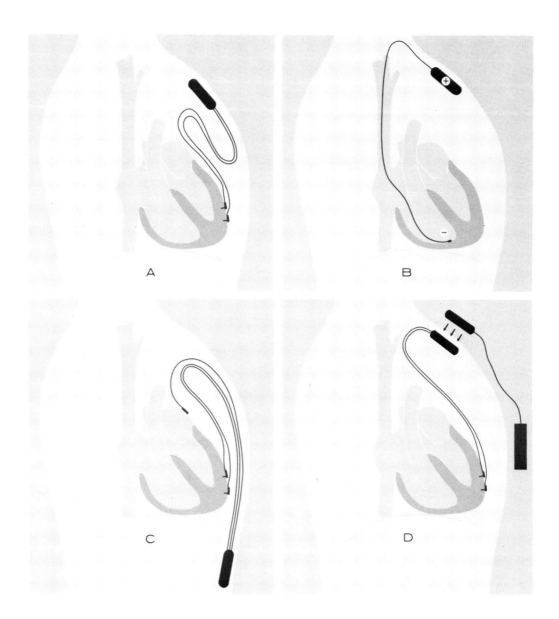

Fig. 3–2. Diagram of pacemaker systems. A, Bipolar myocardial electrodes with the pulse generator in the subcutaneous tissues of the chest wall. B, Unipolar endocardial electrode. Note that the electrode of negative polarity makes contact with the endocardium. C, Synchronous (atrial-programmed pulse generator). Note sensing electrode on left atrium. D, Partially implanted system. Note external transmitting coil placed over implanted receiver. This external appliance could also be an intermittently used charging coil or an activation control for the implanted receiver (see text). (From Chardack, W.M., Gage, A.A., and Federico, A.J.: *In* Davis-Christopher Textbook of Surgery. 11th ed. Edited by D.C. Sabiston. Philadelphia, W.B. Saunders Company, 1977.)

the arrangement may be unipolar, that is, the negative (cathodal) terminal contacts cardiac tissue and the electrical circuit is completed by the metallic housing of the pulse generator (Fig. 3–2B). The relative merits of bipolar and unipolar stimulation are discussed in more detail in Chapter 4. There is little to choose between these two modalities. Current consumption is identical in both configurations, although the voltage requirement is slightly lower for a unipolar system. Bipolar arrangements are inherently redundant and more resistant to interferences by external electrical fields. A unipolar configuration facilitates the monitoring of the pulse generator's output pulse because it produces a greater pacemaker artifact on the surface electrocardiogram.

Myocardial electrodes require a thoracotomy, an upper abdominal surgical approach, or a combination of these, under general anesthesia. The endocardial electrode can be installed under local anesthesia and usually is threaded through the cephalic or external jugular vein into the right ventricular apical trabeculations.

Myocardial electrodes were the first to be used clinically and initially consisted of insulated multistranded stainless steel wires which served as the leads. The bare tips of the wires were buried in a myocardial tunnel,[2,3] or the conductor terminated in two stainless steel pins emerging from a silicone platform and penetrating the myocardium.[4]

The flexing stresses on the leads and electrodes from cardiac motion are severe, approximately 30 million cycles per year. In addition, there are stresses on the leads from motion of the body, especially when the pulse generator is placed in the abdominal subcutaneous tissues as was the case in the early years of clinical application. Breakage and disruption of the lead electrode was then a common occurrence.

In 1961, a helical coil spring was introduced,[5] consisting of a platinum-iridium coil insulated by a silicone rubber sleeve (Fig. 3–3A). The bare coil protruding from a platform served as the electrode tip. This tip was pushed into a bare area of the left ventricular myocardium and held in place by sutures. The stability of this structure was much better than that of the wires, but the results still left much to be desired.

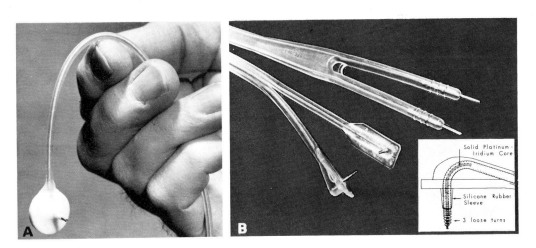

Fig. 3–3. A, Original platinum-iridium helical coil spring myocardial electrode described by us.[5] (From Chardack, W.M., Gage, A.A., and Greatbatch, W.: Correction of complete heart block by a self-contained and subcutaneously implanted pacemaker. J. Thorac. Cardiovasc. Surg., *42*:814, 1961.) B, Subsequent reinforced modification (manufactured by Medtronic, Inc., Model 5814). (From Chardack, W.M.: *In* Gibbon's Surgery of the Chest, 3rd ed. Edited by D.C. Sabiston and F.C. Spencer. Philadelphia, W.B. Saunders Company, 1976.)

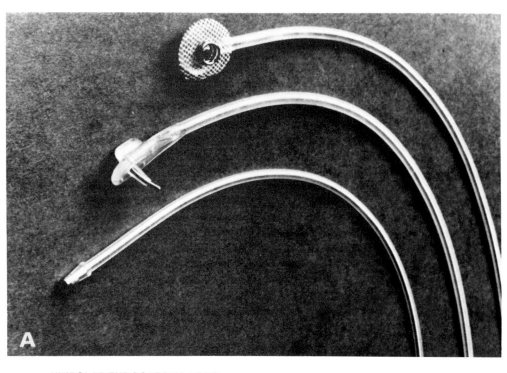

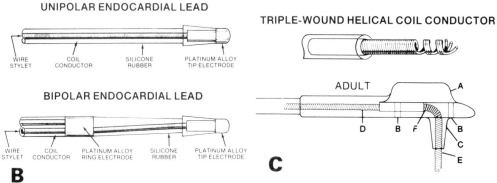

UNIPOLAR ENDOCARDIAL LEAD

WIRE STYLET   COIL CONDUCTOR   SILICONE RUBBER   PLATINUM ALLOY TIP ELECTRODE

BIPOLAR ENDOCARDIAL LEAD

WIRE STYLET   COIL CONDUCTOR   PLATINUM ALLOY RING ELECTRODE   SILICONE RUBBER   PLATINUM ALLOY TIP ELECTRODE

B

TRIPLE-WOUND HELICAL COIL CONDUCTOR

ADULT

C

Fig. 3–4. Commonly used electrode leads. A, Top, screw-in electrode; middle, myocardial electrode; lower, endocardial electrode, unipolar with flanged tip. B and C, Details of construction. (Manufactured by Cardiac Pacemakers, Inc., St. Paul, Minnesota.)

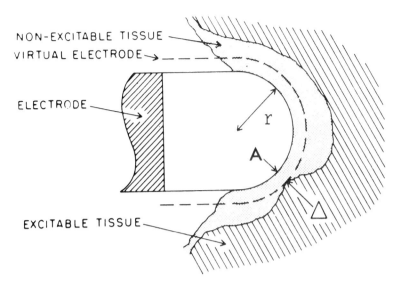

NON-EXCITABLE TISSUE

VIRTUAL ELECTRODE

ELECTRODE

r

A

EXCITABLE TISSUE

Fig. 3–5. Chronic pacing situation with endocardial electrode of popular geometry embedded into muscle at apex of right ventricle. The diameter of scar tissue is not known in any given case. However, its approximate dimension (0.5 to 1.0 mm) is known and calculations lead to conclusion that a decrease in the radius of the hemisphere below the diameter at point A would not yield greater electrode efficiency. (After Parker, B., Furman, S., Hurzeler, P., and Escher, D.[8])

Subsequently, this lead electrode was reinforced with a heavier sleeve. The space between the turns of the coil was filled with silicone rubber and a reinforcing pin was placed into the electrode tip (Figs. 3–3B, 3–4). Since introduction of these reinforcements, the mechanical, as well as the electrical, stability of this electrode has been excellent for periods well in excess of a decade. Clinical usage of this electrode has declined following the introduction of the endocardial lead electrodes in the mid-1960s. Good results have also been reported with coil electrodes made of stainless steel or of Elgiloy,* a nickel cobalt alloy.[6] Because of electrolytic corrosion, most metals other than platinum can be used only in a unipolar mode, i.e., as the cathodal electrode on the heart.

Recently, a sutureless platinum-iridium corkscrew lead electrode was introduced. It has enjoyed increasing popularity and will be dealt with in detail in Chapter 10.

Endocardial lead electrodes are exposed to lesser flex stresses than myocardial ones, and because their installation does not require thoracotomy and general anesthesia, they have become the more widely used lead system. Their structure, bipolar or unipolar, shown in Figures 3–4, 3–6, and 3–7, consists of coil springs (single or multiwound) and ribbon spirals made of stainless steel or other flex resistant alloys. The electrode tip itself is usually made of platinum to minimize current losses caused by polarization.

In recent years, reduction of the size and surface of the electrode has been emphasized as an important factor in saving current and prolonging battery life.[7] Optimal electrode surfaces have been calculated. There is a relationship between the current drain and the thickness of the fibrous tissue reaction surrounding every electrode. Little is achieved by reducing the radius of the electrode tip (generally a hemisphere, a cylinder, or a ring) below the diameter of the fibrous tissue reaction

---

* Elgin Watch Company.

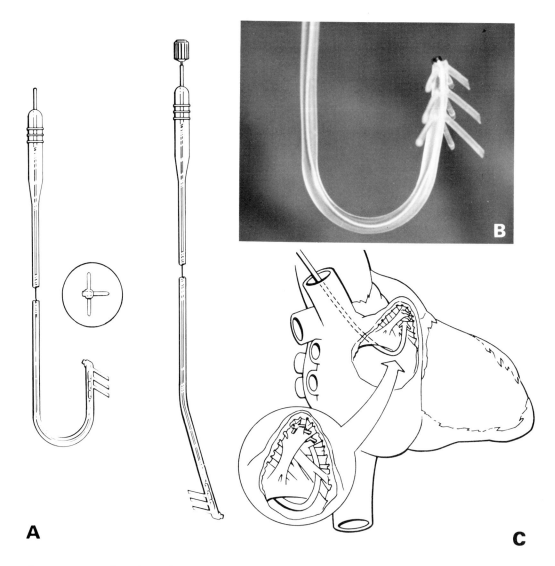

Fig. 3–6. A, J-shaped atrial electrode. (From Citron, P., et al.: Clinical experience with a new transvenous atrial lead. Chest, 73:193, 1978.) B, Diagrammatic representation of electrode implanted. C, Photograph of tined electrode tip. (Manufactured by Medtronic, Inc., Minneapolis, Minnesota.)

(Fig. 3–5).[8,9] An electrode surface commonly used is from 5 to 12 mm.[2] Electrodes with extremely small surfaces can achieve greater current savings but require higher voltages and have led to problems in adequate sensing of the intracardial electrogram, a stringent requirement that must be met with ventricular-programmed pulse generators.[10]

The lead electrode structures described were intended primarily for use on or in the ventricle. The general principles of their construction have also been applied to lead electrodes to pace the atrium, to retrieve atrial potentials, or both. In the case of the epicardial atrial electrodes, the pins were usually shortened, or a clip-on type of electrode was used. In order to adapt the endocardial approach to the atrium and to achieve retention of the electrode in the atrial appendage, J-shaped leads have been designed (Fig. 3–6).[11] The underlying principle is a J-shaped lead which is kept straight, or nearly straight, by an indwelling stylet during placement of the lead. Once the structure is in the atrium, the stylet is withdrawn. The J-shape returns and the electrode hooks into the atrial appendage. Some controversy still exists as to the long-term stability for pacing and/or sensing of atrial endocardial electrodes. Some believe that stable atrial pacing and sensing require an epicardial electrode.

Endocardial electrode lead systems have been widely used because of ease of installation and avoidance of thoracotomy. Their mechanical stability has been good. They have, however, specific drawbacks. The most important is displacement of the lead, which causes increases in current threshold or loss of pacing and/or sensing. The reported incidence of this complication has varied from 7 to 40%. We believe it to be more an intrinsic feature of this approach than a function of the operator's experience. Displacement of the lead tends to occur early and usually during the hospitalization of the patient, but it has also been encountered months and years after installation. In recent years various devices have been developed to achieve fixation and retention of endocardial lead elec-

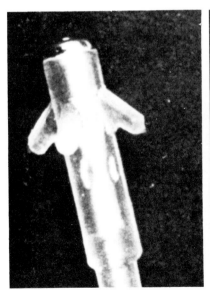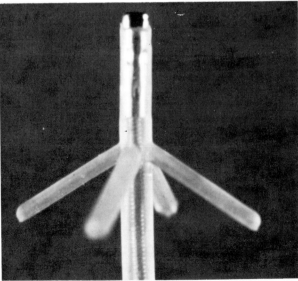

Fig. 3–7. Tined endocardial lead electrodes. Only the enlarged tip is shown. (TENAX, manufactured by Medtronic, Inc., Minneapolis, Minnesota.)

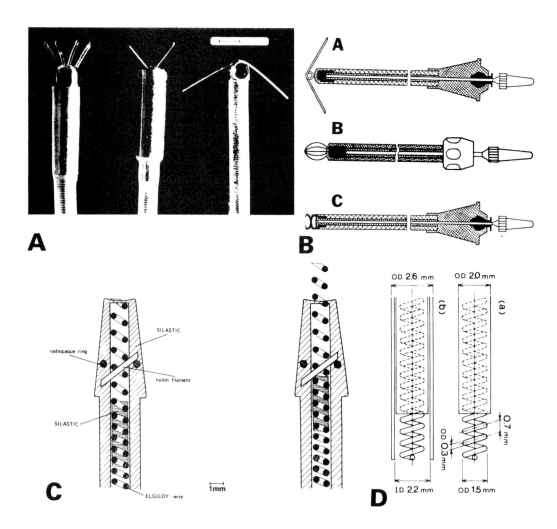

Fig. 3–8.   A variety of designs used to obtain fixation of endocardial electrodes. A, Hook electrodes. From left to right designed by M. Schaldach (1971), W. Irnich (1972), and G. Schmidt (1971). (From Irnich, W.: Engineering concepts of pacemaker electrodes. *In* Advances in Pacemaker Technology. Edited by M. Schaldach and S. Furman. New York, Springer-Verlag, 1975.) B, Wire hooks (A); spreading tip (B); double screw-in (C). (From Bredikis, J.: Permanent cardiac pacing with electrodes with a new type of fixation in the endocardium. Pace, *1*:25, 1978.) C, Screw-in electrode. (From Bisping, H. J., and Rupp, M.: A new permanent transvenous electrode for fixation of the atrium. *In* Cardiac Pacing, Proceedings of the Vth International Symposium, Tokyo, March 14–18, 1978. Edited by Y. Watanabe. Amsterdam, Excerpta Medica, Publisher, 1977.) D, Screw-in electrode. (From Togawa, T., et al.: Experimental and clinical evaluation of a screw-in electrode. *In* Cardiac Pacing, Proceedings of the Vth International Symposium, Tokyo, March 14–18, 1976. Edited by Y. Watanabe. Amsterdam, Excerpta Medica, Publisher, 1977.)

trodes. A number of structures, such as tines, flanges, prongs, and screws, have been used to ensure fixation of the electrode (Figs. 3–7, 3–8). Electrode displacement has been the most commonly observed complication with the older conventional endocardial electrode structures. Long-term observations on the more recent developments with fixation and retention devices are not as yet available.

PULSE GENERATORS

A wide variety of pulse generators are now available. They range from the simple (and historically the first) fixed rate asynchronous pacemaker to a number of sophisticated devices that program themselves automatically from the electrical activity of the heart. Furthermore, the functional parameters of some current pulse generators are noninvasively programmable. Adjustment of stimulus repetition rate, amplitude, or duration is the most important of these.

Pulse generators fall into two broad categories (Table 3–1): *asynchronous devices* which operate independently of cardiac activity and *noncompetitive synchronous devices* which monitor the cardiac electrical activity and deliver (or not) an appropriately timed stimulus. There are approximately 20 major manufacturers of pulse generators in the world. Each offers a number of models. A complete survey of all devices is beyond the scope of this chapter, and only a few representative and innovative designs will be illustrated (Figs. 3–11, 3–14, 3–15).

Asynchronous Pulse Generators

Asynchronous fixed rate pulse generators were introduced in 1960 and remained the most commonly used device until 1966 when noncompetitive pulse generators became available. These early fixed rate devices required a minimum of components (Fig. 3–1) and were inherently insensitive to interference from external electrical fields. Stimuli can be delivered to the atrium (AOO), to the ventricle (VOO), (Fig. 3–9A, B) or to both (DOO).

In the DOO type, the atrioventricular asynchronous pulse generator, two stimuli are applied. The first is delivered to the atrium, and the second, with an appropriate AV delay, to the ventricle. The purpose is to restore atrioventricular synchrony. This requires an additional atrial electrode, two stimuli for each cardiac contraction, and a higher current consumption.

The criticism leveled against fixed rate pulse generators is that they can lead to competitive rhythms in cases of spontaneous ventricular extrasystoles or in cases of temporary or permanent resumption of normal atrioventricular conduction. These events occur frequently in patients with pacemakers (Fig. 3–9C, D). The danger of inducing ventricular fibrillation by pacing stimuli in patients with heart block is generally considered to be remote. There has been no difference in the occurrence of sudden unexplained deaths, conceivably due to induced ventricular fibrillation, in patients with fixed rate pulse generators as compared to a similar group with noncompetitive devices (Table 3–2).[12] As the spectrum of indications has shifted from fixed to intermittent heart block and other arrhythmias, the indications for the use of noncompetitive pulse generators have obviously increased. Conversely, the use of fixed rate pacemakers has decreased and become limited to the few patients known to be in fixed block, who require a replacement pulse generator and who must consider cost.

Programmed Pulse Generators

In current practice, the most widely used pulse generators are of the ventricular-programmed variety. It has been estimated that this type is used in 90% of the patients

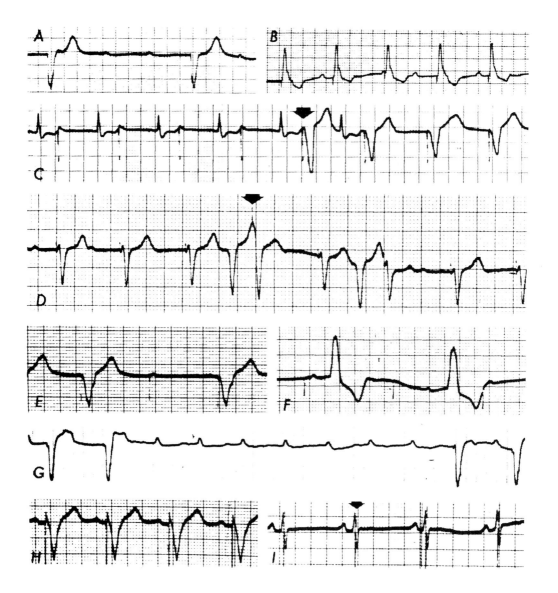

Fig. 3–9. Commonly encountered electrocardiographic patterns in heart block and pacing. *A,* Complete heart block. *B,* Asynchronous pacing (stimulus has no relationship with P wave). *C,* Competitive rhythm. Runs of conducted depolarizations (first five on left) alternate with runs of pacemade beats (last three on right). The arrow shows a pacemade beat interspersed between two conducted depolarizations, leading to a summation of rate. *D,* Competititve rhythm caused by extrasystoles. First three complexes on left are pacemade, the fourth is an extrasystole, and the next pacemaker stimulus (arrow) falls into the vulnerable period after extrasystole. In this particular patient, this phenomenon was innocuous for many years. Extrasystoles during the postoperative period should be suppressed. *E,* Intermittent pacing. Second stimulus from left fails to depolarize. In this case, intermittency was caused by perforation. *F,* Complete failure to pace. None of the three stimuli depolarize. This may be caused by inadequate pulse generator output, electrode displacement, or perforation. *G,* Long period of asystole during interruption of pacing. Note that this occurred even though the driving rate of the pacemaker was slightly below 60. *H,* Complete heart block corrected by synchronous pacemaking. Note constant time relationship between stimulus and preceding P wave. *I,* Resumption of normal conduction during synchronous pacemaking. Pacemaker stimulus (arrow) falls into absolute refractory period. (From Chardack, W. M.: *In* Gibbon's Surgery of the Chest, 3rd ed. Edited by D.C. Sabiston, Jr., and F.C. Spencer. Philadelphia, W. B. Saunders Company, 1976.)

TABLE 3–2

Deaths—Sudden and/or Cause Unknown (Potentially Caused by Ventricular Fibrillation) in 319 Patients (1960 to 1970)

	ASYNCHRONOUS PACEMAKERS	DEMAND PACEMAKERS
No. of patients	205	114
No. of deaths	17	5
% of deaths	8.3	4.5
Patient years at risk	769	188
Death per patient year at risk	1 in 45 years	1 in 38 years

From Chardack, W.M.: *In* Gibbon's Surgery of the Chest, 3rd Edition. Edited by D. C. Sabiston, and F. C. Spencer. Philadelphia, W. B. Saunders Company, 1976.

and is indicated for all primary implantations. External R-wave programmed pacemakers have been known since 1962,[13-15] and the first clinical use of an implantable demand pacemaker was reported in 1966.[16] The purpose of all ventricular-programmed pulse generators is to preclude competitive rhythms caused by normally conducted or ectopic depolarizations and thus avoid the delivery of a pacemaker stimulus into the vulnerable period of the cardiac cycle, the hemodynamic consequences, and reduced efficiency of a competitive rhythm (Fig. 3–9). Two types of ventricular-programmed pulse generators are in use: (1) a ventricular-inhibited device (VVI), also referred to as the true demand pulse generator and the one that has the widest clinical application and (2) a ventricular-triggered variety (VVT).

Ventricular-inhibited Demand Pacemakers

The circuitry of the ventricular-inhibited demand pacemaker detects and responds to any QRS potential that appears at the electrode, endocardial or myocardial. The same electrode is used to retrieve the QRS signal and to carry the output stimulus of the pulse generator. The R-wave signal, appropriately amplified, resets the timing cycle of the demand pulse generator. With the device set to a stimulation frequency of 70 pulses per minute, any ventricular depolarization, ectopic or conducted, which appears before the end of the 857 msec interval (the R-R interval corresponding to a rate of 70 pulses per minute), will suppress the output for another cycle. As long as spontaneous ventricular depolarizations occur at a beat-to-beat rate above 70 per minute, the ventricular-inhibited demand pacemaker remains quiescent and no stimuli appear on the electrocardiogram (Fig. 3–10).

Some devices of this type have a "hysteresis" feature. The escape interval of the pulse generator is longer following a sensed QRS than the interval following an emitted pacing stimulus. This pulse generator does not "cut-in" until the patient's rate drops to a preset value (60 to 65 beats per minute). The advantage claimed for this design is that it will tend to remain quiescent during periods of normal sinus rhythm at rates in the lower range; however, the merit of the hysteresis principle has been questioned.[17]

Accurate sensing of the endocardiac QRS potentials is a cardinal feature of the design of ventricular-programmed pacemakers. This requires filtering and electronic manipulation of the electrical signal to seek out

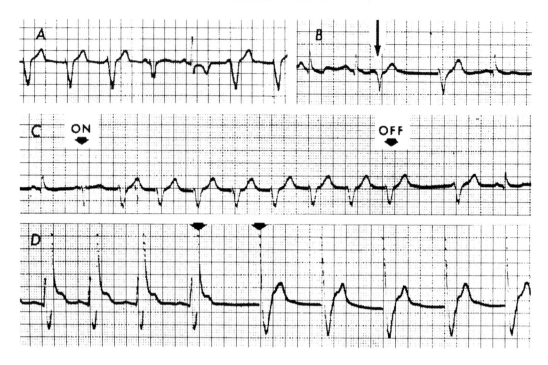

Fig. 3–10. Electrocardiographic patterns with ventricular-programmed pacemakers. *A,* Three pacemade beats on left followed by a fusion beat and a conducted depolarization. The latter suppresses output of pacemaker, which does not appear until preset interval has elapsed. *B,* Normal sinus rhythm—first two complexes on left. At the arrow, a ventricular extrasystole occurs and is followed by a pause that exceeds the programmed cycle of the demand pulse generator. The next depolarization is pacemade, and the last (right) is again a normally conducted beat that suppresses pacemaker output. *C,* Normal sinus rhythm, pacemaker output suppressed, first complex on left. Between arrows, external magnet is applied and device functions as a fixed-rate pulse generator. All depolarizations are pacemade, and when the external control is turned off (arrow, right), a preautomatic pause follows, exceeding the standby interval. The next depolarization is therefore pacemade, and then the normal sinus rhythm (last complex on right) suppresses pacemaker output again. *D,* Ventricular-triggered standby pacemaker. First four depolarizations (left) are conducted, and a pacemaker pulse is directed into the absolute refractory period. Pressure is then applied to the carotid sinus, cardiac rate falls below the standby cycle, and the five depolarizations (beginning at second arrow) are pacemade. (From Chardack, W. M.: *In* Gibbon's Surgery of the Chest, 3rd ed. Edited by D.C. Sabiston, Jr., and F.C. Spencer. Philadelphia, W. B. Saunders Company, 1976.)

potentials of the QRS variety and to discriminate against the sensing of P and T waves. Following the sensing of an endocardial QRS, or after the emission of a pulse, the pulse generator is refractory to another electric input signal (Fig. 3–14). This refractory period should be long enough to prevent the sensing of abnormally large or steep T-waves and short enough to detect early ectopic depolariza-

tion. Following this refractory period, most designs include a brief noise sampling period to prevent interference from external electrical fields. Thus if the sensing circuit detects the presence of repetitive interference potentials, it will revert to a fixed rate mode of pacing instead of having its output suppressed by the interference.

In patients who are in sinus rhythm after a demand pacemaker of the VVI type has been installed, no pacing pulses are emitted as long as the sinus rate remains above the set rate of the pacemaker. Competency of the implanted standby system must therefore be tested from time to time. This is usually accomplished by placing a magnet over the implanted pulse generator. The magnetic field actuates a reed switch in the device which converts it into an asynchronous fixed rate mode of stimulation. Stimuli falling outside the refractory period should then produce electrical parasystole (Fig. 3–10C). In some devices this fixed rate mode has been set to operate at a relatively high rate (80 to 100 pulses per minute), the purpose being to "overdrive" rather than to produce electrical parasystole.

Ventricular-triggered Pacemakers

Ventricular-triggered pacemakers (VVT) have a set escape rate. If spontaneous cardiac activity exceeds this rate, they detect the R-wave and deliver an output pulse after a short delay so that the stimulus falls into the absolute refractory period (Fig. 3–10D). The stimulus artifact is seen on the electrocardiogram and distorts the QRS complex. During normal sinus rhythm, the presence of the artifact does not constitute proof that the stimulus would be above threshold and effective unless the pacing rate can be increased above the normal sinus rate. One specific design (Edwards Pacemaker Systems) emits only a minute stimulus which serves as a tracking signal as long as QRS activity remains above the escape rate of the pulse generator. Since VVT devices deliver a stimulus during periods of normal sinus rhythm, their current consumption is greater than that of ventricular-suppressed devices. Because they are triggered from the QRS signal, they can also be triggered by a small voltage signal applied to the skin, permitting temporary conversion of the system of fixed rate pacing at a higher rate in case this may

be desirable. With rate-programmable devices now available, this particular feature has become obsolete. Ventricular-triggered devices must be protected against interference signals that could lead to a dangerous acceleration of the pacing rate.

Recently a bifocal atrioventricular pulse generator was introduced (DVI).[18] This ventricular-suppressed demand device will pace the atrium as long as atrioventricular conduction remains normal. If AV conduction fails, it will stimulate the ventricle with an appropriate atrioventricular delay. The objective is to combine demand pacing and conservation of atrioventricular synchrony. It requires more complicated electronics, and difficulties with pacemaker-induced arrhythmias have been reported.

Demand pulse generators incorporate sophisticated electronics, since they must be capable of recognizing endocardial potentials differing in amplitude, frequency content, polarity, and rise time. This design objective makes the demand pulse generator more vulnerable to interference by external electrical fields. Unipolar electrode configurations are more difficult to protect than bipolar ones. Up-to-date electronic circuitry and the metallic shielding of the pacemaker do attain the design objectives effectively. However, one must accept the fact that any demand pacemaker will be suppressed by an electrical interference that mimicks a QRS potential or will revert to an asynchronous mode by very strong external electrical interference. Examples of such problems are muscle potentials near the pulse generator, potentials generated by respiratory musculature activity, and intermittent contact of a broken lead. Difficulties in sensing may also arise from inadequate QRS voltages such as may originate in infarcted areas. These problems are of minor clinical significance and are far outweighed by the benefits of the underlying rationale of demand pacemaking, that is, the avoidance of electrical stimulation when it is not needed.

Synchronous P-Wave Atrioventricular Synchronous Pulse Generators (VAT)

Implantable P-wave synchronous pulse generators were introduced in 1963.[19] The concept of restoring the normal mechanism of AV conduction has always aroused considerable interest, since it implies restoration of a normal physiologic mechanism. P-wave synchronous pulse generators require an additional electrode to sense the atrial potential (Fig. 3–2), which is amplified and triggers the pulse generator to deliver a stimulus to the ventricle after a set P-R delay (Fig. 3–9H, I). Atrial-triggered pulse generators must be protected against abnormal atrial electrical activity. To prevent atrial-triggered tachycardias, a blocking circuit with a 2:1 ratio slows the rate of stimulation when atrial signals occur at frequencies between 125 and 150 per minute, and a higher blocking ratio comes into play if the atrial rate increases further. If the atrial electrode fails, atrial potentials become inadequate, or atrial impulse formation slows abnormally, the synchronous pacemaker automatically reverts to an asynchronous mode of pacing at a rate of approximately 70 stimuli per minute.

A discussion of the merits of P-wave synchronous pulse generators (and of AV sequential or AV bifocal devices) must be based on an assessment of the hemodynamics during synchronous and asynchronous pacemaking. With fixed rate pulse generators, there is a limit to which cardiac output can increase in response to high workloads. Maximal performance is of little consequence in a group of patients of a mean age of 70 years, especially since their physical performance is often limited by other factors well below maximum cardiac stress. In regard to the energetics of the heart, a fixed rate compelling cardiac output to increase by an increase of the stroke volume is more efficient than a response by an increase in the rate.[20] It has not been established that the rate response of the atrium is normally optimal, and in fact it has

been found to be inappropriately high in the elderly.[21] The "wisdom" of the mode has been questioned.[22]

Clinical experience in the past two decades has shown that, in most patients, a fixed rate of 70 is compatible with acceptable work performance. In a few, maximal physical performance may be an important objective and require an increase in stroke volume as well as in the rate available only with synchronous pulse generators.

Although improved cardiac performance by proper AV synchronization incident to a properly timed atrial contraction can always be demonstrated experimentally, its loss in most patients does not appear to be clinically significant.[23,24] It is also recognized that at higher pacing rates AV synchrony becomes more important when the pressure work of the left ventricle is abnormally increased or when ventricular function is severely impaired. This leads to the conclusion that AV synchronous pulse generators have their greatest merit in acute situations requiring temporary pacemaking by external pulse generators. The advantages of the system in permanent pacemaking are questionable. Synchronous pacing is contraindicated in the presence of an increase in the frequency of atrial impulse formation. Some patients with synchronous pacemakers have developed angina, decreases in cardiac output, and incipient pulmonary edema at rates above 70 which were still within the normal range of atrial impulse formation.

Although a pacemaker system programmed from the atrium seems an ideal solution, since it is directed at restoration of a normal physiologic state, gains have been more theoretical than practical.

Partially Implanted Pacemakers

Partially implanted systems either transmit the stimulus energy through the intact skin by radiofrequency waves or induction coupling. A number of such devices have been used since 1959 (Fig. 3–2). The advantages of a partially implanted system are that replacement of the pulse generator does not involve another operation, since it is worn outside of the body, and frequency and amplitude of stimulation can be externally adjusted. The drawback of the system is that the patient is required to wear an external appliance, at least temporarily. Partially implanted systems have received less clinical application than fully implanted devices and, with long life and programmable pulse generators now available, they have become obsolete.

Pacemakers powered by rechargeable batteries may be considered partially implanted systems, since part of the system is extracorporeal. Several of these systems have been clinically applied. Because of the small size of the implanted pulse generator, they appear to be attractive for use in the newborn and in the small infant.

Other partially implanted systems include implanted atrial and ventricular pacemakers operating at high frequencies to control tachyarrhythmias. The fully implanted pulse generator is activated and deactivated by an external programmer operated by the physician or the patient.

PULSE GENERATOR RELIABILITY AND POWER SOURCES

Data on the long-term performance of pulse generators were slow to accumulate, since mechanical breakdown of the electrode leads was the predominant failure mode of the system in the early era of pacing. As the electrode problem was resolved, the pulse generator became the factor that limited the life of the system.

Most pulse generator failures have led to limited decreases or increases of the pacing rate or to intermittence or cessation of capture followed by a resumption of an idioventricular rhythm (Fig. 3–9E, F). There have been a number of reported instances in which the mode of failure was

an inordinate increase in the stimulation rate inducing a menacing tachycardia which in some cases led to ventricular fibrillation. The "runaway" pacemaker has been a rare event, but it has occurred even in the fairly recent past with different types and models of pacemakers. It creates an acute emergency and requires disconnection of the malfunctioning device. Prompt resumption of pacing by some other means, such as a prophylactically installed (immediately prior to disconnection) temporary catheter electrode attached to an external pacemaker, is also required. Protection against this mode of failure has been provided in most currently manufactured circuits. The increase in the rate that can be caused by failure of a single component is limited and should not exceed a range of 120 to 140 pulses per minute.

The most important problem of implanted pulse generators has been their limited longevity (15 to 30 months) caused by premature depletion of the mercury-zinc battery; their performance has been far below initial expectations. The responsibility for the unfulfilled prediction of a five-year life is often attributed to an unwarranted optimism by the manufacturers.[25] In fact, the initial estimate of a five-year pulse generator life was made by us and was based on the then available ratings of the mercury-zinc cell which was the only cell available in 1958 and the only cell used in virtually all implanted pulse generators until 1970.[1] The ratings of the cell (1 ampere hour and a shelf life of ten years) had been supplied by the manufacturer.* They had been obtained at room temperature in an ambient atmosphere of relatively low humidity. There had been no conceivable need at that time for long-term tests under conditions prevailing in human tissue, namely, a saline solution at a temperature of 37° C. It quickly became apparent that under those conditions substantial internal

---

* P.R. Mallory Company, Tarrytown, New York.

losses (self-discharge) reduced the pulse generator life to an average of approximately two years.

In the early 1970s, the mercury-zinc cell was improved, and the current drain on it was reduced by shorter pulse duration, more efficient circuitry and improved electrode design, but some characteristics of the cell were difficult to overcome. It uses a liquid electrolyte and as current is produced, the chemical reaction liberates hydrogen gas which must be disposed of. These features made it difficult to achieve hermeticity of the implanted device.

In 1970, alternate power sources came into use, namely, nuclear batteries and lithium cells, both of which can be hermetically sealed.

The Isotopic Cardiac Pacemaker

Nuclear power can provide the energy requirements of a pacemaker system for several decades. The device, first used clinically in 1970 in France,[26] and in 1972 in the United States of America,[27] uses 150 mg of plutonium-238, predominantly an alpha emitter with a half-life of about 87 years (Fig. 3–11). The nuclear fuel is contained by a heavy multilayered capsule and serves as a heat source at a temperature of about 100° C. Heat is transformed into electricity by a bismuth telluride thermopile. The cold source is the outer titanium housing of the pulse generator which is less than 1° C above body temperature. Currently available nuclear pulse generators are of the R-wave ventricular-inhibited type.

Radiation levels on the surface must obviously be negligible, and the fuel must be contained with absolute safety. The fuel capsule, as well as the entire pulse generator assembly, has been tested under conditions simulating a variety of credible accidents, such as vehicle collision, rifle ammunition, airplane crashes, and fire. After several years of extensive clinical testing and an exhaustive environmental impact study, radioisotope pulse generators were cleared by the United States Atomic Energy Commission for general use. Between 1970 and 1977, 2358 radioisotope pacemakers have been implanted throughout the world.[25] No system failure or accident related to the nuclear power source has been reported. In this group, only 14 failures have occurred, and they were related to components in the electronic circuitry. The first generation of radioisotope batteries was designed to last ten years and eight years have now elapsed since the first implant.

Second generation devices (Fig. 3–11) have a design objective of 45 years, and since the behavior of the nuclear power source is predictable, this appears to be a reasonable expectation. A study by the Atomic Energy Commission showed that the radiation effect of the device on essential organs in the patient is of the order of the average natural background radiation (and far below that received by the population in certain states, such as Colorado). The radiation is inconsequential, compared to that involved in routine diagnostic studies. Nevertheless, some have stated that such devices never should have been used in man. We believe that the nuclear-powered pacemaker is completely safe, has had a superb record of performance, and should not be denied to the few patients who require a pulse generator for several decades.

Lithium Systems

A new high energy density solid electrolyte cell using lithium iodine was reported in 1970 and adapted to an implantable pulse generator in 1971.[28] Experimental experience with the lithium iodine system spans nine years; clinical experience with it was first reported in 1974 (Fig. 3–12)[29] and now covers eight years. Although a total of six different battery systems making use of lithium are known to be in existence, we

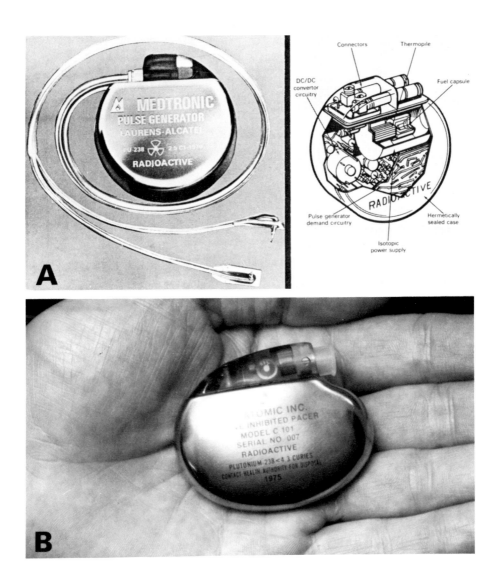

Fig. 3–11. A, First isotopic pulse generator (Medtronic-Laurens-Alcatel VVI)[26,27] equipped with bipolar myocardial helical spring electrodes (Medtronic Model 5814). Weight 170 grams; volume 90 cc. The radioactive fuel is plutonium-238 and the design life of this first unit was 10 years with a potential of 20 years. B, Second generation nuclear-powered pulse generator. It is lighter and smaller (61 grams, 33 cc, 6 cm long) with a design life of 45 years. It has been in clinical use since 1974. (Courtesy David Purdy, Coratomic, Inc., Indiana, Pennsylvania.)

Radiation from these devices is negligible. For instance, the radiation dose to the patient's trunk is approximately 350 mrem per year as compared to an exposure of 5,000 to 30,000 mrem from a single GI series and fluoroscopy.

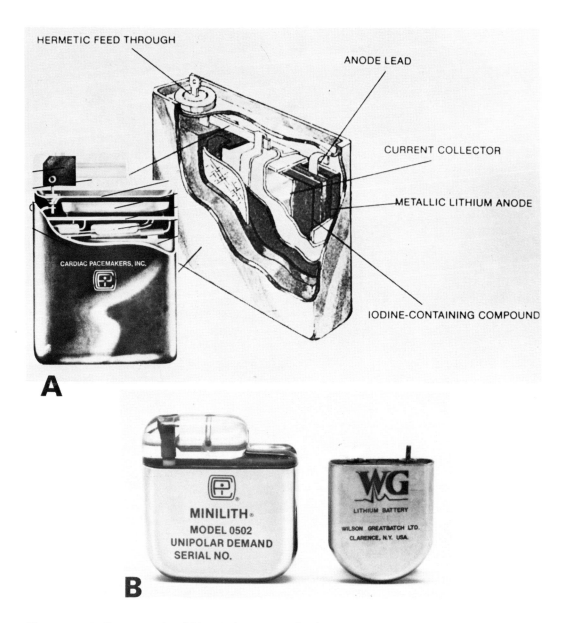

Fig. 3–12.   A, First generation lithium iodine powered pulse generator.[28,29] Dimensions 77 × 56 × 16 mm; weight 165 gm; volume 70 cc; WG 702 cell. (From Chardack, W.M.: Cardiac pacemakers and heart block. *In* Gibbon's Surgery of the Chest, 3rd Ed. Edited by D.C. Sabiston, Jr., and F.C. Spencer. Philadelphia, W.B. Saunders Company, 1976.) B, Second generation lithium pulse generator. Dimensions 49 mm × 52.4 mm × 17.0 mm; weight 93.5 gm; volume 37.7 cc; WG cell 752. (Courtesy Cardiac Pacemakers, Inc., St. Paul, Minnesota.)

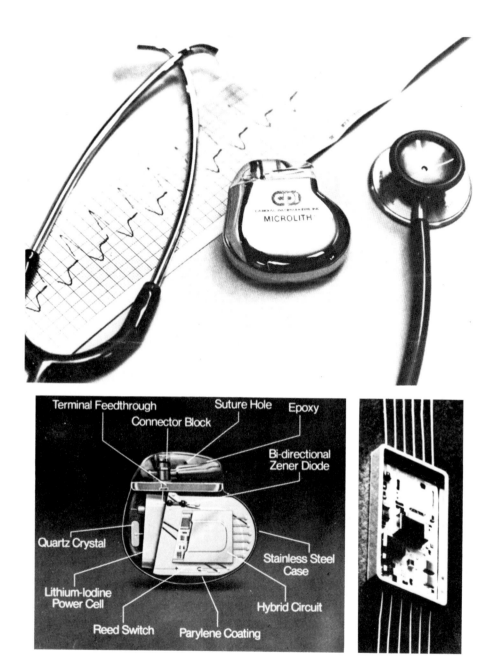

Fig. 3–13. Third generation lithium powered pulse generator. Dimensions 53 mm × 55 mm × 18 mm; weight 75 gms; volume 36 cc; power source WGL lithium-iodine cell; output 5.0 volts, beginning of life. Note triple hermetic seal and construction detail. Available in asynchronous, demand, and programmable demand pulse generators. (Courtesy Cardiac Pacemakers, Inc., St. Paul, Minnesota.)

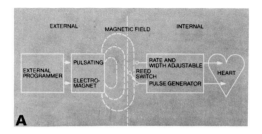

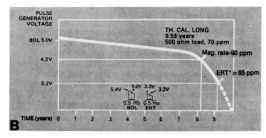

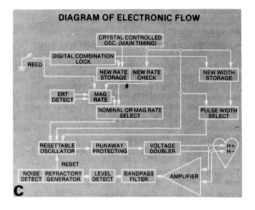

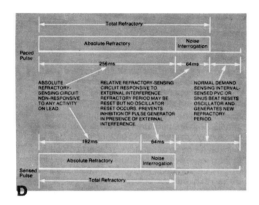

Fig. 3–14. Diagrammatic description of programmable pulse generator (Microlith-P manufactured by Cardiac Pacemakers, Inc., St. Paul, Minnesota). A, Schematic of programming by transmission of a coded signal. B, Typical depletion characteristics of lithium iodine cell, Model 755 (Wilson Greatbatch, Ltd., Clarence, New York). C, Block diagram of electronic circuit. Compare this with 8-component blocking oscillator shown in Figure 3–1. D, Schematic showing absolute refractory and noise interrogation period characteristic of demand pulse generators.

will discuss only the lithium-iodine system because it is the most commonly used and has been under observation for the longest period of time. The reliability of this system in clinical practice has proven to be better than that of the previously used mercury cells.

Several features of the lithium system make it ideal for use in an implantable pulse generator. Its energy density compares favorably, in size and weight, with that of the mercury cell. These characteristics have led to a smaller and lighter pulse generator of a geometry that is more suited to implantation (Figs. 3–12, 3–13). The lithium-iodine system uses a solid electrolyte, no gas is formed during the chemical reaction, and the cell is hermetically sealed. As current is drawn from the battery, resistance within the cell increases and a slow decline in cell voltage occurs. Thus the discharge curve for this system shows a slow linear voltage decrease which tends to accelerate more rapidly when the cell nears depletion (Fig. 3–14). This end-of-life depletion takes place over a period of months and lends itself to end-of-life indicators in the electronic circuitry, such as a decrease of the pacing rate, a change of pulse width, or both. The capacity of this battery system varies somewhat depending on size, weight, and cell design, but after eight years of actual experience, it is credible to expect a pulse generator life of ten years and with further improvements a 20-year pulse generator is possible. Since the mean age of patients requiring an implantable pulse generator has remained at 70 years, even though the spectrum of clinical indications has changed, the lithium-iodine or equivalent systems should satisfy the requirements for a lifetime pacemaker in about 90% of the patient population.

The lithium-iodine system can be hermetically sealed without difficulty. The electronic microcircuit is in a second separate hermetically sealed container, and the metallic housing of the pulse generator acts as a third hermetic seal (Figs. 3–12, 3–13).

The original electronic circuitry was a simple two-transistor, transformer-coupled, blocking oscillator (Figs. 3–1, 3–15). The next generation of pulse generators were demand pacemakers with printed circuit boards and transistors. These were followed by hybrid integrated circuits and then by monolithic integrated circuits with hundreds of transistors (Fig. 3–15), capacitors, and resistors, all screened onto silicone chips with individual elements too small to be seen with the naked eye. In electronic engineering, simplicity is directly related to reliability. This would lead one to conclude that the more complicated circuits would be less reliable; however, the screening of components makes human error in assembly nearly impossible. In addition, the ease at which these tiny silicone chips can be hermetically sealed allows the present pacemaker to be considerably more reliable than its discrete component predecessor.

At the present time, random electronic failures occur in a small fraction of 1% of devices per year, and reliability of the electronic circuitry has increased considerably in the past 20 years. It must be realized by the physician and the patient, however, that random failure will always occur at some finite, albeit very low, incidence. The observed incidence of failures now compares favorably with that of other prostheses implanted in the body and also with the adverse reactions occurring during the administration of many drugs.

A number of other power sources have been used experimentally and clinically in implantable pulse generators. Rechargeable battery systems have been dealt with. For the sake of completeness, mention should be made of biologic fuel cells and radioactive power sources using a beta voltaic system converting beta radiation from promethium-147 directly into electricity. None of these systems has seen wide clinical usage.

PROGRAMMABILITY

The concept of adjusting the output of implantable pacemakers, pulse amplitude, or repetition rate or both, dates back to 1960, the year of the first clinical applications. Noninvasive programming of a high and low rate was then described.[2] It aimed at a higher pacing rate during physical exercise. Invasive programming by insertion of a needle of triangular cross section was accomplished in the early 1960s.[30] The needle-penetrated potentiometers were palpable on the periphery of the pulse generator, and rate, and output amplitude could be adjusted. A much more sophisticated system using an external programmer to choose between four output current amplitudes and a limited number of rates was introduced in 1972.*

A second generation device of recent manufacture uses variations in a magnetic field to transmit a coded digital signal to the implanted pulse generator (Figs. 3–13, 3–14). The rate is programmable from 30 ppm to 119 ppm in steps of 1 ppm. Instead of programming the pulse amplitude, the duration of the stimulus can be adjusted from 0.1 to 1.9 msec in steps of 0.1 msec. The output width is 0.05 when the controller is set to the zero position.

Noninvasive programming of the pulse width through an external rotating magnet was reported initially in 1970.[31] The device then in use was quite unsophisticated in comparison to the one shown in Figures

---

* Omnicor, Cordis Company, Miami, Florida.

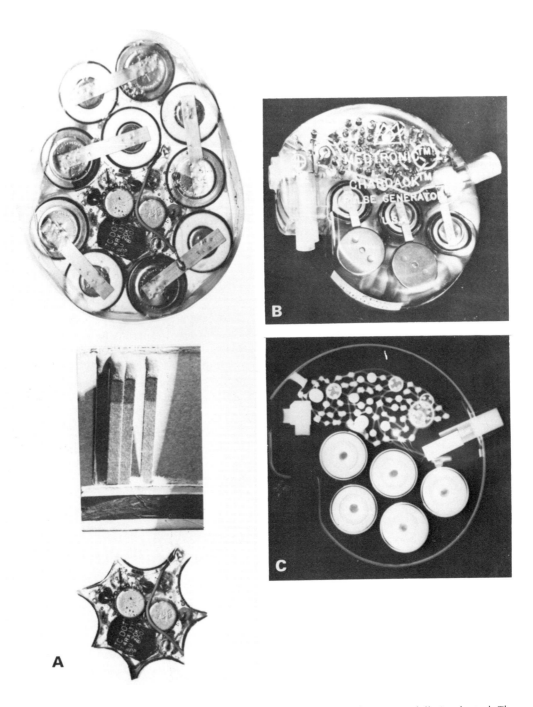

Fig. 3–15. Pictorial history of pacemaker technology. A, First pacemaker successfully implanted. The circuitry, embedded in epoxy, has 1 transformer, 2 transistors, 8 resistors, and 2 capacitors (lower left) and 10 mercury cells. B, Typical demand pacemaker (late 1960,[5] manufactured by Medtronic, Inc.) containing approximately 40 discrete components assembled on a circuit board (or cord wood construction) and only 5 mercury cells. C, X-ray picture of pacemaker. Protrusion on right is a potentiometer permitting invasive adjustment of rate or amplitude.

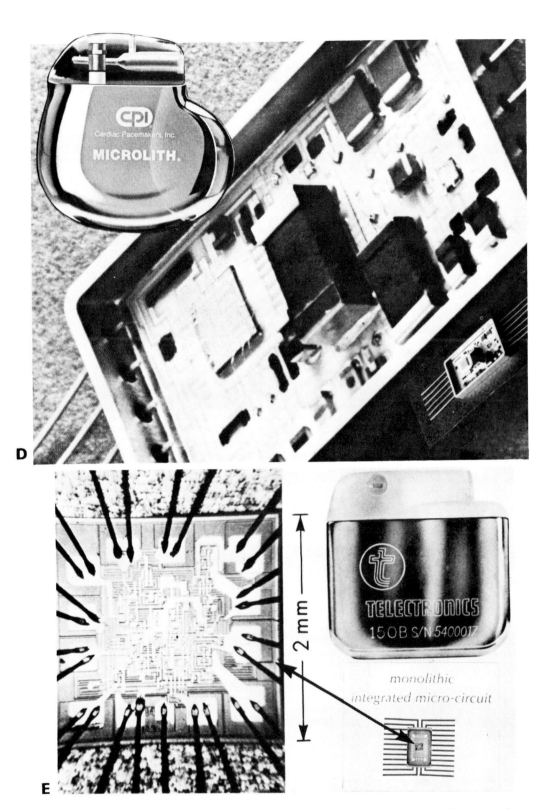

Fig. 3–15 (continued). D, Contemporary pacemaker using a hermetically sealed hybrid. Actual size shown in lower right corner (Courtesy Cardiac Pacemakers, Inc., St. Paul, Minnesota.) E, Contemporary pacemaker using a fully integrated circuit. A myriad of components is contained in the small chip, shown in actual size (lower right: 2 × 2 mm), in its hermetically sealed can, and magnified (lower left). (Courtesy Telectronics, Inc., Buffalo, N.Y.)

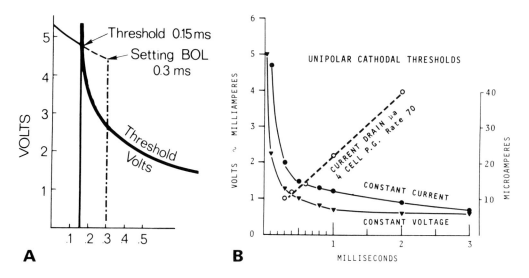

Fig. 3–16. A, Typical threshold curve with nominal 5.2 output pulse. Threshold several weeks after implantation is at 0.15 msec pulse duration. Setting of 0.3 msec provides 100% margin above threshold requirement. B, Strength duration curve obtained by constant current and constant voltage stimuli. Obtained from myocardial electrode (unipolar cathodal) three years after implantation. It is more efficient to stimulate at 5 milliamperes at a pulse duration of 0.3 msec (2 times threshold) than at 2 msec and 2 milliamperes. Drain on batteries depends upon current × time and not on energy (that is current × voltage × time). Note that current drain (microamperes) decreases linearly with pulse width. Data on current drain were obtained from a four-cell pulse generator set to a rate of 70. These data were obtained in 1970. Note that today's circuits are much more efficient, and at a pulse width setting of 0.3 msec, drains well below 10 microamperes should obtain in 90% of patients. (After Chardack, W.M., et al.: Magnetically actuated pulse width control for implantable pacemakers. Ann. Cardiol. Angeiol. (Paris), 20:345, 1971.)

3–13 and 3–14, but it emphasized the advantages of programming pulse width rather than amplitude. The physiologic basis for this type of programming is shown in Figure 3–15 depicting a typical strength duration curve. Since the threshold is dependent on current (produced by voltage) and pulse duration, either one of these parameters can be adjusted to obtain a stimulus pulse that exceeds the threshold requirement by an appropriate margin of approximately 100%. Adjustment of the pulse width yields two important advantages. It is more efficient, since it entails no energy loss in the electronic circuitry. More importantly, the duration of the pulse generator artifact as it appears on the body surface lends itself to an absolute and highly accurate readout by a relatively sim-

ple and inexpensive monitoring device. Adjustment of the pulse amplitude entails loss of energy in the circuitry. Recognition of the pacemaker artifact as it appears on the body surface requires the use of an oscilloscope and lends itself only to a relative measurement. For this reason, when output amplitude is programmed, the programmer's setting must be taken at face value, since the accuracy of the setting cannot be verified by an absolute measurement.

Our experience in the past eight years with noninvasive pulse width adjustment* has shown that in 355 patients with a variety of electrodes, 90% had a threshold of 0.15 msec or less (at an output voltage of

---

* Medtronic pulse generators Model 5931 and Model 5961. Medtronic, Inc., Minneapolis, Minnesota.

5.2) and therefore could be paced with a pulse width set between 0.25 and 0.3 msec. Under these circumstances, current drain on the pulse generator is low (Fig. 3–16) and even lower with the more efficient circuitry of current devices (Fig. 3–13). At settings between 0.25 and 0.3 msec, a pacing rate of 70 beats per minute, and constant pacing, a pulse generator longevity of 11 years is a conservative estimate. We conclude that programmability of the pulse duration is a most valuable feature which achieves important savings in current drain and lends itself to easy monitoring and to a periodic check of the patient's threshold requirements and of the underlying spontaneous cardiac electrical activity.

Programmability of the rate appears to be of value but only in a small number of cases.[32] Postimplantation changes in the heart rate may be of benefit when one wishes to increase the rate to control tachyarrhythmias and suppress ectopic activity or to decrease the rate to control angina (reducing cardiac work and increasing diastolic coronary flow). Clinical experience has shown that these situations arise rarely, but if they do occur, the availability of a noninvasive method to change the rate is of importance, since it may avoid the replacement of a pulse generator by one of a different rate.

Programmability of the refractory period, the sensitivity of QRS detection, the AV delay, and the pacing mode are under development. A good deal of evaluation will be required to appraise the merit of the programmability of these features. It must be emphasized that clinical experience with programmable pacemakers is still limited. Cases of misprogramming have already been reported. We know from experience that problems with electromechanical systems take time to become manifest and final judgment of the benefits of this advanced and exciting technologic development should be reserved until it can be backed by hard data from actual experience.

PERSPECTIVES

Since their introduction, implantable pacemakers have led to complete rehabilitation of patients with atrioventricular block, and their survival is close to that of a normal comparable population,[33,34] whereas before pacing the one-year mortality rate was 50 to 60%. In addition, pacing is applied to a variety of other rhythm disorders. It is true that these results have been achieved at the cost of many repeat operations caused by failure of the electrode or the pulse generator and often because the original estimates of battery life were not borne out.

Some components of the pacemaker system can be evaluated by accelerated testing. The batteries cannot, at least not with acceptable confidence. To have delayed therapy until the "perfect" system had been designed and tested would have meant that over a period of ten years countless lives would have been lost, not to mention the disability of the survivors. Also, such a course of "omission" would have gone unnoticed.

Most pacemaker malfunctions have not constituted a great risk to life, even though they have required repeated interventions. There has been considerable emphasis in the lay press on the number of deaths caused by "faulty" pulse generators. The number of documented instances is a small proportion of the hundreds of thousands of devices that have been implanted. The General Accounting Office made a survey of these occurrences in the United States over a three-year period (1972 to 1975). Only 10 documented instances came to light, with an additional 18 suspected but not proved. Another survey, covering 40,000 patients in 1975, revealed a documented incidence of 19 cases, or 0.06% of the pacemaker population.[35] This incidence is insignificant compared to the long-term mortality encountered with cardiac valve replacements, many other surgical procedures, or even adverse reactions from a variety of drugs.

The media in recent years also focused on the high cost of medical care, and the pacemaker has frequently been indicted as a high cost technologic item. Nothing could be further from the truth. The total cost of pacemaking per patient day has been assessed at approximately $3.00/day in the United States (1975)[36] and at a low of 60¢/day in Great Britain (1976).[37] Compare this to a cost of $12,000 to $20,000 per year for a patient on kidney dialysis or one with a kidney transplant whose rehabilitation is far from complete.

Much has been said about the high cost of pacemaker therapy to the patient and the economy. Little has been said about the contribution to the economy of therapy which restores productivity through the avoidance of morbidity and mortality, in purely monetary terms, not even considering intangibles like the value of human life and suffering on which a dollar value cannot be placed. The pacemaker is a good case in point. The mean age of the patients is 70 years. Few patients will return to a productive life and become contributors (in terms of dollars) to the economy. This would lead one to conclude that the economic impact of pacemaker therapy might be one of high cost. In fact, analysis shows that the contribution to the economy resulting from the treatment of the small percentage of young people who are returned to productive work far outweighs the treatment cost of the elderly. It has been calculated that the total treatment cost of the patient population, in the United States of America in 1976 was exceeded three times by the net benefits resulting from the contribution made to the economy by the rehabilitation of younger patients. This "high cost technology therapy" has not been a drain on the economy but has made a positive contribution to it.[38]

Reliability problems with pacemakers have also contributed to the enactment of the Medical Device Act investing the Food and Drug Administration of the United States of America with regulatory authority over medical devices of all kinds. This has led to an increase in the cost and the time involved in the development and the manufacture of medical devices, but it is questionable whether the legislation has improved the quality and reliability of pulse generators.[39] Indeed, the greatest number of devices recalled recently have involved pulse generators manufactured according to standards set by and under the supervision of the regulatory agency.

We conclude that cardiac pacing systems have been vastly improved since their inception. The reliability and longevity of current devices have been increased. The indications for their use have been broadened. The operative risk of this therapy is as low as that of cardiac catheterization, the beneficial results are immediate, and the rewards in terms of reduction of mortality and morbidity are great.

REFERENCES

1. Chardack, W.M., Gage, A.A., and Greatbatch, W.: A transistorized, self-contained, implantable pacemaker for the long-term correction of complete heart block. Surgery, 48:643, 1960.
2. Kantrowitz, A., et al.: The treatment of complete heart block with an implanted controllable pacemaker. Surg. Gynecol. Obstet., 115:415, 1962.
3. Zoll, P.M., et al.: Long-term electrical stimulation of the heart for Stokes-Adams disease. Ann. Surg., 154:330, 1961.
4. Hunter, R.W., Roth, N.A., and Bernardez, D.: A bipolar myocardial electrode for complete block. Lancet, 79:509, 1959.
5. Chardack, W.M., Gage, A.A., and Greatbatch, W.: Correction of complete heart block by a self-contained and subcutaneously implanted pacemaker. J. Thorac. Cardiovasc. Surg., 42:814, 1961.
6. Nathan, D.A.: Synchronous electronic ventricular pacing. J.A.M.A., 199:109, 1967.
7. Furman, S., Garvey, J., and Hurzeler, P.: Pulse duration variation and electrode size as factors in pacemaker longevity. J. Thorac. Cardiovasc. Surg., 69:382, 1975.
8. Parker, B., Furman, S., Hurzeler, P., and Escher, D.: Electrode geometry and the evolution of long-term endocardial threshold. Conference Eng.

Med. Biol., 27th, Philadelphia, 1974. Proceedings Chevy Chase, Md., Alliance for Eng. in Med. and Biol., 1974.

9. Irnich, W.: Consideration in electrode design for permanent pacing. In Cardiac Pacing. Edited by H. J. Thalen. Assen, The Netherlands, Van Gorcum & Co., Publisher, 1973, p. 268.

10. Hughes, H.C., Brownlee, R.R., and Tyers, G.F.O.: Failure of demand pacing with small surface area electrodes. Circulation, 54:128, 1976.

11. Citron, P., et al.: Clinical experience with a new transvenous atrial lead. Chest, 73:193, 1978.

12. Zoll, P.M., and Weintraub, M.J.: Safety of competition from fixed rate pacemakers. In Cardiac Pacing. Proceedings of the Vth International Symposium, Tokyo, March 14–18, 1976, Edited by Yosho Watanabe. Amsterdam, The Netherlands, Excerpta Medica, Publisher, 1977.

13. Nicks, R., Stening, G.F.H., and Hulme, E.C.: Some observations on the surgical treatment of heart block in degenerative heart disease. Med. J. Aust., 2:857, 1962.

14. Zacouto, F.: Cardiorythmeur intracorporel a inhibition externe. Soc. Francaise Cardiol., 20 Octobre 1963, p. 1296.

15. Lemberg, L., Castellanos, A., Jr., and Berkovits, B.V.: Pacemaking on demand in A-V block. J.A.M.A., 191:106, 1965.

16. Parsonnet, V., et al.: Clinical use of an implantable standby pacemaker. J.A.M.A., 196:104, 1966.

17. Friedberg, H.D., and Barold, S.S.: Editorial. On hysteresis in pacing. J. Electrocardiol., 6(1):00–2, 1973.

18. Berkovits, B.V.: Bifocal demand pacing. Digest 9th International Conference in Medical and Biological Engineering, Melbourne, August 24, 1971.

19. Nathan, D.A., et al.: An implantable synchronous pacemaker for the long-term correction of complete heart block. Am. J. Cardiol., 11:362, 1963.

20. Chardack, W.M.: Heart block treated with an implantable pacemaker—past experience and current developments. Progr. Cardiovasc. Dis., 6:507, 1964.

21. Furman, S.: Fundamentals of cardiac pacing. Am. Heart J., 73:261, 1967.

22. McNally, E., and Benchimol, A.: Medical and physiological considerations in the use of artificial cardiac pacing. Part I, Am. Heart J., 75:380, 1968; Part II, Am. Heart J., 75:679, 1968.

23. Braunwald, E.: Symposium on cardiac arrhythmias with comments on the hemodynamic significance of atrial systole. Am. J. Med., 37:655, 1964.

24. Burchell, H.B.: A clinical appraisal of atrial transport function. Lancet, 1:775, 1964.

25. Parsonnet, V.: Cardiac pacing and pacemakers VII. Power sources for implantable pacemakers Part I and Part II. Appraisal and reappraisal of cardiac therapy. Am. Heart J., 94:517, 1977.

26. Laurens, P., and Piwnica, A.: Stimulateur cardiaque isotopique, recherche sur la securite et la fiabilite a long terme. Arch. Mal. Coeur, 63:906, 1970.

27. Gage, A.A., Chardack, W.M., and Federico, A.J.: Isotopic cardiac pacemaker. Arch. Surg., 109:671, 1974.

28. Greatbatch, W., et al.: The solid-state lithium battery:a new improved chemical power source for implantable cardiac pacemakers. IEEE Trans. Bio-Med. Eng. BME, 18 (5):317, 1971.

29. Lillehei, C.W., et al.: A new solid state long life lithium powered pulse generator. Ann. Thorac. Surg., 18:479, 1974.

30. Chardack, W.M., et al.: Two years' clinical experience with the implantable pacemaker for complete heart block. Dis. Chest., 43:225, 1963.

31. Chardack, W.M., et al.: Magnetically actuated pulse width control for implantable pacemakers. Ann. Cardiol. Angeiol. (Paris), 20:345, 1971.

32. MacGregor, D.C., et al.: The utility of the programmable pacemaker. Pace, 1:254, 1978.

33. Soots, G., et al.: Zur u berlebenszeit von patienten mit herzschrittmachern. Wschr., 117:537, 1975.

34. Furman, S.: Controversies in cardiac pacing. In Cardiology. Edited by Eliot Corday. Philadelphia, F.A. Davis Co., 1977, pp. 301–317.

35. Parsonnet, V.: Round table discussion in Cardiac Pacing. Proceedings Vth International Symposium. Tokyo, March 14–18, 1976. Edited by Yoshio Watanabe. Amsterdam, The Netherlands, Excerpta Medica, Publisher, 1977.

36. Stoney, W.S., et al.: Cost of cardiac pacing. Am. J. Cardiol., 37:23, 1976.

37. Norman, J.: Pacemakers: the long-term cost. Lancet, 1:88, 1976.

38. Chardack, M.H., B.S. (Econ.): Senior thesis, unpublished data.

39. Skalnik, B.: Pacemakers and the Medical Device Amendments of 1976. Pace, 6:36, 1978.

SELECTED READINGS

Electrical control of cardiac activity is a recent and still ongoing development involving the disciplines of surgery, cardiology, electrophysiology, electronics, and bioengineering. A good overview can be gained from a review of the proceedings of the five international symposia on cardiac pacing which have been held every three years beginning in 1963. The proceedings of four of these symposia are in the English language and the last two are cited as selected references. They contain contributions by numerous authors covering every technical and clinical aspect of cardiac pacing.

The views of the authors are set forth in more detail in:

Chardack, W.M., Gage, A.A., and Federico, A.J.: *In* Davis-Christopher Textbook of Surgery. Edited by D.C. Sabiston, Jr. Philadelphia, W.B. Saunders Company, 1977.

Chardack, W.M.: Cardiac pacemakers and heart block. *In* Gibbon's Surgery of the Chest, 3rd Ed. Edited by D.C. Sabiston, Jr. and F.C. Spencer. Philadelphia, W.B. Saunders Company, 1976. (The bibliography in this chapter is up to date to 1975 and provides further documentation of the views of the author.)

The historical developments in the field of electrical stimulation of the heart have been covered in:

Schechter, D.C.: Background of clinical cardiac stimulation. N. Y. State J. Med., *71–72*:2575, 1971–1972. (This article is a detailed account of the history of electrical stimulaton of the heart.)

Glenn, W.W.L.: (Ed.): Cardiac pacemakers. Ann. N.Y. Acad. Sci., *111*:813, 1964.

Furman, S. (Ed.).: Advances in cardiac pacemakers. Ann. N.Y. Acad. Sci., *167*:515, 1969.

Thalen, H.V. (Ed.): Cardiac Pacing. Proceedings Fourth International Symposium on Cardiac Pacing, Groningen, The Netherlands, April, 1973. Van Gorcum and Co., The Netherlands, 1973.

Cardiac Pacing. Proceedings Fifth International Symposium on Cardiac Pacing. Tokyo, Japan, 1976. Amsterdam, The Netherlands, Excerpta Medica, 1977.

4

Physiologic Basis of Cardiac Pacing

SEYMOUR FURMAN

The cardiac pacemaker is the most successful electronic device implanted in the body and has been used in some 300,000 persons worldwide. It is, at present, one of the mainstays of modern cardiac therapy. Many cardiac arrhythmias have become permanently controllable by electrical cardiac stimulation since the initial development of external transcutaneous pacing in 1952, the later development of wired external transthoracic and transvenous pacing, and finally, the implantable transvenous and transthoracic pacemakers.

Three bases have made widespread outpatient pacemaker therapy possible. The first was the development of a wholly implantable device, initially unsuccessfully powered by a rechargeable nickel-cadmium battery and later in a successful version by a mercury-zinc battery which became the universal power source for implanted cardiac pacemakers until recently and which, even in 1977, was the power source of approximately half the pacemakers implanted.

The second basis was the development of long-term pacing by the transvenous route which allowed the extension of pacemaker therapy to virtually anyone, whatever the state of well-being. Transthoracic pacing, which had been obviously successful, nevertheless was not as freely applied to the elderly or debilitated. Transvenous implantation with local anesthesia and little physiologic disturbance has filled the need for a universally useful technique.

The third basis was the development of pacemakers able to sense and respond to atrial and/or ventricular activity and be noncompetitive with spontaneous cardiac function. These developments opened pacemaker therapy to the patient with intermittent heart block and a wide variety of other arrhythmias, such as the sick sinus syndrome, which together account for half of the patients paced. Fixed complete heart block, the classic indication for cardiac pacing, has decreased to about one fifth. It was recognized years ago that many patients who demonstrated complete heart block on one occasion had frequent episodes of intermittent AV conduction.

At present, the pacemaker field is undergoing renewed ferment. Over the past four years a new power source, the lithium cell, has been introduced; it is capable of prolonged longevity, unknown except for the nuclear pacemaker of preceding years. It permits hermetic sealing of the power source and circuit on a widespread, practical basis and provides a pacemaker that in any one of a variety of fabrications and power sources will last for the lifetime of one half to two thirds of all patients.

A simultaneous development has been the change in the electronic industry's capability for the production of sophisticated, miniaturized, and long-lasting circuitry. The discrete circuit of condensers, transistors, and resistors is now old-fashioned and has been replaced by hybrids, which have a few older components along with the newer small, single unit circuits. These circuits alone offer higher reliability and complexity, greater longevity, and far smaller size. They have increased efficiency, and decreased current drain to allow batteries of small capacity and size but long shelf life to last far longer than the much bulkier batteries of an earlier era.

In general, the more complex and the more the capability of a circuit, the greater the battery drain. New pacing modes are under development and older modes, only marginally successful because of major battery drain and short life, have now become more useful because of reduced stimulation and circuit energy requirements. Because of these changes in pacemaker circuitry, power source, and hermetic sealing, there has been overall reduction in volume and weight by 50 to 70% and increase in longevity from an average of two and one-half to three years to a realistic projection of several times that duration. Electrode changes in the past few years have made transthoracic pacing easier and have equally made transvenous pacing by active fixation electrodes more secure and more readily possible.

The major thrust of cardiac pacing in the last few years has been the addition of pacing for the sick sinus syndrome and other arrhythmias to that for complete or intermittent heart block. Approximately one third of all patients now undergoing pacing have sick sinus syndrome. A variety of other bradycardias or tachycardias not related to complete or intermittent heart block further increase the proportion. This finding, though well recognized only in the past few years, was heralded by the first patient subjected to prolonged transvenous pacing. He had bradycardia, asystole, and recurrent Adams-Stokes seizures but did not have classic complete heart block; rather he had rheumatic mitral valve disease, chronic atrial fibrillation, and a very slow ventricular response. The immediate cause of asystole was hypokalemia which at that time was unappreciated as the cause of his bradycardia.

Patients undergoing implantation of a permanent cardiac pacemaker average 72 years of age (Fig. 4–1), over one half with arteriosclerotic heart disease, one fifth with hypertension, and one tenth with diabetes mellitus. Rheumatic heart disease accounts for approximately 5% of those implanted and acute myocardial infarction for another 5%. Approximately 1% of implants are required because of heart block produced as a complication of cardiac surgery (Table 4–1).

The indications for implantation of a cardiac pacemaker are presently being extended into two major directions. The first is the treatment prophylactically of the patient who has undergone electrophysiologic study with demonstration of a prolonged H-V interval or other findings indicative of impending AV dissociation. These may occur following acute myocardial infarction or a syncopal attack of otherwise undetermined origin. The second area is management of reentry tachycardias of the macro and micro variety and other ventricular and supraventricular tachycardias by a combination of bursts of rapid atrial pacing, bursts of rapid ventricular pacing, the establishment of a ventricular or atrial rate in combination with medication to suppress

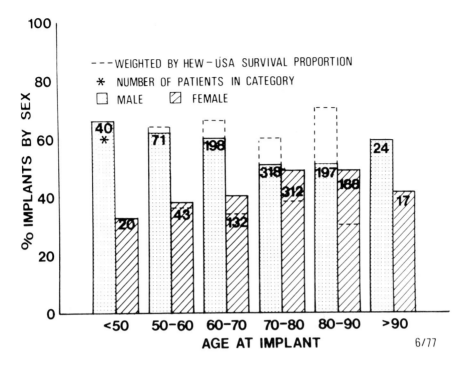

Fig. 4–1. Percentage of pacemaker implants by age and sex between 1962 and 1976 for 1,560 patients implanted at Montefiore Hospital and Medical Center. The bar graphs are weighted by the relative proportion of men and women in the overall population at each age group, as well as by the number of pacer patients who appear in this group. Because of the number of men and women in the 80- to 90-year group it is approximately twice as likely that a surviving male will require a pacemaker implant than a female.

TABLE 4–1

Pacer Implants: Rhythm Disturbance

Sinus node dysfunction	36%
Brady-tachy syndrome	20%
Sinus arrest	11%
Sinus bradycardia	5%
Atrial fibrillation with ventricular rate below 50	4.1%
Complete heart block	18%
Acquired	17%
Congenital	1.0%
Intermittent heart block	35%
Wolff-Parkinson-White syndrome	1.0%
Other ventricular arrhythmia	2.5%
Drug-induced bradycardia	1.0%
Malfunction of implanted pacer	1.0%

myocardial irritability, and the stimulation of the heart during a "window" for termination of tachycardia by competitive pacing either at rapid or physiologic rates. These latter two indications are assuming ever greater importance in the management of tachycardias and of patients with minimally *manifested* AV conduction disturbances.

PROGRAMMABLE PACEMAKERS

One of the most significant recent developments, and one certain to assume far greater future importance, is that of noninvasive programming of pulse generator function. Minimal or even noninvasive variation of pacemaker output and rate is not new. Some of the earliest pacemakers allowed operation of one or two potentiometers either via a percutaneous needle to vary output and rate or via a small subcutaneous incision to approach a resistor, short circuit of which would double the output of the implanted unit. Other units had a magnetic switch which allowed the selection of one or another of two different rates. Both of these techniques were of limited value as the bulk of patients then implanted with pacemakers had fixed complete heart block, and it was not then appreciated that reduction of output would increase pulse generator longevity.

It rapidly became apparent that a single rate, usually 70 beats per minute, was adequate for almost all circumstances of activity. Other variability included the noninvasive addition of counter voltage against the pacer output to allow measurement of stimulation threshold. Still another approach was the magnetic activation of a pacemaker mode in which it continually reduced its output by 0.35 volts from maximum to zero so that the approximate threshold could again be determined. By 1970 a unit existed with a potentiometer activated by an external magnet in which rate was fixed, but pulse duration and, therefore, pacemaker output could be varied. This unit has been associated with a prolonged longevity when used at a short pulse duration.

At present, five different programmable pacemakers are commercially available, and more are expected. All allow the variation of pacemaker rate. Several also allow noninvasive variation of output. These latter pacemakers allow the increase of longevity if the pulse duration or other output factor is reduced so that battery drain is decreased, as presently available lithium batteries have little internal leakage and reduction of output can be directly related to prolongation of longevity. Rate variation is of relatively little importance in patients with fixed complete heart block, but in patients with sick sinus syndrome, or similar conditions, rate variation assumes greater importance.

For patients with inoperable coronary disease a slow pacemaker rate is useful in conjunction with administration of beta blocking agents such as propranolol to reduce myocardial oxygen consumption and cardiac rate. In the elderly, extreme sinus bradycardia may be as slow as 20 to 25 per minute, though the same patient may be substantially asymptomatic at a rate of 50 per minute. A variable rate pacemaker allows protection against the slower rate without imposing a more rapid rate than would be physiologically desirable.

Of even greater interest is the impending availability of programmability of pulse duration, output voltage, sensitivity, refractory period, and pacemaker rate, perhaps in the same unit. Programming will aid the reduction of electromagnetic interference by a reduction of sensitivity and of sensing a poor electrogram by increase of sensitivity. The more distant future will see programmability for control of tachycardias.

THRESHOLD OF CARDIAC STIMULATION

Understanding of the threshold of cardiac stimulation is the basis of electrode and pulse generator design, pulse generator output, and implant technique. A pacemaker that is not able to stimulate the heart can do nothing else therapeutic. The selection of pulse generator output is affected by the threshold characteristics of the electrode. The balance of power source longevity and the output needs to stimulate are affected by a variety of factors.

1. Proximity of the electrode to stimulatable tissue.
2. The maturity of the electrode, i.e., the time it has been in a single position.
3. Pulse duration.
4. Polarity—unipolar or bipolar—and size of the anode.
5. Electrode surface area.
6. The metal of fabrication.
7. Drug effects and electrolyte balance.

Electrode Position

Electrode position is controlled by the surgeon, and the intraoperative selection of the best site is most important. Each electrode, whether myocardial or endocardial, has specific threshold limits within which almost all implants will fall. Current and voltage thresholds rise rapidly with separation from viable myocardium, and such separation can be recognized by high threshold. During normal maturation a layer of nonstimulatable tissue forms, increasing the effective electrode size because of separation of the metal from sensitive tissue. This fibrous layer increases as a function of the geometry of the electrode but always stabilizes, and it is this stabilization that retains thresholds within limits so that it does not rise indefinitely and above the output of any pulse generator (Fig. 4–2).

A significant recent development is that of the active fixation endocardial electrode. All earlier endocardial electrodes had been allowed to become passively attached to the endocardium by the development of an investing fibrous layer. The active fixation

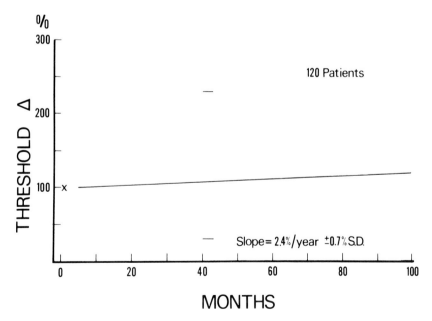

Fig. 4–2. Follow-up of 120 patients with implanted pacers for at least five years demonstrated an overall stability of threshold. The symbol X represents average initial chronic threshold for entire group, arbitrarily assigned 100%. Thereafter mean threshold increased by 2.4% ± 0.7% per year. Widest scatter for any individual is represented by two short horizontal lines. Even 100 months after first pulse generator replacement, threshold remains essentially stable.

electrodes have a small metal screw or metal or nylon wires or "barbs" projecting from the tip which grasp the endocardium and reduce the possibility of early displacement. Early experience has been highly promising. Other designs that may be equal or superior are in preparation.

Electrode Maturity

The *acute* threshold is ascertained during implantation. Following stabilization, several weeks after implant, it is chronic. Between the two, threshold rises, first to a peak about a week after implant and then descends to a stable level two to three times above acute (Fig. 4–3).

The maturing process varies inversely with electrode size so that smaller, more efficient electrodes increase threshold proportionally more than larger electrodes. An electrode with 8 mm² surface area increases current threshold four times between acute and chronic. Electrodes with larger surface areas have a smaller ratio so that an electrode of 50 mm² surface area has a chronic/acute ratio of only 2.3. Nevertheless, the lower acute and chronic thresholds of small electrodes are more significant than their greater chronic-to-acute threshold ratio. An 8 mm² electrode has a chronic threshold of 0.91 ± 0.52 mA, and the 50 mm² electrode has a chronic threshold of 3.62 ± 2.09 mA (both at 1 msec pulse duration). The latter has been a wholly unacceptable threshold at any time during the development of pacemaker technology and certainly is at present.

After the initial increases, indefinite threshold stability can be anticipated. Efforts to construct pulse generators with prolonged longevity are based on the implicit assumption that such threshold stability exists. The only reasons for replacement of a chronically functioning electrode are:

1. Irreparable lead fracture.
2. Irreparable insulation failure.
3. Infection.

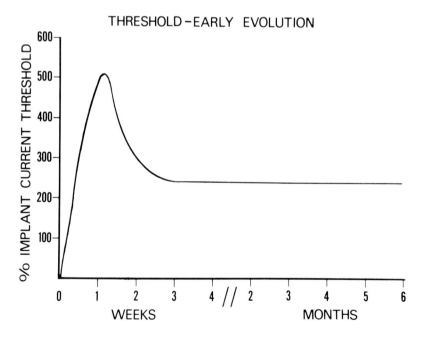

THRESHOLD–EARLY EVOLUTION

Fig. 4–3. In contrast with chronic threshold, acute current threshold increases variably, as much as ten times implant level, but usually far less. Typically, it reaches a chronic level two to three times acute threshold (graphic display is diagrammatic).

4. Electrode corrosion caused by a direct current leak from the pulse generator, a defect possible even in some modern designs.
5. The most uncommon progressive threshold rise above the output capacity of a generator.

The last is almost always caused by undetected poor initial placement, as repositioning either a transvenous or myocardial electrode usually results in permanent stability.

Pulse Duration

Threshold varies as a function of impulse duration, though somewhat differently for each parameter. The strength-duration curve is the major basis for understanding cardiac stimulation threshold. Current, voltage, charge (the product of current and time), and energy [the product of current, voltage, and time ($E = IVT$)] all vary as a function of pulse duration. Minimum consumption of the capacity of the pacemaker power source is sought and accomplished without loss of safety margin by analysis of the strength-duration curve.

CURRENT. Current at threshold from a constant current generator is parallel to the abscissa from about 1.0 msec (rheobase). Threshold values rise as pulse duration shortens below about 0.7 msec.

VOLTS. Rheobase is reached at 1.0 msec.; at shorter durations threshold rises.

CHARGE AND ENERGY. The two derived functions, charge and energy, show a different pattern. Charge is the most useful single function to comprehend longevity of the generator, as it describes threshold in the same terms in which chemical battery capacity is measured (milliampere hours or ampere hours) and its consumption is in-

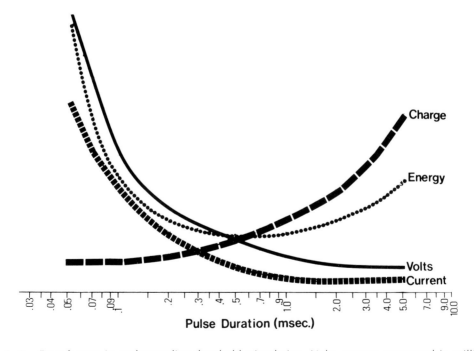

Fig. 4–4. Four factors in understanding threshold stimulation. *Volts, current* (measured in milliamperes), *charge* (measured in microcoulombs), and *energy* (measured in microjoules) are lowest at a pulse duration of 0.5 msec, which is therefore the most efficient pulse duration. Nevertheless, as charge is the most important single factor, its consumption continues to decrease with still shorter pulse durations.

versely related to battery longevity. Charge expended at threshold decreases with shortened pulse duration, as the decline in time is far more rapid than increase in current required.

The most efficient pulse duration for energy consumption lies between 0.25 and 1.0 msec where the curve is lowest, flat, and parallel to the abscissa. At shorter and longer pulse durations, energy and current consumption at threshold rises. Voltage output of a chemical battery is fixed, and reduction of voltage supplied to the electrode is less efficiently accomplished for conservation of capacity than reduction of pulse duration or current flow (Fig. 4–4).

IMPEDANCE. Impedance to the flow of electrical energy varies directly with pulse duration, lower at short pulse durations and higher at longer duration, so that short pulse duration (i.e., 0.1 to 0.5 msec) has an added advantage over the longer duration.

Electrode polarization associated with high output and long pulse duration is a buildup of charge opposing further flow of current. On an oscillogram it appears as a rising voltage during a constant current stimulus, increasing with pulse duration and current density but reaching a maximum which is specific for each metal.

Electrode Surface Area

The surface area of stimulating electrodes is directly and linearly related to the current threshold of stimulation. The shape of the stimulating surface plays a role, but its clinical significance is not clear. Electrodes with smaller surface areas have lower current and charge thresholds than do larger electrodes, and the current density threshold (mA/mm^2) remains relatively constant over a wide range of surface areas. Voltage threshold also decreases with surface area, though not so greatly as do current and charge. These phenomena exist both at implant (acutely) and chronically.

The chronic-to-acute threshold ratio de-pends upon the size and shape of the electrode and the thickness of the nonexcitable fibrous tissue which separates the electrode from the excitable myocardium. Spherical electrodes have the highest chronic threshold factor and cylindrical electrodes have the smallest. An electrode of surface area as low as 4 mm^2 has been used clinically and has been successful, though such smaller electrodes may have corrosion problems at conventional pulse generator output levels.

Anodal and Cathodal Stimulation

Threshold of stimulation is determined during diastole when ventricular sensitivity

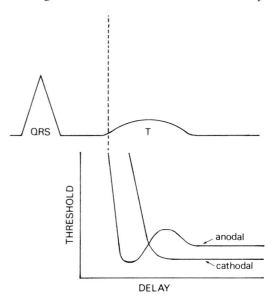

Fig. 4–5. Relation between anodal and cathodal current threshold, as a function of interval after end of absolute refractory period (dotted line). Initially, the heart is sensitve only to anodal stimulation, then more sensitive to anodal than cathodal, and finally during most of diastole it is more sensitive to cathodal than anodal stimulus. Bipolar electrode with equal size anode and cathode (e.g., a myocardial implant) will stimulate from anode or cathode depending on stimulus amplitude and timing. The earlier the cardiac response the greater the possibility of onset of ventricular fibrillation.

has returned to a stable level prior to another QRS complex. During that period the myocardium is more sensitive to cathodal than anodal stimuli and, for a constant current stimulus, equally sensitive to cathodal and bipolar stimuli. Cardiac sensitivity to stimulation changes significantly during and immediately after the QRS complex during the relative refractory period. The phenomenon of pacemaker-induced ventricular fibrillation, in which the stimulus falls into the vulnerable period of the cardiac cycle, has been observed during bipolar stimulation in all published instances except one and is related to the anode of a bipolar electrode (Fig. 4–5). The threshold for pacemaker stimulus induced ventricular fibrillation decreases during myocardial ischemia, infarction, metabolic imbalance, and drug intoxication.

Electrode Metal

The metal for a pacemaker electrode must be:

1. Electrochemically inert.
2. Nontoxic.
3. Resistant to electrolytic destruction.
4. Of low electrical resistance.

The electrode should not go into solution during passage of an electrical current, at least at the conventional pacing pulse duration and output levels. Any salt formed during pacing should be nontoxic. If a metal meets these criteria only as a cathode, then it may be used only for unipolar pacing. Three metals have been successfully used for permanent pacing:

1. Platinum with 10% iridium.
2. Elgiloy, an alloy of cobalt, iron, chromium molybdenum, nickel, and manganese.
3. A silver and stainless steel combination.

The threshold is a function of the reactivity of the metal and the overvoltage developed during passage of a current for cardiac stimulation. The more noble a metal, the lower this overvoltage and consequently the lower the voltage and current pacing threshold. Platinum-iridium has consistently lower thresholds than the more reactive metal, Elgiloy. Nevertheless, all three metals have been quite successful for long-term pacing, and the difference in threshold is inconsequential as a practical matter.

Drug Administration and Electrolyte Balance

Changes in electrolyte concentration have an effect on stimulating threshold. Potassium administration reduces threshold briefly, whereas potassium and insulin in combination increase threshold. Hypertonic sodium chloride increases threshold. Increasing P_{O_2} has little effect; slight hypoxia increases threshold and marked hypoxia reduces threshold. Increase of P_{CO_2} increases threshold and a decrease has little effect.

Glucocorticoids and epinephrine and ephedrine decrease threshold. Isoproterenol, aldactone, propranolol, verapamil, quinidine, and ajmaline all increase threshold. Digitalis, morphine, lidocaine, and procainamide have little effect. All of these agents, at the usual therapeutic levels, have little sustained effect on threshold and can usually be disregarded. Even where a pronounced immediate effect occurs, sustained administration is usually accompanied by a gradual return to baseline cardiac sensitivity.

Unipolar and Bipolar Pacing

Unipolar or bipolar cardiac stimulation refers to the number of electrodes attached to the portion of the heart to be stimulated. Atrial bipolar or unipolar and ventricular bipolar or unipolar stimulation exist. The presence of two electrodes, one in the atrium and the other in the ventricle with a common ground electrode, remote from the heart, is not bipolar pacing or sensing but rather unipolar. Whether the pacemaker is called unipolar or bipolar depends on the location of *both* electrodes. More important, all stimulation is really bipolar, as current flows from the negative terminal which must be attached to the heart and returns to the generator via the positive terminal which may be the ring of the bipolar endocardial electrode, a second intramyocardial elecrode identical to the negative lead (as in a thoracotomy implant) or a portion of the pacemaker case.

The stimulus that drives the heart via the cathode will reach the pulse generator anode equally whether the anode is within the myocardium, the ventricle, or elsewhere in the body. The *current* threshold of cardiac stimulation is, therefore, a function of the stimulation aspects of the cathode, and it is equal for unipolar and bipolar configuration. The *voltage* threshold varies as a function of the resistance of the lead system. For example, the ring of a bipolar electrode is a much smaller and, therefore,

a higher resistance contact than the case of a pulse generator. The large surface area of the anode of the unipolar generator provides a lower resistance pathway and a lower voltage threshold. The difference is not great. Although more bipolar than unipolar electrodes have been implanted, by far more manufacturers have provided unipolar pacemakers, and these now dominate the field (Table 4–2).

UNIPOLAR AND BIPOLAR SENSING

The unipolar electrogram is the result of the passage of the depolarization wave

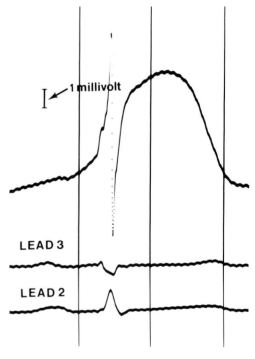

Fig. 4–6. Typical unipolar ventricular electrogram timed for its events against lead 2 and 3. The pacemaker is triggered by intrinsic deflection, the vertical rapid indicator of the passage of current past the electrode. The elevated S-T segment is the "current of injury." When the electrode becomes chronic, the S-T segment becomes isoelectric. Intrinsic deflection changes little in amplitude but decreases by about 40% in rate of development (dv/dt).

TABLE 4–2

Unipolar/Bipolar Pacing (Permanent Leads)

	UNIPOLAR	BIPOLAR
1. Implantation		
Transthoracic	Easier	
Transvenous	Easier	
2. Threshold		
Current	Equal	Equal
Voltage	Lower	
3. Durability	Equal	Equal
4. Sturdiness	Equal	Equal
5. QRS sensing	Greater	
6. VF liability		Greater
7. Follow-up	Easier	
8. ECG analysis	Easier	
9. EMI		Resistant
10. Repair	Easier	

front past the intracardiac electrode (Fig. 4–6). The subcutaneous, remote electrode is too far removed for any signal it detects to play any significant role in the net bipolar signal. Over 2000 electrograms recorded during pacemaker implant and pulse generator replacement were analyzed for the following:

1. Configuration, i.e., morphology of the depolarization wave, the QRS complex.
2. The amplitude of the complex.
3. The rate of development (slew rate) or change in voltage as a function of time (dv/dt) of the ''intrinsic deflection,'' (ID), and the vertical straight line portion of the intracardiac signal which triggers the pacemaker.
4. The presence of injury and repolarization waves, the analogs on the peripheral ECG or the ST segments and T waves.

Additional signals occasionally appearing are far field and represent electrical activity distant from the electrode, i.e., skeletal muscle potentials, the contraction of the other ventricle, external electromagnetic interference, and occasionally stimuli from another electrode, as in AV sequential pacing system (Fig. 4–7).

The bipolar signal results from the subtraction of the signals from both cardiac

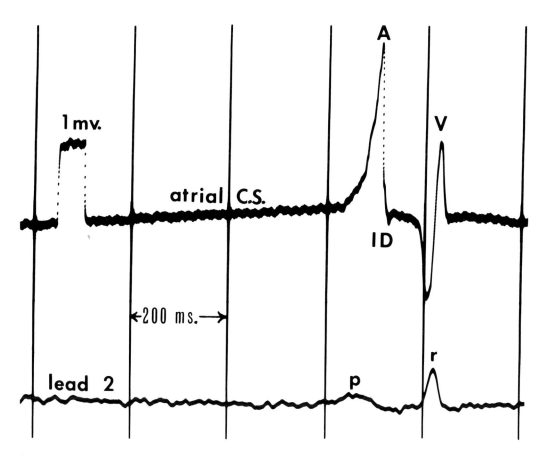

Fig. 4–7. Far-field signal may be the QRS complex when sensing the P wave from the atrial appendage or coronary sinus. Bipolar electrodes sense far-field signals far less than unipolar.

poles. Each individually presents a unipolar configuration; the interaction of the two produces the bipolar signal. If the bipolar axis is at right angles to the depolarization pathway the two signals are identical and simultaneous at each pole. These will cancel, producing a small or zero bipolar result. In this circumstance conversion from bipolar to unipolar increases the net signal. A parallel electrode orientation causes delay of the same signal at one pole relative to the other and can result in an augmented bipolar signal greater than either unipolar component. The delay also produces a signal with two intrinsic deflections compared to the single intrinsic deflection of the unipolar electrogram. During transvenous pacing the net bipolar signal also depends on the signal on the proximal electrode. If that electrode contacts contractile tissue, the ID will be large; if it is separated from viable tissue, the ID will be of small amplitude and the rate of rise slow. In that instance the signal will be poor, and the net bipolar signal will be a reflection of the signal from the electrode tip.

Comparison of a group of ventricular electrode bipolar and tip signals, simultaneously recorded, shows that bipolar sensing has the following characteristics:

1. Intrinsic deflections are increased or decreased, more widely variable compared to unipolar signals, but without a significant difference of the mean of bipolar and unipolar electrograms, i.e., the scatter of bipolar is greater, largely because of a second signal, which does not appear in unipolar electrograms.
2. The duration of the intrinsic deflection is significantly shortened, by a mean of 28%.
3. The injury currents are attenuated by 37%.
4. The T waves are attenuated by 34%.
5. The far-field effects are substantially reduced.

The first of these five qualities is equal for both unipolar and bipolar electrodes; for the last four the advantage is with the bipolar configuration.

The sole disadvantage of the bipolar configuration is the wider scatter of signals and the possibility of ID attenuation if the electrodes are oriented at exactly a right angle to the wave propagation. Overall, 2% of bipolar signals are too small to be sensed (when the unipolar analogous signal would be adequate) and they are smaller than the unipolar tip signal in a total of 51%. In 43% the bipolar ID is larger than the unipolar and in 6% the two are equal. Bipolar S-T

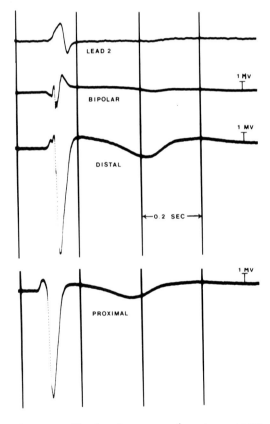

Fig. 4–8. Bipolar electrogram from transvenous electrode timed against lead 2. In this instance, large proximal and distal (or tip) electrograms are of almost equal amplitude and oriented so that two signals subtract and produce a bipolar signal smaller than either.

segment elevation and distant potentials are smaller than those for the unipolar electrode in 96%.

The bipolar electrode cancels far-field, electromagnetic, and injury signals, as these "noises" arrive simultaneously and at equal amplitude at both poles. The ID otherwise almost always affects the poles unequally and/or nonsimultaneously and is augmented rather than diminished. The effect is improvement in signal-to-noise ratio, caused only by the geometry of the sensing electrode, independent of circuit factors (Fig. 4–8).

Conventional wisdom has held that bipolar sensing has been inferior to unipolar sensing because of the much longer unipolar dipole from the intracardiac cathode to the subcutaneous anode. Conversion of a bipolar to a unipolar system has been recommended to improve poor sensing. Evaluation of a series of simultaneously recorded unipolar and bipolar signals from the same bipolar electrode, with the unipolar signal referenced to the usual position of the subcutaneous anode, has shown that the belief of bipolar sensing inferiority is not well founded.

Though unipolar pacemakers have been more widely implanted and in greater numbers than bipolar, the possibility of greater dispersion of electromagnetic interference in the world may increase the relative safety of bipolar compared to unipolar electrodes. In that circumstance be aware that bipolar and unipolar pacing are virtually equivalent.

The factors outlined in this chapter are of prime importance to the comprehension of the remainder of this book. Knowledge of the physiology and technology of cardiac pacing is critical. The practitioner overlooks basic principles at his peril and that of his patient. The question of which electrode to use, large or small, unipolar or bipolar, and whether by thoracotomy or transvenously, arises daily. The utility of programmability of output to ascertain post-implant threshold, increase output to accommodate a high threshold or decrease output to prolong longevity is of great value. The cardiac electrograms describe generator sensing requirements, circumstances in which sensing may be satisfactory or poor, and the possible methods of management.

SELECTED READINGS

Barold, S.S., and Gaidula, J.J.: Failure of demand pacemakers from low-voltage bipolar ventricular electrograms. J.A.M.A., *215*:923, 1971.

Chamberlain, D.A., et al.: Sequential atrioventricular pacing in heart block complicating acute myocardial infarction. N. Engl. J. Med., *282*:577, 1970.

Chardack, W.M., et al.: Magnetically actuated pulse width control for implantable pacemakers. Ann. Cardiol. Angeiol., *20*:345, 1971.

Chardack, W., Gage, A.A., and Greatbatch, W.: A transistorized, self-contained, implantable pacemaker for the long-term correction of complete heart block. Surgery, *48*:643, 1960.

De Caprio, V., Hurzeler, P., and Furman, S.: A comparison of unipolar and bipolar electrograms for cardiac pacemaker sensing. Circulation, *56*:750, 1977.

Dekker, E., Buller, J., and van Erven, F.A.: Unipolar and bipolar stimulation thresholds of the human myocardium with chronically implanted pacemaker electrodes. Am. Heart J., *71*:671, 1966.

Fisher, J.D., et al.: Cardiac pacing and pacemakers. II. Serial electrophysiologic-pharmacologic testing for control of recurrent tachyarrhythmias. Am. Heart J., *93*(5):658, 1977.

Fisher, J., Furman, S., and Escher, D.J.W.: Pacemaker failures characterized by continuous direct current leakage. Am. J. Cardiol., *37*:1019, 1976.

Fontaine, G., et al.: Bilan d'une étude statistique par ordinateur du seuil de stimulation endocavitaire avant l'implantation d'un pacemaker. Presse Med., *79*:2215, 1971.

Fowler, N.O., Fenton, J.C., and Conway, G.F.: Syncope and cerebral dysfunction caused by bradycardia without atrioventricular block. Am. Heart J., *80*:303, 1970.

Friedberg, C.K., Donoso, E., and Stein, W.G.: Nonsurgical acquired heart block. Ann. N.Y. Acad. Sci., *111*:835, 1964.

Furman, S.: The present status of cardiac pacing. Surg. Gynec. Obstet., *143*:645, 1976.

Furman, S., Hurzeler, P., and De Caprio, V.: The ventricular endocardial electrogram and pacemaker sensing. J. Thorac. Cardiovasc. Surg., *73*:258, 1977.

Furman, S., and Schwedel, J.B.: An intracardiac pacemaker for Stokes-Adams seizures. N. Engl. J. Med., *261*:943, 1959.

Greatbatch, W., et al.: Polarization phenomena relating to physiological electrodes. Ann. N.Y. Acad. Sci., *167*:722, 1969.

Hunter, S.W., et al.: A new myocardial pacemaker lead (sutureless). Chest, *63*:430, 1973.

Irnich, W., Bleifeld, W., and Effert, S.: Permanente transvenose Elektrostimulation des Herzens mit einer myokardial-fixierten Elektrode. Thoraxchirurgie, *20*:440, 1972.

Kahn, A., Morris, J.J., and Citron, P.: Patient-initiated rapid atrial pacing to manage supraventricular tachycardia. Am. J. Cardiol., *38*:200, 1976.

Luceri, R.M., et al.: Threshold behavior of electrodes in long-term ventricular pacing. Am. J. Cardiol., *40*:184, 1977.

Mehra, R., Furman, S., and Crump, J.F.: Vulnerability of the mildly ischemic ventricle to cathodal, anodal, and bipolar stimulation. Circ. Res., *41*:159, 1977.

Morse, D., et al.: Preliminary experience with the use of a programmable pacemaker. Chest, *67*:544, 1975.

Moss, A.J., and Rivers, R.J., Jr.: Termination and inhibition of recurrent tachycardias by implanted pervenous pacemakers. Circulation, *50*:942, 1974.

Naclerio, E.A., and Varriale, P.: "Screw-in" electrode: new method for permanent ventricular pacing. N. Y. State J. Med., *74*:2391, 1974.

Parsonnet, V., et al.: The fate of permanent intracardiac electrodes. J. Surg. Res., *6*:285, 1966.

Preston, T.A.: Anodal stimulation as a cause of pacemaker-induced ventricular fibrillation. Am. Heart J., *86*:366, 1973.

Smyth, N.P.D., et al.: The significance of electrode surface area and stimulating thresholds in permanent cardiac pacing. J. Thorac. Cardiovasc. Surg., *71*:559, 1976.

Timmis, J.C., Gordon, S., and Helland, J.: Enhanced electrode stability: the endocardial screw. Abstract, Vth International Symposium on Cardiac Pacing, Tokyo, March 14–18, 1976.

Wellens, H.J.J.: Programmed Electrical Stimulation of the Heart in the Study and Treatment of Tachyarrhythmias. Leiden, J.E. Stenfert Krose, 1971.

Zipes, D.: Electrophysiological mechanisms involved in ventricular fibrillation. Circulation (Suppl. III), *11*:120, 1975.

Zoll, P.M.: Resuscitation of the heart in ventricular standstill by external electrical stimulation. N. Engl. J. Med., *247*:768, 1952.

5

The Cardiac Conducting System

G. DOYNE WILLIAMS

The first written description of the motion of a heart removed from a living animal is ascribed to Galen (A.D. 129–199). He also observed the pulsatile loss of blood when an artery was cut and observed "the arteries must be porous, since they take part in the process of respiration and pulsation. At their diastole they take in air, and at their systole they expel sooty matter."

The Dark Ages provided no further significant written accounts of cardiac activity until Da Vinci (1452–1519) noted that the "heart moves by itself." Despite the continuing availability of these and other important clues, early scientists repeatedly failed to recognize that the heart beats to circulate the blood, this fact not being established until 1628 by Harvey.

The purpose of the heartbeat having been established, the mechanism of the initiation of the rhythm remained to be described. The mysteries of electric phenomenon and the equally mysterious spontaneous rhythmic contractions of excised hearts and portions thereof provided early students of medicine with a strong suggestion that the two were somehow related.

Galvani's experiments of 1791 in which contractions of excised hearts and muscles could be produced by electrical stimulation suggested an "electrical origin of life." This led logically to studies linking the origin of the heartbeat to electrophysiologic processes. Aldini (1819) achieved brief periods of renewed cardiac activity by applying transthoracic shocks to decapitated criminals and reportedly successfully resuscitated a child with cardiac arrest following a fall from a high window.

Pioneer work on the conduction system of the heart was initiated in 1883 by Gaskell who studied turtle hearts. He recognized the coordination between the atrial and ventricular contractions and suggested (in direct contradiction to teachings of the time) that a bridge of something other than fibrous tissue must exist between the atria and ventricles. This conductive connection was subsequently described by His and Kent in 1893 in independent reports. Tawara named it the atrioventricular node (AV node) in 1906, and also added the previously described Purkinje fibers to the ventricular portion of the conducting system.

In 1907 Keith recognized the specialized tissue at the superior vena caval-atrial junction as the usual site for the initiation of the heartbeat and named it the sinoatrial node.

ANATOMY

Primitive cardiac muscle cells possess three major properties: automaticity, the ability to initiate an electrical impulse; conductivity, the ability to conduct the electrical impulse; and contractility, the ability to shorten and do work. These properties, all of which are found in primitive myocardial cells, have become the principal properties of individually specialized myocardial cells through evolution. One group of cells has become the "pacemaker cells," and they have essentially lost the ability to contract. They are found in the sinus node, AV node, and His-Purkinje system. Other cells have specialized further to lose contractile and most automatic properties and, in addition, are able to conduct impulses at a much reduced rate, a property used to advantage in the AV node. The third group of cells primarily contract and perform the actual work of the atria and ventricles. They can, however, when required (in failure of normal excitatory cells) initiate the heartbeat at a slower rate.

THE SEQUENCE OF CONDUCTION OF THE HEART BEAT

The heart will respond to the most rapidly occurring available stimulus, which is usually the sinus node. The sinus node is the major pacemaker of the heart and is appropriately located in a most superior position at the junction of the superior vena cava with the right atrium. The node is elliptical and approximately 15 mm in length and is located 1 mm or less beneath the epicardium. A constant feature of the node is its relationship to a large central artery. The framework of the sinus node is of dense collagen which is arranged about the central artery. Within the dense collagen are many centrally located large pale "P" or pacemaking cells. Also scattered throughout the collagen network are pale, small Purkinje fibers which are quite dense near the central artery where they tend to encircle the vessel. The sinus node fibers become Purkinje tracts at the margin of the node.

The central artery of the sinus node, commonly termed the "sinus node artery," may arise from one of three locations. Its origin from the right coronary artery is anatomically identified as the right sinus node artery (42%). If it arises from the proximal 10 mm of the circumflex branch of the left coronary artery, it ascends on the anterior wall of the left atrium to reach the inner atrial muscle bundle through which it usually courses enroute to the sinus node and is termed the "left sinus node artery" (30%). It may also be called the posterior node artery and in this case would arise from the proximal 50 mm of the circumflex coronary artery. It makes its course intramurally much like the left sinus node artery through the interatrial muscle bundle to the superior vena caval junction but differs by its course over the lateral wall of the left atrium between the attachments of atrial appendage and left superior pulmonary vein (22%). The relationship of the sinus node and its artery was more of academic interest in the past. Recently, however, with the advent of extensive atrial reconstruction in the correction of congenital cardiac defects, damage to the sinus node artery has become a prominent feature of serious arrhythmias.

The possibility of a relationship between the pulsations of the intranodal artery and the size of the vessel at any given time in the cardiac cycle and the actual pacemaking function of the sinus node has been suggested. Drugs that decrease the caliber of the artery are associated with accelerated activity of the sinus node and those that increase the caliber of the artery with a slowing of the intrinsic beat. Electronically it has been suggested that the pulse in the sinus node artery provides the coupling for two independently functioning oscillators, the sinus node and the AV node, and this interaction tends to stabilize the sinus mechanism.

Removal of the influence of the higher pacemakers (loss of sinus node function) results in impulse formation from a lower center, usually the NH region of the AV node, which has an intrinsic rate of 40 to 55 beats per minute. Failure of this system leads to pacemaking from Purkinje fibers of the ventricles at a rate of 25 to 40 beats per minute. The importance of these less rapid lower pacemaking foci was first demonstrated by Stannius in 1852 in the frog heart by placing tight ligatures between first the sinus venosus and the atria and then between the atria and the ventricle. Sinoatrial impulses occur normally at 60 to 100 beats per minute in humans and are conducted across the atria to the AV node by way of the internodal tracts. Best recognized on a functional and not an anatomic basis, three such tracts are described (Fig. 5–1). The anterior tract (Bachmann's bundle) conducts from atria to ventricles as well as providing right to left atrial communicating fibers. The middle internodal tract (Wenckebach) and posterior tract (Thorel) conduct only from sinoatrial to AV node. These tracts have assumed much greater significance in recent years, as more complex surgical techniques for congenital cardiac defects have increased the possibility of damage to these pathways resulting in bothersome and sometimes fatal arrhythmias.

The internodal pathways converge on the AV node which is located just above the coronary sinus on the posterior wall of the right atrium adjacent to the tricuspid valve orifice. The AV node can be conveniently thought of as the only normal entrance point for impulses coming from the atria, from either normal or ectopic foci, to reach the ventricles across the fibrous barrier.

Structurally, the AV node is in some ways similar to the sinus node. Many entwining fibers of nervous tissue are present, but less collagen is seen than in the sinoatrial node. The node is morphologically similar throughout its length with no visible anatomic basis for producing the upper, middle, and lower nodal mechanisms which are described on the electrocardiogram. Near the AV node lie many autonomic ganglions presumably of vagal influence. The AV node receives its blood supply 90% of the time from the right coronary artery and is thus frequently affected by posterior myocardial infarction involving the right coronary artery and its branches.

Descending fibers from the AV node form the AV bundle (bundle of His) which passes through the central fibrous body and then to the posterior border of the membranous interventricular septum and onto the top of the muscular septum. At this point a slender bundle of fibers (the right bundle branch) descends to enter the right ventricular subendocardium. The left bundle branch is not well defined and consists of a large number of fibers emerging from the left side of the common bundle throughout much of its course and entering the left ventricle in a subendocardial position. Because of the diffuse nature of the conducting system to the left ventricle it is much more difficult to produce left bundle branch block either by disease or surgical injury than it is to produce right bundle branch block. The bundle branches (both right and left) reach the ventricular musculature through terminal branchings known as Purkinje fibers. Histologically, it has been difficult to show that those fibers identifiable as Purkinje fibers go to all areas of the myocardium and thus could act as the sole transmission of the impulses to the myocardium. It is more likely that other fibers which possess conductive characteristics but resemble normal myocardial fibers also act in the transmission of signals to the ventricles.

Normally only those impulses through the AV node and its bundle branches reach

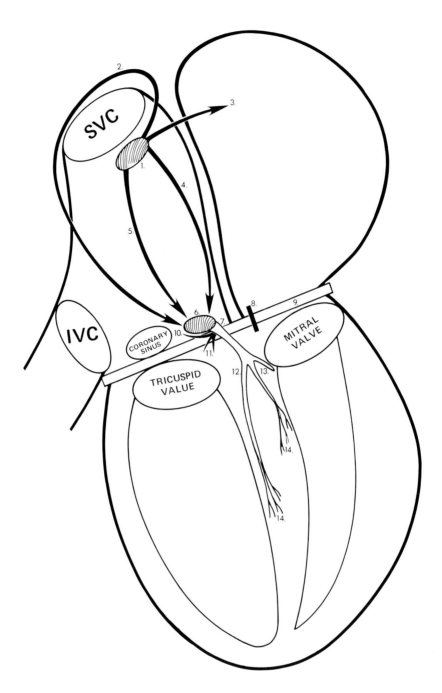

Fig. 5–1. Cardiac conducting system: 1, sinus node; 2, posterior internodal tract; 3, left atrial extension of Bachmann's bundle; 4, Bachmann's bundle (anterior internodal tract); 5, middle internodal tract; 6, AV node; 7 AV bundle; 8, bundle of Kent; 9, fibrous barrier; 10, James fibers; 11, Mahaim fibers; 12, right bundle branch; 13, left bundle branches; 14, Purkinje fibers.

the ventricles. Other pathways exist, however, and become functional under certain conditions. The most commonly recognized extra pathway, the bundle of Kent, directly connects the atria and ventricles across the fibrous barrier and provides rapid communications of impulses avoiding the AV nodal delay and gives rise to the preexcitation arrhythmia known as the Wolff-Parkinson-White syndrome. Less well known are the bypass fibers of James, which conduct impulses directly from the atrium to the upper AV bundle around the AV node, and the Mahaim fibers conducting from the upper AV bundle to the ventricles.

THE ELECTROCARDIOGRAM

Measurable electrical current accompanying motion of the heart was demonstrated by Ludwig and Waller with the capillary electroscope in 1887 and clinically applied by Einthoven with a string galvanometer system in 1903. Einthoven recorded and identified the electrical events associated with depolarization and repolarization of the cardiac components and assigned identifying letters (Fig. 5–2). Sinoatrial node discharge is not recorded on the surface electrocardiogram, but the resulting atrial muscular depolarization is and becomes the P-wave. No electrocardiographic activity is seen as the impulse transverses the AV node (the tissue masses involved are too small for measurable surface electrogram activity), but passage of the impulse to the ventricular myocardium and its subsequent depolarization are recorded as the QRS complex. This is followed by the T-wave of ventricular repolarization. (The repolarization wave of the atria is small and lost in the QRS complex.) Occasionally in the normal electrocardiogram an additional wave, the U-wave following the T-wave, is seen. Its significance is not understood at this time.

The surface electrocardiogram as described above exhibits only a portion of the electrical events accompanying the heartbeat. An additional technique, His bundle recording or an "intracardiac electrogram" can also provide valuable information. His recordings require fluoroscopic positioning of a bipolar intracardiac electrode with contacts on either side of the AV

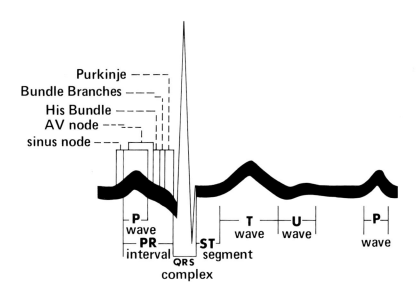

Fig. 5–2. Normal scalar electrocardiogram.

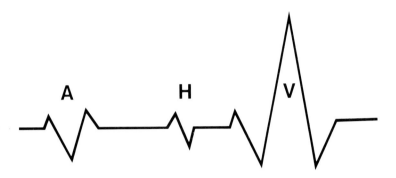

Fig. 5–3. His bundle recording.

node in the right atrium. This technique provides detailed information regarding passage of the impulse from the sinoatrial node through the AV node, an event recorded on the surface electrocardiogram simply as a P-wave with P-R interval. The His recording, however, breaks the P-R interval down into two important components, the A to H interval and the H to V interval (Fig. 5–3). This permits definition of delayed AV conduction as within (prolonged A to H interval) or distal to the AV node (prolonged H to V interval).

HEART BLOCK

Disease involving the conduction system may result in interruption of impulse formation, termed pacemaker failure, or of impulse propagation, referred to as conduction delay or block. Abnormalities of impulse formation involve functions of the sinus node, since it is the dominant or primary pacemaker. Dysfunction of the sinus node may be manifested by (1) persistent sinus bradycardia, (2) intervals of sinus arrest as evidenced by absent P-waves in which no escape rhythm arises or a lower ectopic pacemaker eventually takes over after several seconds, (3) paroxysmal or chronic atrial fibrillation due to temporary or permanent suppression of the sinus, and (4) tachycardia alternating with bradycar-

dia. All of these rhythm disturbances have been referred to as the sick sinus syndrome.

Abnormalities of impulse transmission result either in delay of conduction or failure in further propagation, and either of these events may be termed block. As stated earlier, the P-R interval of the electrocardiogram represents a period in which the impulse traverses the conduction system from the sinus node to the ventricular myocardium. Block occurring below the bifurcation of the bundle in one or all of the fascicles results in recognizable alterations in the QRS complex and constitutes the well-defined entities of bundle and fascicular block. PR prolongation without abnormality in the QRS complex implies block in the conduction tissue beginning below the sinus node and extending distally to the area of bundle bifurcation. The following terminology is used in defining AV block with regard to the scalar ECG.

First degree AV block is defined as a PR interval of 0.21 seconds or more without blocked beats: it is therefore a delay.

Second degree AV block requires blocked beats. One form of second degree AV block originally described by Wenckebach and subsequently classified by Mobitz as Type I, is an AV delay characterized by progressive PR prolongation until an atrial beat (P wave) is not conducted. The progression of PR prolongation occurs in decreasing increments between each P-R interval so that the R-R intervals progressively shorten until the nonconducted beat occurs.

Type I block is a conduction delay in which the impulse arrives progressively earlier until it becomes completely blocked. Type I AV block can occur anywhere in the conduction system but is characteristically found in the AV node where physiologic decremental conduction is always present. Hence, Mobitz I or Wenckebach AV block usually signifies an AV nodal site of block that is temporary and reversible and often due to enhanced vagal tone.

Mobitz Type II AV block is present when blocked beats occur with conducted beats that have a constant P-R interval. His bundle studies have determined that this form of block occurs below the His bundle and results in a prolonged H-V interval. This form of block, unlike Type I, is ominous because it implies significant disturbance in conduction below the AV node. It often occurs in conjunction with bundle branch or bifascicular block.

Third degree AV block is complete AV block with the total absence of AV conduction. With complete blockage of transmission of normal impulses lower pacemaker foci drive the ventricles. To follow a general rule, the lower the level of block, the slower the rate, and the wider the QRS complex.

FASCICULAR BLOCKS

The traditional view of the common bundle dividing into left and right bundles has been considerably modified in recent years. We now recognize a right bundle emerging from the bundle of His to supply the musculature of the right ventricle and two (or more) bundles, an anterior and a posterior, arising from the bundle of His for the left ventricle. The divisions of the bundle of His are known as fascicles. Block may involve either the right or left bundle branch. Right bundle branch block combined with either left anterior or posterior fascicular block is known as bifascicular block.

Right bundle branch block (RBBB) is identified on the ECG by a QRS complex of 0.12 sec or more with a late slurred R-wave in V_1 or V_2 and a wide slurred S-wave in V_5 and V_6. Left bundle branch block (LBBB) is recognized as a wide slurred R-wave in V_5 or V_6 and a wide slurred S-wave in V_1 or V_2. Anterior fascicular block is recognized electrocardiographically by marked left axis deviation (LAD) to $-45°$ or more; the initial forces are directed rightward and inferiorly (small Q-waves in lead 1 and AVL, small R-waves in leads 2, 3, and AVF), and the terminal forces superiorly and leftward so that the initial and terminal forces are approximately 180° apart in the frontal plane. This pattern is a result of the delay in anterior superior forces in the sequence of ventricular depolarization.

Posterior fascicular block, in an analogous fashion, results in a delayed activation of the inferior wall so that the initial forces are leftward and superiorly directed (small Q-waves in leads 2, 3, and AVF and small R-waves in lead 1 and AVL). Terminal forces are directed toward the right, resulting in marked right axis deviation (RAD) to 110° or greater. Bifascicular block or right bundle branch block with either anterior or posterior fascicular block is readily recognized on the ECG as RBBB + LAD or RBBB + RAD, respectively. Trifascicular block is always present when bifascicular block is accompanied by Mobitz Type II block, since intermediate block must be present in the remaining conduction fascicle. Progression to complete heart block is most likely.

ABNORMAL CONDUCTION

Disturbances responsible for abnormalities of impulse formation or conduction are basically of two types: functional, those that are reversible and are not associated with anatomic lesions; and organic, those that are irreversible and correlated with recognized pathologic processes. Drugs such as digitalis, propranolol, quinidine, and procainamide, as well as increased vagal tone, depress normal impulse formation and conduction, particularly at the sinus and AV node, resulting in functional bradyarrhythmias and AV block. Propranolol, quinidine, and procainamide depress conduction below the AV node as well. These agents must be withdrawn before evaluating any patient with disturbances in conduction or impulse formation. Intrinsic disease of the conducting system usually results in morphologic changes detected by careful postmortem studies.

Disease of the conduction system can be separated into (1) pathologic processes that specifically disrupt the conduction system or contiguous structures and (2) disruption of conduction tissue incident to pathologic processes that primarily affect cardiac tissue. Autopsy specimens demonstrating fibrous replacement of the right bundle and one or more fascicles of the left bundle with normal coronary arteries have been reported. These studies have emphasized that the fibrotic process is in general selective for peripheral branches of the conduction system; complete AV block develops subsequent to progressive fascicular block rather than immediately involving the common bundle or AV node. The etiology of this pathologic state is unknown. Because of its appearance in older patients it probably represents degenerative changes of the conduction system associated with aging. The term *sclerodegenerative process* has been suggested by Lenegre to describe this finding. In addition, cardiac sclerosis that involves contiguous structures may affect the conducting system secondarily. Progressive calcification and fibrosis of either a rheumatic mitral or aortic valve, for example, may extend to involve the adjacent conducting system.

Coronary artery disease is another common cause of abnormality of the conduction system. Although most cases are caused by atherosclerotic coronary artery disease of the common variety, James has emphasized that small vessel disease such as occurs in thrombotic thrombocytopenic purpura, polyarteritis nodosa, and Friedreich's ataxia may also involve the conduction system. The conduction system may be implicated in one of two ways—a myocardial infarction or transient ischemia. Anterior myocardial infarction due to occlusion of the left anterior descending coronary artery may result in RBBB or RBBB + LAD (bifascicular block). Complete heart block may be the result of widespread necrosis of the anterior and posterior walls of the heart. Right coronary artery occlusion may cause sinus node dysfunction. This is usually transient and due to altered autonomic tone or transient ischemia.

The sick sinus syndrome is often caused by progressive and generalized coronary disease rather than by acute infarction. When the posterior descending coronary artery which supplies the inferior surface of the left ventricle and the AV node is occluded, there is often transient AV block, usually first degree or Type I second degree block. Permanent AV block as a result of posterior infarction is uncommon, but may occur when a small infarction involves the common bundle. Severe pump failure and a high mortality are usually associated with complete AV block incident to anterior wall infarction.

Cardiomyopathies may also be the cause of conduction system disease. Idiopathic myocardial hypertrophy and other forms of primary cardiomyopathy are more common than the secondary cardiomyopathies. The latter category includes amyloidosis, hemachromatosis, scleroderma, myotonia dystrophica, and Friedreich's ataxia. Bundle branch block, particularly of the left bundle, occurs frequently, but progression to complete AV block is uncommon.

Operative injury to the conduction system as a consequence of hemorrhage, infarction, or suture penetration into the AV node or common bundle may result in temporary or permanent AV block. This is most likely to occur with large ventricular septal defects, such as repair of tetralogy of Fallot, or with large defects in the membranous septum. In uncomplicated ventricular septal defects without dextro position or corrected transposition, the main bundle lies along the inferior surface of the defect.

Cardiac mapping has shown that the conduction system lies along the superior edge of the defect in cases of corrected transposition of the great vessels. Unusual conducting system pathways are also seen in single ventricle. Myocardial mapping has become an essential part of the surgical procedure in these complex cases in order to avoid permanent AV block.

In the past surgical procedures limited to the atrial level were not felt to be serious threats to the conduction system. Recent studies have demonstrated that most atrial arrhythmias following cardiac surgery can be traced to injuries of the atrial conduction system. A large secundum atrial septal defect may be closed with large widely placed sutures, which encompass many, if not all, of the internodal conductive pathways in the interatrial septum. In addition, the incision made in the lateral wall of the right atrium to approach the defect may itself divide one of these pathways. Recently, patching instead of direct suturing of large atrial septal defects (ASD) has become more common. This will allow closure of the defect with closely placed sutures near the edge of the defect and minimal involvement of the atrial septum. The incidence of significant atrial arrhythmias following ASD closure has, as a result, become negligible.

Until recently, serious atrial arrhythmias commonly have accompanied Mustard repairs for transposition of the great vessels. Many children have little SA nodal activity postoperatively and an AV nodal subsidiary pacemaker is quite common. Recent studies have shown that injury to the SA nodal artery or direct trauma to the node during atrial incision or sewing in the atrial baffle is a common cause for these arrhythmias. Strict attention to detail when making the atrial incision and sewing in the patch so as to avoid the areas where the SA node and nodal artery are known to lie has reduced the incidence of postoperative arrhythmias.

Permanent AV block in the older adult is a serious problem, but modern pacemaking techniques make it a tolerable inconvenience for many patients. Production of complete AV block surgically in the infant, however, is a much more serious matter. It therefore behooves the pediatric cardiac surgeon to have a thorough knowledge of the anatomy of the specialized conduction system in all congenital cardiac anomalies and to employ techniques that will avoid injury to this system.

SELECTED READINGS

Hurst, W.J., and Logue, R.B. (editors): The Heart. New York, McGraw-Hill Book Company, 1978.

Katz, A.M.: Physiology of the Heart. New York, Raven Press, 1977.

McAlpine, W.A.: The Heart and Coronary Arteries. New York, Springer-Verlag, 1975.

Noble, D.: The Initiation of the Heartbeat. Oxford, Clarendon Press, 1975.

Williams, G.D., et al.: Electric control of the heart. Curr. Probl. Surg., February-March, 1974.

6

Indications for Permanent Cardiac Pacing

PHILIP VARRIALE
JOSEF NIZNIK
EMIL A. NACLERIO

The scope and clinical application of cardiac pacing have rapidly evolved and expanded since its inception nearly two decades ago. The many cardiac arrhythmias and conduction disturbances currently amenable to pacemaker therapy include those which are well established and others for which the role of pacing is less certain and controversial.

In this chapter the indications for permanent pacing are presented and discussed in accordance with the specific electrocardiographic dysfunctional patterns and their correlative clinical features. The role of other diagnostic procedures, such as bundle of His recordings and rapid atrial pacing, is included, since these assessments are often necessary to validate the need for pacemaker therapy.

SINUS NODE DYSFUNCTION AND RELATED DISORDERS

Sick Sinus Syndrome

The varied disorders of sinus node function, more clearly recognized in the past decade, may give rise to a wide spectrum of distinct electrocardiographic arrhythmias and associated symptomatology principally related to cerebral ischemia and disturbed cardiac performance. Sick sinus syndrome (SSS), introduced in 1968 by Ferrer, has become the accepted term describing the clinical and electrocardiographic findings that characterize sinus node dysfunction. At the present time SSS represents the most frequent indication for permanent cardiac pacing.

Sick sinus syndrome occurs most commonly in the elderly, but may appear at any age. It has been suggested as a cause of sudden death in children and young athletes. The pathophysiologic mechanisms responsible for sinus node dysfunction may include impaired automaticity, disordered impulse conduction to the atrium, or disturbances in autonomic regulation. Pathologic dysfunction of the sinus node may generate an inappropriately slow or unstable sinus rhythm, usually less than 50 beats/min, or facilitate tachycardia, nearly always of the supraventricular variety. In approximately 60% of patients with SSS, functional abnormalities of the AV node or intraventricular conduction system coexist.

The underlying anatomic pathologic process of SSS is not always apparent. In the elderly without obvious coronary artery disease it may result from senile degeneration or idiopathic sclerodegenerative lesions within or around the SA node. Other causes include coronary artery disease, myocarditis, surgical trauma, pericarditis, or collagen disease.

The diagnosis of SSS is initiated and often established by the recognition of certain ECG manifestations. These include the following patterns:

1. Severe sinus bradycardia, usually persistent, sometimes episodic and not drug-induced (Fig. 6–1).
2. Long pauses in sinus rhythm caused by sinus arrest, sinus pause, or sinoatrial (SA) block (Fig. 6–2).
3. Atrioventricular (AV) junctional escape rhythms with or without unstable sinus activity.
4. Brady-tachyarrhythmia syndrome (BTS) characterized by episodic tachyarrhythmias, usually supraventricular, interrupting sinus bradycardia.

When considering SSS, it is important to exclude a variety of extrinsic factors that may be responsible for the apparent sinus node dysfunction. Drugs such as digitalis, propranolol, quinidine, and reserpine may produce severe sinus bradycardia and/or SA block, easily reversed upon withdrawal of the inciting agent. On the other hand, drug-induced sinus node disorders caused by small amounts of digitalis or propranolol can unmask and suggest SSS and presage its onset.

The majority of patients with SSS have a constellation of signs and symptoms that are often attributable to hypoperfusion of vital organs such as the brain, heart, and kidney. The major manifestations of cerebral ischemia include episodes of dizziness, lightheadedness, syncope, slurred speech, or paresis. When these occur in the elderly, they are frequently erroneously interpreted as the consequence of a minor cerebrovascular accident. Less apparent symptoms

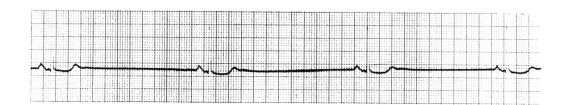

Fig. 6–1. Symptoms of dizziness and presyncope were present in elderly patient who had severe sinus bradycardia with almost persistent ventricular rates below 35 beats/min. Symptoms disappeared with permanent pacing.

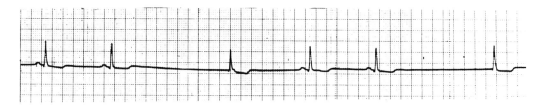

Fig. 6–2. Sinus bradycardia associated with disturbances of sinus node discharge—sinus arrest or pause—and long asystolic periods is a relatively common ECG pattern of SSS.

include fatigue, personality changes, irritability, and intermittent forgetfulness. The cardiac manifestations of SSS, although less common than cerebral symptoms, include angina pectoris, cardiac failure, and palpitations incident to bradyarrhythmia and/or tachyarrhythmia.

Brady-tachyarrhythmia syndrome (BTS) is a distinct and common manifestation of advanced SSS (Fig. 6–3). It is readily identified by the frequent alterations between episodic tachyarrhythmia (usually atrial fibrillation, flutter, or tachycardia and, less often, ventricular tachycardia) and severe sinus bradycardia. The characteristically abrupt rhythm changes tend to generate a variety of discomforting symptoms, including syncope. Drug therapy alone is often unsuccessful in the control of tachycardic arrhythmias and may aggravate the bradycardic component. Permanent pacing allows easier management of BTS, particularly when combined with drug therapy.

Permanent cardiac pacing is clearly indicated for patients whose disturbing symptoms are obviously generated by the manifest ECG abnormalities of sinus node dysfunction, that is, for patients with symptomatic sick sinus syndrome (SSSS). As a general rule, permanent pacing is not recommended for patients with sinus node dysfunction or bradyarrhythmia unless these arrhythmias are associated with impaired cardiac function or the usual symptoms of SSS.

For many patients the history and routine ECG recordings will at best arouse suspicion of SSS. The ECG findings in early or mild SSS and their relation to the existing symptoms can remain elusive and may not be easy to assess with certainty. This group includes patients, particularly the elderly, with symptoms of lightheadedness, dizziness, or syncope of uncertain origin who have normal electrocardiograms or evidence of only modest sinus bradycardia (rates of 50 to 60 beats/min).

It is now recognized, however, that patients with SSS can manifest normal sinus rhythm during asymptomatic periods and overt sinus node dysfunction only sporadically. Another group of patients with suspected SSS develop marked or persistent sinus bradycardia and/or SA block following relatively small amounts of digitalis or propranolol and mild neurologic symptoms only incident to this drug-induced bradyarrhythmia.

Further diagnostic investigation in these patients with suspected SSS is necessary to support the need for pacing therapy. A diagnostic evaluation should include the following:

1. **AMBULATORY OR DYNAMIC ECG MONITORING (HOLTER MONITOR).** This essential procedure is widely used and involves an extended continuous ECG recording using a portable tape recorder for a period of 12 to 24 hours. This monitoring technique is considered the best diagnostic

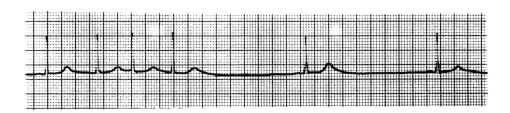

Fig. 6–3. Brady-tachyarrhythmia syndrome is characterized by brief or prolonged periods of atrial tachyarrhythmia (in this example atrial fibrillation) that alternate with slow sinus rate. A variable period of asystole often follows termination of the tachyarrhythmia. Syncope may ensue if this asystolic period is sufficiently prolonged.

tool for the detection of a large variety of ECG abnormalities indicative of sinus node dysfunction when none is documented on repeated or random ECG rhythm strips. Holter monitoring represents the initial and perhaps the ultimate approach in the search for intermittent and difficult to capture ECG abnormalities of SSS.

2. **PROVOCATIVE ELECTROPHYSIOLOGI-CAL TESTS.** It may be desirable to proceed with provocative testing in certain patients when ECG abnormalities of SSS remain marginal or uncertain. These testing methods should not be considered as absolute criteria but rather as indirect evidence of SSS.

Rapid atrial pacing or, rarely, pharmacologic agents are used for provocative testing. Pacing of the atrium at rates that produce overdrive suppression permits an assessment of sinus node automaticity and suppressibility. The postpacing pause for each paced rate to 150 pulses/min at increments of 10 pulses/min allows determination of the so-called *sinus node recovery time* (SNRT). An interval of 1.6 seconds or more between the last paced stimulus and the first spontaneous sinus beat at any pacing rate for 30 to 60 seconds duration is considered abnormal.

The *corrected sinus node recovery time* (CSNRT), determined as a difference between the postpacing pause and control sinus cycle length, is considered a more specific measurement for sinus node dysfunction. An interval greater than 525 msec is considered abnormal. Calculated sinoatrial conduction time (SACT) using a programmed atrial extra-stimulus technique, although less useful and specific, is also utilized as a test for sinus node integrity.

Intravenous atropine (1 mg) or isuprel (1 to 2 μg/min) has been proposed as a method to evaluate sinus node function. Failure to increase the sinus rate beyond 90 beats/min in sinus bradycardia may be considered compatible with a diagnosis of sick sinus syndrome.

Atrial Fibrillation with Slow Ventricular Rate

Untreated chronic atrial fibrillation with slow ventricular rates (30 to 50 beats/min) is considered to be an expression of advanced sinus node dysfunction, particularly if a stable sinus mechanism does not resume after electrical cardioversion (Fig. 6–4). Atrial fibrillation with a retarded ventricular response suggests impaired and multiple concealed conduction within the AV node. The role of permanent pacing in these patients is self-evident when this arrhythmia is responsible for the symptoms of cerebral ischemia or aggravated cardiac failure.

Hypersensitive Carotid Sinus Syndrome

This entity represents a distinct cause of dizziness or syncope, whose mechanism

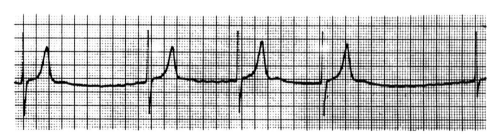

Fig. 6–4. Atrial fibrillation with inordinately slow ventricular rate below 40 beats/min not related to drug therapy may occur in elderly patient with associated symptoms of cerebral ischemia or cardiac failure. Permanent pacing permits easier management of congestive heart failure and relieves symptoms.

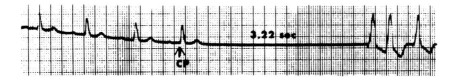

Fig. 6–5. Hypersensitive carotid sinus syndrome is a rare cause of syncope but sometimes responsible for an elderly patient's neurologic symptoms. Mild carotid sinus stimulation (indicated by arrow) characteristically produces an asystolic period longer than 3 seconds. Asystole is terminated by pacemaker beat induced by temporary pacing catheter in right ventricle.

relates to carotid sinus hypersensitivity (Fig. 6–5). The accepted criteria for this syndrome include a postcarotid stimulation period of asystole greater than 3 seconds or a systolic or a diastolic decrease in arterial blood pressure of at least 50 mmHg. Many of these patients often have manifestations of diabetes mellitus, coronary artery disease, and/or hypertension. A permanent demand cardiac pacemaker is recommended for effective control of the hypersensitive carotid sinus syndrome if medical measures fail to control symptoms.

ATRIOVENTRICULAR CONDUCTION ABNORMALITIES

Complete AV Block (Third Degree AV Block)

Complete AV block is an advanced and serious conduction disturbance characterized by the failure of supraventricular impulses, usually atrial, to reach the ventricles. In 3° AV block, the ventricles are activated by an escape rhythm arising within the His bundle or distal intraventricular conduction system. The site of conduction disturbance is usually related to one or more specific portions of the specialized AV conduction system: (1) AV node, (2) His bundle, and (3) intraventricular conduction system.

An ECG readily identifies complete AV block, but a His bundle recording is re-quired to definitively localize the site of block. The manifest slow ventricular rate may be responsible for symptoms of cerebral hypoperfusion or cardiac failure or may predispose to life-threatening ventricular arrhythmias. With few exceptions, permanent pacing is clearly indicated for all patients with acquired chronic complete AV block.

COMPLETE AV NODAL BLOCK. As a result of AV nodal block, an escape rhythm, usually narrow QRS complex, originates from the His bundle and conducts synchronously to both ventricles via the intraventricular conduction system. The His bundle electrogram accurately identifies AV nodal block by an H potential that precedes each escape beat. Complete AV nodal block is most commonly seen in adults who manifest digitalis toxicity or have inferoposterior myocardial infarction. It is usually transient during infarction, and normal conduction frequently returns if the patient survives. Chronic complete AV nodal block is rare but requires permanent pacing if it is associated with symptoms or an excessively slow ventricular rate. Other causes of complete AV nodal block are infiltrative diseases, degenerative calcific extension from a calcified mitral annulus, or total ischemic necrosis involving the AV node.

Congenital complete heart block, encountered in infants and children, is anatomically characterized by an absent AV node, deficient AV node, or an impaired atrio-AV nodal communication.

Permanent pacemaker insertion is indicated if syncope or signs and symptoms of congestive heart failure incident to AV block or a wide QRS complex beyond 120 msec are present (Chapter 13).

COMPLETE HIS BUNDLE BLOCK. This type of complete AV block requires a His bundle recording for diagnostic confirmation, since the surface ECG usually demonstrates a narrow QRS escape rhythm. So-called split His bundle potentials (H − H¹) characterize an intra-Hisian block. In the His bundle electrogram, the distal His potential below the site of block precedes the escape beat that conducts to the ventricles. His bundle block occurs more frequently in women and usually generates a slow ventricular rate ranging between 30 to 50 beats/min.

The lesions responsible for this conduction defect may be consequent to coronary artery disease, hypertension, calcific aortic stenosis, or a sclerodegenerative process associated with aging termed Lev's disease. In the latter state, sclerocalcific material within the cardiac skeleton involves the His bundle encased within the central fibrous body. Permanent cardiac pacing is indicated for all symptomatic patients with complete His bundle block. Permanent pacing for patients who are asymptomatic is not entirely certain but probably is indicated in view of the unfavorable prognosis.

COMPLETE TRIFASCICULAR BLOCK. Complete intraventricular conduction system block is the cause for the most commonly encountered type of acquired complete AV block (Fig. 6–6). It is characterized by a block distal to the His bundle, an idioventricular escape rhythm without a preceding H potential, and a ventricular rate frequently less than 40 beats/min.

The major pathologic lesion in most patients with this acquired form of AV block is degenerative and less often the result of ischemic necrosis. Lev's disease involving the pars membranacea and summit of the ventricular septum may envelop and impair conduction within the proximal intraventricular conduction system. Lenegre's disease, an idiopathic degeneration affecting middle aged patients, nullifies the more distal portion of the trifascicular conduction system.

Symptoms of cerebral ischemia, including Stokes-Adams attacks (Fig. 6–7), are conspicuously present. Congestive heart failure and other manifestations of impaired pump performance secondary to a slow and

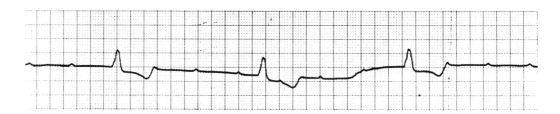

Fig. 6–6. Slow idioventricular escape rhythm frequently appears when acquired complete AV block develops distal to His bundle. This pattern is an absolute indication for a permanent pacemaker.

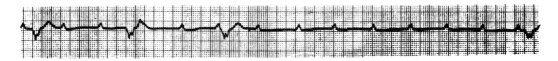

Fig. 6–7. Complete AV block due to complete trifascicular block is commonly associated with slow and unstable ventricular escape rhythm. Prolonged ventricular asystole leading to Stokes-Adams attacks and even sudden death is not unusual.

unstable ventricular rate may occur. Implantation of a permanent cardiac pacemaker is indicated in all patients with acquired complete trifascicular block whether symptoms exist or not.

Second Degree AV Block

WENCKEBACH AV BLOCK (MOBITZ TYPE I AV BLOCK). Wenckebach AV block is often benign, of transient duration, and usually not an indication for permanent pacing. It is almost always characterized as an incremental conduction delay within the AV node or progressive prolongation of the AH interval and eventual block of an atrial impulse without a His bundle potential. In the adult population it is seen most commonly as a self-limited conduction disturbance during acute inferoposterior infarction or as a manifestation of digitalis toxicity. It may also occur in young healthy adults or trained athletes and is considered as a benign manifestation of heightened vagal tone. Permanent pacing is not indicated in adult patients with chronic Wenckebach AV nodal block unless cardiac failure or symptoms of cerebral ischemia occur as a result of a slow and unstable ventricular rate. In children or adolescents, Wenckebach AV nodal block leads to complete AV block on occasion and will require pacing therapy.

MOBITZ TYPE II AV BLOCK. This form of AV block is characterized by a constant PR interval and sudden failure of AV conduction of an atrial impulse (Fig. 6–8). Paroxysmal advanced AV block with or without life-threatening ventricular tachyarrhythmias may ensue, leading to syncope and even sudden death (Fig. 6–9). The site of block rarely relates to an intra-Hisian lesion and manifests normal QRS complexes during conduction. More commonly, Mobitz Type II is recognized by a fixed bundle branch or bifascicular block during conduction and intermittent loss of ven-

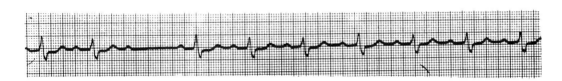

Fig. 6–8. Infrequent AV block of atrial impulse that occurs in association with conducted beats showing fixed bundle branch block pattern and prolonged but constant PR interval (in this example 0.26 sec) is consistent with Mobitz Type II AV block. His bundle electrogram demonstrated prolonged HV interval and block distal to recorded His bundle potential.

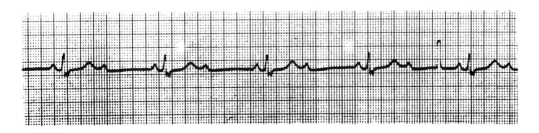

Fig. 6–9. 2:1 AV block with right bundle branch block of conducted beat is advanced and high degree AV block and a common precursor of complete AV block. Site of AV block was distal to His bundle potential on electrographic recording.

tricular response when AV block occurs in the remaining functioning fascicle of the intraventricular conduction system. When AV block is distal to the His bundle, the atrial electrogram is followed by a His bundle potential. All patients with this electrophysiologic derangement, whether symptomatic or not, require permanent cardiac pacing because of the increased proclivity toward complete AV block and its serious consequences.

CHRONIC BUNDLE BRANCH BLOCK

The role of pacing in patients with combined intraventricular conduction defects termed bifascicular block or incomplete bilateral bundle branch block without documented second degree or advanced paroxysmal AV block remains unresolved and controversial. This problem is particularly relevant for patients who have symptoms of syncope or episodic dizziness of uncertain origin or abnormally prolonged infranodal conduction time as determined by His bundle studies. Patients with the following ECG patterns should receive special consideration as potential candidates for permanent pacing:

1. RBBB + LAH—right bundle branch block combined with block of the anterior or superior division of the left bundle (left anterior hemiblock).
2. RBBB + LPH—right bundle branch block combined with block of the inferior or posterior division of the left bundle branch (left posterior hemiblock).
3. Bundle branch block (either RBBB or LBBB) associated with first degree AV block.
4. Alternating bundle branch block.

Recent clinical studies have shown that patients with such ECG patterns maintain a precarious state of AV conduction. With the passage of time, the risk of developing

trifascicular block and transient or prolonged complete AV block or asystole is well documented. Three significant conclusions have evolved from these experiences:

1. Combined intraventricular conduction defects are the most frequent precursor of established or intermittent complete AV block.
2. The formidable risk of developing Mobitz Type II AV block or complete AV block in patients with bifascicular or chronic bundle branch block appears to be a function of the time duration of this ECG abnormality.
3. Prolongation of the HV interval to more than 70 msec in patients with chronic bundle branch block is an independent risk factor for progression to high grade AV block.

In accordance with these considerations, a realistic and practical clinical approach is proposed for patients with chronic bundle branch block to assess the need for treatment with permanent pacing. This is based upon the presence or absence of symptoms at the time bundle branch block is recognized.

Symptomatic Chronic Bundle Branch Block

The following approach is applicable for patients with combined intraventricular conduction defect who have unexplained syncope, recurrent dizziness, or lightheadedness without ECG evidence of AV block. At the outset, it is essential to exclude other causes of these prevailing symptoms. These causes include neurologic disorders, occult gastrointestinal bleeding, orthostatic hypotension, aortic stenosis, hypertrophic cardiomyopathy, paroxysmal tachyarrhythmias, sinus node dysfunction, and vagally induced syncope.

Continuous ECG monitoring for 24 hours is warranted if pertinent diagnostic information is not ascertained from the clinical and laboratory examination. A His bundle study is then performed if an incriminating electrical disturbance is not manifest by ECG monitoring. A His bundle electrogram will provide crucial diagnostic information and will assist the physician to arrive at a rational therapeutic decision. It has been suggested that a prolonged HV interval of 70 msec or longer identifies the patient who has an unusually high risk for advanced AV block.

In most clinics, prophylactic insertion of a permanent pacemaker is indicated in patients with chronic bundle branch block and an abnormally prolonged HV interval in whom no other factor can be determined as the cause of the existing neurologic symptomatology. In patients with less prolonged or normal HV interval, permanent pacing is recommended when symptoms continue to recur without explanation. The elimination of symptoms by pacing strongly favors the existence of undetected intermittent AV block as the true origin of symptoms in these patients.

Asymptomatic Chronic Bundle Branch Block

The indication for prophylactic cardiac pacing in patients with asymptomatic chronic bifascicular block is even less certain and highly controversial. Nonetheless, several investigators have advocated permanent pacing for selected asymptomatic patients with a distinct likelihood of developing complete AV block or asystole and the high risk of sudden death.

In a recent study by Vera and co-workers, 48 out of 50 patients with chronic bifascicular block and evidence of complete trifascicular block or Mobitz Type II block had HV intervals of 65 msec or more. On the basis of this experience, the authors recommend prophylactic permanent pacing for asymptomatic patients with bifascicular block and an abnormally prolonged HV interval because of the apparent implication

of an impending AV block. Narula observed a mortality incidence of 23% per year for patients 70 years or older with a prolonged infranodal conduction time of 70 msec or more when cardiac pacing was not instituted. This compared to a mortality incidence of 10% per year for similar patients who received prophylactic cardiac pacing. Scheinman and co-workers focused upon the prognostic value of infranodal conduction time. The incidence of sudden death in patients with chronic bundle branch block associated with an HV interval of 70 msec or more was 17%, and progression to advanced AV block was 21%. In this prospective study, by contrast, sudden death and progression to second or third degree AV block remained less than 3% when HV prolongation was less than 70 msec.

Despite these studies, most clinics have adopted a conservative approach and closely follow asymptomatic patients with chronic bifascicular block and an abnormally prolonged HV time at frequent intervals. Presently we feel that a definitive statement for prophylactic permanent pacing in asymptomatic patients with chronic bundle branch block and prolonged infranodal conduction time is not warranted until further prospective studies establish the predictability of complete AV block and the mechanism of sudden death in these patients.

RECURRENT TACHYARRHYTHMIAS

Various permanent cardiac pacing techniques have been employed with increasing frequency for the prevention and termination of supraventricular and ventricular tachycardias. Electrical pacing designed for the termination of arrhythmias is often used as a last resort for a limited number of patients who have an incessant, often life-threatening, refractory arrhythmia, do not respond to drug therapy alone, or have unacceptable or toxic side effects from drug therapy.

Prevention of Tachyarrhythmias

Conventional modes of permanent pacing may often prevent supraventricular and ventricular arrhythmias that tend to arise when the basic sinus mechanism is slow. This has been well appreciated for the variety of arrhythmias in the brady-tachyarrhythmia syndrome that occur in the setting of a retarded sinus rate. The rate support of cardiac pacing, moreover, allows a more vigorous pharmacologic suppression of tachyarrhythmias when pacing alone is not completely successful.

Atrial overdrive pacing using an atrial demand pacemaker is an efficient technique of pacing that is often effective in the suppression of certain resistant supraventricular and ventricular tachycardias (Fig. 6–10).

An intact AV conduction system and an optimal pacing rate that provides the most effective control of recurrent arrhythmias must be established for each patient with temporary pacing prior to long-term overdrive suppression. The advent of rate-programmable pulse generators enables noninvasive modification of the prescribed pacing rate for arrhythmia control. After pacemaker implantation an appropriate pacing rate may be selected and changed with an externally controlled programmer to enhance control of the inherent rhythm disturbance.

The bifocal or QRS-inhibited AV sequential pacemaker is a more physiologic pacing technique for the control of many resistant arrhythmias when AV conduction is impaired. Control of ventricular premature

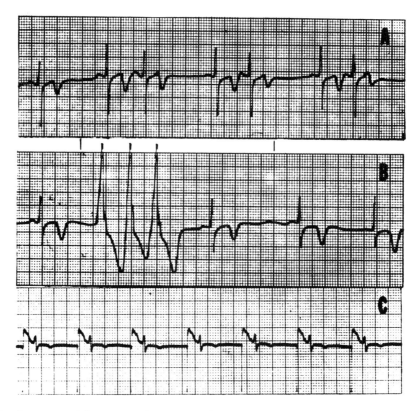

Fig. 6–10. Frequent atrial premature beats (A) and bursts of ventricular tachycardia (B) were resistant to a variety of drug regimens, and slowing of sinus node was further aggravated. Intact AV conduction permitted atrial demand pacing (C) that successfully suppresssed arrhythmic disturbances and symptoms.

systoles with long compensatory pauses or intermittent ventricular tachycardia can be more effectively established with this pacing method. Additionally, appropriate adjustment of the AV sequential interval may inhibit many AV or ventriculoatrial (VA) reentrant or reciprocating tachycardias.

Rate control by electrical pacing for slow or even normal heart rates can prevent recurring atrial or ventricular arrhythmias by several mechanisms:

1. A shortened cycle length induced by cardiac pacing may eliminate atrial or ventricular premature beats that initiate reentrant or reciprocal tachycardias or prevent automatic ectopic beats to emerge.
2. The critical electrophysiologic disparity of the dual pathways of a reentrant circuit involving varying conduction and refractory properties can be altered by faster pacing rates and/or adjustment of the AV sequential interval. These electrophysiologic changes induced by pacing may then dispose to inhibition of AV or VA reciprocating conduction.
3. Arrhythmic activity may be controlled by improvement in cardiac performance or hemodynamics incident to cardiac pacing, particularly when atrial demand or AV sequential pacing is used.

Termination of Tachyarrhythmias

SUPRAVENTRICULAR TACHYCARDIAS. Several pacing techniques have been introduced and applied for the conversion of recurrent, drug-resistant supraventricular tachycardias and tachycardias associated with or without manifest Wolff-Parkinson-White syndrome. Implanted pacemakers that provide bursts of rapid atrial stimulation (RAS) for overdrive suppression have been most successful and increasingly employed in recent years (Fig. 6–11).

A newer development has been the patient-activated radiofrequency triggered pacemaker. This system consists of an implantable receiver and external transmitter that provides an adjustable pacing rate up to 400 pulses/min. Atrial leads are placed pervenously into the right atrial appendage or secured epicardially at thoracotomy. The pacemaker receives its power from the handheld, patient-triggered transmitter through radiofrequency coupling. It must be emphasized that this technique represents a last resort modality of treatment and is applicable only for a highly select group of patients in whom the refractory arrhythmia is recurrent, disabling, often life-threatening, and resistant to conventional drug therapy. Prior sophisticated electrophysiologic studies are mandatory to determine the efficacy and safety of this pacing technique. Therapeutic pacing is not indicated in reentrant supraventricular tachyarrhythmia if atrial fibrillation with an excessive ventricular response incident to accelerated AV conduction is induced during rapid atrial stimulation.

VENTRICULAR TACHYCARDIA. Termination of recurrent, life-threatening, drug refractory ventricular tachycardia by bursts of rapid ventricular pacing at rates from 190 to 300 pulses/min for several seconds' duration has been reported in several studies involving a small number of patients. A recent technique employs an implantable pacemaker that is manually activated by the application of a magnet for rapid stimulation to provide 8 to 12 pulses for 2 to 3 seconds.

Many serious objections have been raised about rapid ventricular pacing using an implantable pacemaker for the conversion of ventricular tachycardia. Pacemaker activation with bursts of rapid ventricular pacing pulses will probably require the presence of a physician in the event defibrillation becomes necessary. Not infrequently, despite pacing, the ventricular tachycardia continues to recur. At the present time, rapid ventricular pacing using an

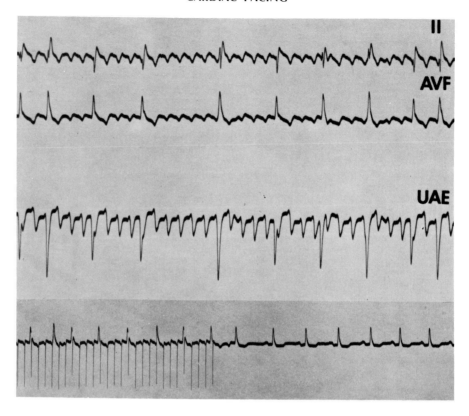

Fig. 6–11. Atrial flutter with variable AV conduction is recorded in the standard limb leads II and AVF and confirmed by intra-atrial unipolar electrographic recording (UAE). Rapid atrial pacing at 400 pulses/min and 7 mA pulse amplitude for approximately 8 seconds converted this arrhythmia to sinus rhythm (bottom tracing).

implantable pacemaker must be considered experimental and indicated for the rare patients whose tachycardia is not otherwise controlled.

SPECIAL SITUATIONS

Permanent cardiac pacing is used in a variety of situations such as following acute myocardial infarction, open heart surgery, and cardiac pacing in infants and children. The latter two subjects are discussed in Chapters 12 and 13.

Acute Myocardial Infarction

The indications for permanent pacing following acute myocardial infarction are highly controversial. In recent years a number of studies have focused upon the role of prophylactic permanent pacing following acute myocardial infarction in a subgroup of patients who have an increased risk of late sudden death. Patients who survive a transient advanced AV block, including Mobitz Type II AV block in association with bifascicular or bundle branch block in the setting of acute myocardial infarction, have a one-year mortality rate of 60 to 85% following hospital discharge. Several studies advocate the use of prophylactic permanent pacing in this group of patients because of a significant improvement in this ominous prognosis.

Prophylactic pacing has also been recommended for patients who survive myocardial infarction and have bundle branch block or bifascicular block with a prolonged HV interval of 70 msec or more. It is reasonable to state that further controlled clinical studies and well-documented observations in a large patient population will be required to determine the ultimate goal of permanent pacing in this group of high risk patients.

It is well recognized that patients who develop bundle branch block, multiple fascicular blocks, or transient advanced AV block of the His-Purkinje system during acute myocardial infarction have a poor immediate prognosis and a formidable hospital mortality rate ranging between 30 and 75%. The role of temporary cardiac pacing in this group of patients with serious conduction disorders is discussed in Chapter 9.

SELECTED READINGS

Atkins, J.M., et al.: Ventricular conduction blocks and sudden death in acute myocardial infarction. Potential indications for pacing. N. Engl. J. Med., 288:281, 1973.

Atkins, J.M., et al.: Prognosis of right bundle branch block and left hemiblock: A new indication for permanent pacing. Am. J. Cardiol., 26:624, 1970.

Befeler, B., and Castellanos, A., Jr.: His bundle recordings, bundle branch block and myocardial infarction. Ann. Intern. Med., 86:106, 1977.

Biddle, T.L.: et al.: Relation of heart block and left ventricular dysfunction in acute myocardial infarction. Am. J. Cardiol., 39:961, 1977.

Breithardt, G., Seipel, L., and Loogen, F.: Sinus node recovery time and calculated sinoatrial conduction time in normal subjects and patients with sinus node dysfunction. Circulation, 56(No. 1):43, 1977.

Col, J.J., and Weinberg, S.L.: The incidence and mortality of intraventricular conduction defects in acute myocardial infarction. Am. J. Cardiol., 29:344, 1972.

Conde, C.A., et al.: Effectivenesss of pacemaker treatment in the bradycardia-tachycardia syndrome. Am. J. Cardiol., 32:209, 1973.

Denes, P., et al.: H-V interval in patients with bifascicular block (right bundle branch block and left anterior hemiblock): clinical, electrophysiological correlations. Am. J. Cardiol., 35:23, 1975.

DePasquale, N.P., and Burns, M.S.: Natural history of combined right bundle branch and left anterior hemiblock (bilateral bundle branch block). Am. J. Med., 54:297, 1973.

Dhingra, R.C., et al.: The significance of second degree atrioventricular block and bundle branch block. Circulation, 49:638, 1974.

Dreifus, L.S., et al.: Use of atrial and bifocal cardiac pacemakers for treating resistant dysrhythmias. European J. Cardiol., 3/4, 257–266, 1975.

Engel, T.R., Bond, R.C., and Schaal, S.F.: First-degree sinoatrial heart block: Sinoatrial block in the sick sinus syndrome. Am. Heart J., 91:303, 1976.

Fenig, S., and Lichstein, E.: Incomplete bilateral bundle branch and A-V block complicating acute anterior wall myocardial infarction. Am. Heart J., 84:38, 1972.

Ferrer, M.I.: The sick sinus syndrome in atrial disease. J.A.M.A., 206:645, 1968.

Ferrer, M.I.: The sick sinus syndrome. Circulation, 42:635, 1973.

Fisher, J.D., et al.: Cardiac pacing and pacemakers. II. Serial electrophysiologic-pharmacologic testing for control of recurrent tachyarrhythmias. Am. Heart J., 93 (5): 658, 1977.

Fisher, J.D., Mehra, R., and Furman, S.: Termination of ventricular tachycardia with bursts of rapid ventricular pacing. Am. J. Cardiol., 41:94, 1978.

Fruehan, C.T., et al.: Refractory paroxysmal supraventricular tachycardia: Treatment with patient-controlled permanent radiofrequency atrial pacemaker. Am. Heart J., 87:229, 1974.

Furman, S.: Cardiac pacing and pacemaker. I. Indications for pacing bradyarrhythmias. Am. Heart J., 93(4):523, 1977.

Gann, D., et al.: Prognostic significance of chronic versus acute bundle branch block in acute myocardial infarction. Chest, 67:298, 1975.

Johnson, R., et al.: Chronic overdrive pacing in the control of refractory ventricular arrhythmias. Ann. Intern. Med., 80:380, 1974.

Jordon, J.L., Yamagnichi, I., and Mandel, W.J.: Studies on the mechanism of sinus node dysfunction in the sick sinus syndrome. Circulation, 57:217, 1978.

Kahn, A., Morris, J.J., and Citron, P.: Patient-initiated rapid atrial pacing to manage supraventricular tachycardia. Am. J. Cardiol., 38:200, 1976.

Kaplan, B.M., et al.: Tachycardia-bradycardia syndrome (so-called "sick sinus syndrome"). Am. J. Cardiol., 31:497, 1973.

Kulbertus, H., and Collignon, P.: Association of right bundle-branch block and left superior or inferior intraventricular block. Its relation to complete heart block and Adams-Stokes syndrome. Br. Heart J., 31:435, 1969.

Lasser, R.P., Haft, J.I., and Friedberg, C.K.: Relationship of right bundle-branch block and marked left axis deviation (with left parietal or peri-infarction block) to complete heart block and syncope. Circulation, 37:429, 1968.

Lenegre, J.: Etiology and pathology of bilateral bundle branch block in relation to complete heart block. Progr. Cardiovasc. Dis., 6:409, 1964.

Lev, M.: Anatomic basis for atrioventricular block. Am. J. Med., 37:742, 1964.

Lichstein, E., et al.: Findings of prognostic value in patients with incomplete bilateral bundle branch block complicating acute myocardial infarction. Am. J. Cardiol., 32:913, 1973.

Lister, J.W., et al.: Rapid atrial stimulation in the treatment of supraventricular tachycardia. Chest, 63:995, 1973.

Maur, K.V., et al.: Hypersensitive carotid sinus syncope treated by implantable demand cardiac pacemaker. Am. J. Cardiol., 29:109, 1972.

Moss, A.J., and Rivers, R.J.: Termination and inhibition of recurrent tachycardias by implanted pervenous pacemakers. Circulation, 50:942, 1974.

Narula, O.S., et al.: Atrioventricular block: localization and classification by His bundle recordings. Am. J. Med., 50:146, 1971.

Narula, O.S.: His Bundle Electrocardiography. Philadelphia, F.A. Davis Company, 1975, pp. 437–449.

Pittman, D.E., et al.: Rapid atrial stimulation: Successful method of conversion of atrial flutter and atrial stimulation. Circulation, 46:788, 1972.

Ritter, W.S., et al.: Permanent pacing in patients with transient trifascicular block during acute myocardial infarction. Am. J. Cardiol., 38:205, 1976.

Rosen, K.M., et al.: Cardiac conduction in patients with symptomatic sinus node disease. Circulation, 43:836, 1971.

Scanlon, P.J., Pryor, R., and Blount, S.G., Jr.: Right bundle branch block associated with left superior or inferior intraventricular block. Circulation, 42:1135, 1970.

Scheinman, M.M., Weiss, A., and Kunkel, F.: His bundle recordings in patients with bundle branch block and transient neurological symptoms. Circulation, 48:322, 1973.

Scheinman, M.M., et al.: Prognostic value in infranodal conduction time in patients with chronic bundle branch block. Circulation, 56:240, 1977.

Steiner, C., et al.: Electrophysiologic documentation of trifascicular block as the common cause of complete heart block. Am. J. Cardiol., 28:436, 1971.

Strauss, H.C., et al.: Electrophysiologic evaluation of sinus node function in patients with sinus node dysfunction. Circulation, 53:763, 1976.

Varriale, P., and Kennedy, R.J.: Right bundle branch block and left posterior hemiblock: vectorcardiographic and clinical features. Am. J. Cardiol., 29:459, 1972.

Vera, Z., et al.: Prolonged His-Q interval in chronic bifascicular block. Relation to impending complete heart block. Circulation, 53:46, 1976.

Voss, D.M., and Magnin, G.E.: Demand pacing and carotid sinus syncope. Am. Heart J., 79:544, 1970.

Waxman, M.B., et al.: Self-conversion of supraventricular tachycardia by rapid atrial pacing. Pace, 1:135, 1978.

Waugh, R.A., et al.: Immediate and remote prognostic significance of fascicular block during acute myocardial infarction. Circulation, 48:765, 1973.

Wise, J.R.: Patient-activated atrial pacing in the treatment of recurrent supraventricular tachycardia. Chest, 65:212, 1974.

Young, D., et al.: Wenckebach atrioventricular block (Mobitz type I) in children and adolescents. Am. J. Cardiol., 40:393, 1977.

7

His Bundle Electrocardiography and Intracardiac Stimulation

JOSEPH ANTHONY C. GOMES
ANTHONY N. DAMATO

The recording of His bundle activity and the simultaneous use of intracardiac stimulation technique in man has considerably enhanced our knowledge of impulse formation and impulse transmission. In recent years these techniques have been amply utilized in (1) studying the electrophysiologic characteristics of the atrioventricular (AV) transmission system;[1-12] (2) localizing AV conduction delay and block;[13-35] (3) the evaluation of patients with bundle branch blocks,[27,33,36-42] sick sinus syndrome,[43-45] and Wolff-Parkinson-White syndrome;[46-49] (4) delineating the mechanisms in supraventricular tachyarrhythmias;[50-53] (5) assessing the effects of antiarrhythmic agents on the AV conduction system;[54-61] and (6) clarifying the selection of therapeutic modalities in treating patients with various abnormalities of the conducting system.[14,20,21,41,42,44,60,87-89,99,100,125] The purpose of this chapter is to review the role of His bundle electrocardiography and intracardiac stimulation techniques in assessing abnormalities of the AV conducting system and the sinus node.

ANATOMIC AND PHYSIOLOGIC CONSIDERATIONS

A proper understanding of disturbances in AV conduction requires consideration of the normal anatomy and physiology of the human conducting system. The cardiac conducting system has the propensity of impulse generation and impulse transmission. Normally, the electrical stimulation of the heart is initiated in the sinoatrial (SA) node which is located at the junction of the superior vena cava and the right atrium. The SA node is supplied by the sinus node artery which is a branch of the right coronary artery in 55% of subjects or a branch of the left circumflex artery in 45% of subjects.[62] The SA node is comprised of a tripartite cellular population consisting of P cells, transitional cells, and working myocardial cells.[63] The P cells are specialized pacemaker cells capable of spontaneous phase 4 depolarization (automaticity). The latter is an inherent property of all potential pacemaker cells in the heart.

After the electrical impulse is generated in the SA node, the impulse is conducted through specialized conducting tracts and/or atrial musculature to depolarize the AV node. The AV node measures 5 to 7 mm in length and 2 to 5 mm in width and is situated beneath the right atrial endocardium above the insertion of the septal leaflet of the tricuspid valve and anterior to the ostium of the coronary sinus.[64,65] The AV node is supplied by the AV node artery, which is a branch of the right coronary artery in 90% of human hearts or of the left circumflex in 10%. Since the right coronary artery supplies the AV node in the majority of subjects, the AV node often sustains ischemic injury in association with occlusion of the right coronary artery. An important physiologic characteristic of the AV node is to slow or delay transmission of atrial impulses and thus decrease conduction velocity.[66] In fact, delay at the AV node makes up the major part of the P-R interval on the surface electrocardiogram. The inability to sustain a 1:1 ventricular response in atrial fibrillation, atrial flutter, and during rapid atrial pacing is due to delay and block of atrial impulses within the AV node. Like the SA node, the AV node is richly supplied by the autonomic nervous system and is highly sensitive to changes in autonomic tone. Vagal stimulation slows AV nodal conduction, whereas vagolytic drugs such as atropine accelerate AV nodal conduction.[54] Similarly, extrinsic or intrinsic sympathetic stimulation or inhibition will respectively enhance or delay AV nodal conduction time.

From the AV node the impulse is conducted through the His-Purkinje system or the infranodal conducting system comprised of the bundle of His, the bundle branches, and the peripheral Purkinje network to depolarize the ventricular myocardium. The His bundle is composed of Purkinje fibers coursing either in the base of the membranous septum or along the left side of the crest of the intraventricular septum.

Only recently has it been recognized that in some patients the His bundle may traverse the right side of the interventricular septum. Massing and James observed right-sided His bundle in 5 of 32 normal human hearts.[67] Dual blood supply from the posterior descending coronary artery and the left anterior descending coronary artery makes the His bundle less susceptible to ischemic injury.

The right bundle branch is often a direct continuation of the His bundle coursing down the anterior aspect of the right side of the interventricular septum until it reaches the anterior papillary muscle of the right ventricle where it divides into the peripheral Purkinje fibers that ultimately terminate in the myocardium. It receives its major blood supply from the left anterior descending coronary artery and can often sustain damage from occlusion of the LAD.

The left bundle branch is a relatively short structure about 1.5 mm in cross section coursing from right to left through the inferior margin of the interventricular membranous septum. Anatomic studies have demonstrated that the human left bundle branch (1) may divide into two discrete divisions without proximal interconnections:[68] the anterosuperior fascicle which courses along the anterior septum in close proximity to the RBB along the apex and anterior free wall of the left ventricle and the posterior inferior fascicle that courses along the diaphragmatic and posterobasal portion of the septum and the left ventricular (LV) free wall; (2) divides into three rather than two fascicles;[69] and (3) is a diffuse fanlike structure.[70] Rosenbaum proposed the trifascicular concept of the bundle branch system in man and defined electrocardiographic criteria for block in one or more fascicles of the trifascicular system.[68] However, recent studies by Massing and James have indicated that the left bundle is rarely, if ever, organized into two separate fascicles or radiations.[67] Nonetheless, the proposal of the left bundle branch system as a functional bifascicular system serves a clinically useful electrocardiographic concept. Although the trifascicular concept of the bundle branch conducting system will be adhered to in the discussion of bundle branch conduction defects, it should be pointed out that the presence of left anterior and left posterior hemiblock need not connote anatomic block in isolated left bundle fascicles in the true sense of the word.

HIS BUNDLE STUDIES IN AV CONDUCTION ABNORMALITIES

The P-R interval of the surface ECG tracing reflects conduction time of an electrical impulse from the atrium to the ventricular myocardium.[71] However, the electrical activity of the conducting tissue interposing between the atria and the ventricular myocardium is not recordable on the P-R interval. Consequently, analysis of the P-R interval limits our knowledge regarding the precise site of delay and/or block within the AV transmission system. In recent years the widespread application of the catheter technique for extracellular recording of the electrical activity of the His bundle (HB) and various other portions of the specialized conducting system has made it possible to precisely define and quantitate the anatomic site of delay and block in AV conduction.

In our laboratory the methods for studying the AV transmission system include (1) His bundle recordings, (2) the effects of incremental and acute interrupted atrial pacing on the AV conducting system, (3) premature atrial stimulation, (4) ventricular pacing and premature stimulation, and (5) the effects of alteration in autonomic tone on the AV conducting system. It should be noted that some of these methods are of academic and research interest only; thus in the discussion to follow only those methods with clinical implication shall be dealt with.

His Bundle Recordings

The technique of recording activity from the HB has been previously described in detail and will be mentioned only briefly in this section.[72] A J-shaped tripolar or quadripolar catheter is percutaneously introduced by the Seldinger technique into a femoral vein, generally the right, and under fluoroscopy and ECG monitoring is advanced into the right ventricular cavity across the tricuspid valve. The electrodes of the catheter are connected to AC input of ECG amplifiers. When the catheter is freely floating in the right ventricular (RV) cavity across the tricuspid valve, two deflections are clearly visible. The A deflection, which corresponds to atrial activity, and the V deflection, which corresponds to ventricular activity. The catheter is gradually withdrawn to a level just across the tricuspid valve until another biphasic or triphasic deflection is seen between the A and V deflections (Fig. 7-1) which corresponds to the electrical activity of the HB.

Whenever the femoral approach is not feasible, the electrode catheter is introduced into an antecubital vein.[73] If a balloon type of catheter is employed, then fluoroscopy may not be required.[74]

An HB electrogram is recorded at frequency settings of 40 to 500 Hz. The intracardiac electrogram is primarily composed of three distinct deflections. These deflections correspond to the activation of the low atrial septum (A wave), the bundle of His (H), and the ventricular myocardium (V) (Fig. 7-1). The A-H interval is measured from the onset of the atrial electrogram to the onset of the HB deflection. This interval, which reflects AV nodal conduction time, normally measures 60 to 140 msec. The H-V interval is measured from the onset of the HB deflection to the earliest point of ventricular activation either on the surface ECG or the intracardiac V electrogram. The H-V interval may also be referred to as the H-Q interval. The H-V

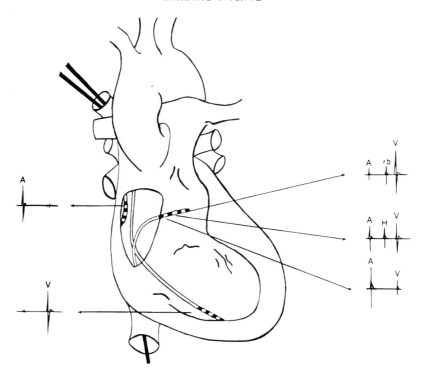

Fig. 7–1. Intracardiac electrograms obtained with three quadripolar catheters positioned in region of high right atrium, right ventricular apex, and across tricuspid valve. Using proximal poles for recording, bipolar electrograms from region of high right atrium (A) and right ventricle are obtained (left). Distal poles are utilized to stimulate respective chambers. For recording activity from the bundle of His, a J-shaped quadripolar catheter is percutaneously introduced into a femoral vein and positioned across tricuspid valve. Electrograms recorded by using bipolar combinations are demonstrated on the right. Combination of two distal poles records right bundle (rb) deflection, whereas combination of two middle poles records proximal His bundle deflection. Combination of proximal poles records large A deflection and a small V deflection but no His bundle deflection.

interval reflects His-Purkinje conduction time and measures from 30 to 55 msec.

Atrial Pacing and Premature Atrial Stimulation

For atrial pacing studies, we introduce a quadripolar electrode catheter into an antecubital vein; under fluoroscopic guidance and ECG monitoring, the catheter is positioned against the lateral wall of the right atrium at its junction with the superior vena cava. The proximal poles of the catheter are utilized for recording a high atrial electro-

gram and the distal poles for pacing the region of the high atrium. To stress the AV conducting system, the atria are electrically stimulated, starting at a rate slightly faster than the sinus rate. The pacing rate is kept constant for about 30 seconds until the next rate (in increments of 10 beats) is begun. Incremental atrial pacing is done up to rates of 200 to 220 beats/minute or up to the onset of anterograde AV nodal Wenckebach or higher grades of AV block. Atrioventricular nodal (A-H) and His-Purkinje (HV) conduction times are measured for each rate. Normally as the atrial rate is increased, there is progressive prolongation of the

A-H interval, reflecting progressive delay in AV nodal conduction time, whereas the H-V interval stays constant. In most normal subjects type I, AV nodal Wenckebach block or higher grades of AV nodal block are observed at atrial pacing rates of > 140 beats/minute. We also use the method of interrupted acute atrial pacing at rapid rates but at rates that do not produce AV nodal block. Unfortunately atrial pacing has not been a significantly useful method for stressing the His-Purkinje system (HPS).

Premature atrial stimulation is done by pacing the atria at a fixed basic cycle length and introducing a programmed premature atrial stimulus at increasing prematurity until atrial muscle refractoriness is encountered. The method is useful in studying ventricular aberration, refractory periods of the AV conducting system, and in the initiation of paroxysmal supraventricular tachycardias. However, data acquired by this method have little, if any, clinical implications in patients with AV conduction delay or block.

Alteration of Autonomic Tone

To assess the effects of alteration in autonomic tone on the AV conduction system, we (1) routinely do carotid sinus massage and (2) when necessary, study the effects of intravenous atropine and/or isoproterenol.

ABNORMALITIES IN AV CONDUCTION

Atrioventricular conduction abnormalities have been classified into first degree, second degree, high degree, and third degree or complete heart block and bundle branch blocks.

First Degree Heart Block

First degree heart block results in prolongation of the P-R interval on the surface ECG (> 0.20 sec).[75,76] This form of block may be due to conduction delay within the AV node, the bundle of His, and the bundle branch Purkinje system.[14,15,28,32,77] Delay in AV nodal conduction is the most common cause of first degree AV block which is reflected on the HB electrogram as a prolonged A-H interval, whereas the H-V interval is normal in duration (Fig. 7-2). In patients with first degree AV nodal block atrial pacing results in further prolongation of the A-H interval with occurrence of type I AV nodal Wenckebach block or higher grades of AV block at relatively slower heart rates (Fig. 7-2). If first degree AV block is associated with a normal QRS complex duration, it almost always denotes conduction delay within the AV node. Rarely, however, delay within the HB itself may result in first degree heart block with a normal QRS complex.[30] A His bundle electrogram (HBE) is essential for diagnosing first degree AV block due to delay within the HB. Enhanced vagal tone, atrial pacing, myocarditis, AV nodal disease, acute inferior wall myocardial infarction, and drugs such as digitalis and propranolol are the commonest causes of first degree AV nodal block.

In and of itself first degree heart block due to AV nodal delay does not require any specific therapy. Often exercise, atropine, or enhanced sympathetic tone results in improvement in AV nodal conduction. Neither is the presence of first degree AV block a contraindication for the administration of digitalis or propranolol. However, it is to be noted that patients with first degree AV nodal block run the risk of developing higher grades of AV nodal block after the administration of digitalis or propranolol.

Conduction delay within the HB itself or the bundle branch Purkinje system is a relatively uncommon cause of P-R prolongation. This form of delay is most often seen in the presence of bundle branch block (BBB) and is reflected by intra-Hisian delay or a prolonged H-V interval on the HBE. The presence of first degree AV block in the

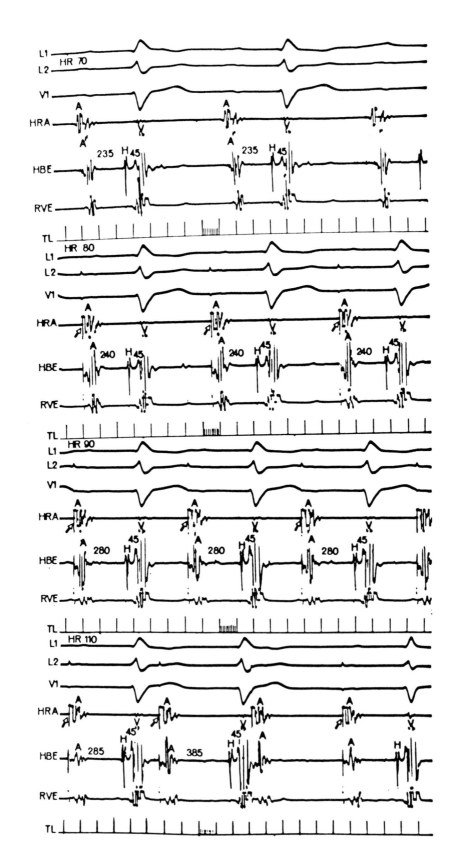

presence of BBB should alert the clinician to the presence of AV nodal or His-Purkinje delay or both and requires an HBE for definitive diagnosis. Studies of first degree heart block in the presence of BBB have shown a prolonged H-V interval in 50 to 68% of patients with right (R) BBB and left anterior hemiblock (LAHB); in 73 to 86% of patients with RBBB and left posterior hemiblock (LPHB) and in 56 to 76% of patients with left (L) BBB.[78]

No specific therapy is required in patients with first degree AV block due to delay in conduction within the HPS or the combination of AV nodal and His-Purkinje delay. Nonetheless, these patients should be carefully followed; if higher grades of block do occur within the HPS, then a permanent pacemaker is indicated.

Second Degree AV Block

Second degree AV block may be subclassified into type I or Wenckebach block and type II AV block.

TYPE I SECOND DEGREE AV BLOCK. This form of block is commonly referred to as the Wenckebach phenomenon. It is electrocardiographically characterized by a progressive prolongation of the P-R interval until a P wave is nonconducted to the ventricle. The classic feature of Wenckebach periodicity is a progressive diminution of the increments of P-R interval prolongation so that the R-R intervals become progressively shorter. The ECG pattern of type I second degree AV block may

result from conduction delay and block within the AV node, the bundle of His, and the bundle branch Purkinje system.

TYPE I SECOND DEGREE AV BLOCK WITHIN THE AV NODE. On the HB recording, type I second degree block within the AV node is characterized by progressive prolongation of the A-H interval until the atrial deflection is not followed by a HB deflection (Fig. 7–3). The classic feature of Wenckebach periodicity within the AV node is the progressive diminution in the increments of the A-H interval resulting in progressively shorter R-R intervals. Typical Wenckebach cycles, however, have been found to be less common than the atypical form, particularly when conduction ratios are 5:4 or greater. In one study, the first A-H interval as shortest was observed as the most common feature occurring in 98% of cycles analyzed, whereas progressive diminution of the increments of the R-R intervals was less common and occurred in only 35% of cycles.[79] Often the greatest increment in A-H interval may occur with the last conducted beat of the cycle, whereas at other times the increase in A-H intervals may be minimal prior to the nonconducted beat.

Type I second degree block within the AV node is the most common form of type I second degree block. It is encountered most often in association with atrial pacing, digitalis toxicity, the administration of propranolol, and in acute inferior wall myocardial infarction. When type I second degree AV block is the result of digitalis toxicity, withholding the drug and administering small doses of atropine may be all

Fig. 7–2.   First degree A-V block (due to A-V nodal conduction delay) and the response to incremental atrial pacing. From top to bottom, L_1, L_2, V_1 = ECG leads; HRA = high right atrial electrogram; HBE = His bundle electrogram; RVE = right ventricular electrogram; TL = time lines generated at 10 and 100 msec. Top panel: During sinus rhythm, AV nodal conduction time is prolonged (A-H interval = 235 msec) whereas His-Purkinje conduction time is within normal limits (H-V interval = 45 msec). Bottom panels: At atrial pacing rates of 80 and 90 beats/minute, there is progressive prolongation of A-H interval (240 and 280 msec, respectively), whereas the H-V interval remains constant. A-V nodal Wenckebach block occurs at atrial pacing rates of 110 beats/minute.

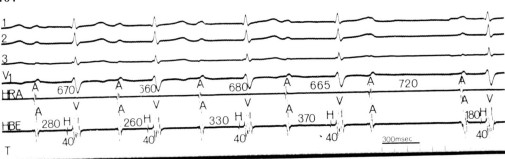

Fig. 7–3. Type I second degree A-V block with 5:4 A-V conduction ratio. A-H interval of first conducted beat measures 280 msec, whereas that of second conducted beat measures 260 msec. There is, however, a progressive prolongation of A-H intervals of third and fourth conducted beats. The fifth and nonconducted atrial impulse (5:4 AV conduction ratio) is blocked above bundle of His. Note that A-H interval (180 msec) of conducted beat following nonconducted beat is abbreviated.

that are necessary to achieve 1:1 AV conduction. However, if the ventricular rates are slow (< 40 beats/min) and if the patient is in congestive heart failure or severely hypokalemic, a temporary pacemaker may be indicated. Type I second degree AV block within the AV node in association with inferior wall myocardial infarction is generally a temporary phenomenon seen within the first 24 to 48 hours of the acute process. Often small doses of atropine result in 1:1 AV conduction or conversion to

a longer Wenckebach conduction ratio. A temporary pacemaker is recommended if the block progresses to higher grade AV block, the patient is symptomatic, and the course is complicated by ventricular arrhythmias.

TYPE I SECOND DEGREE AV BLOCK WITHIN THE HPS. Type I second degree AV block occurring within the HPS may be due to conduction delay and block within the HB itself or within the bundle branch Purkinje system. The precise identification of these

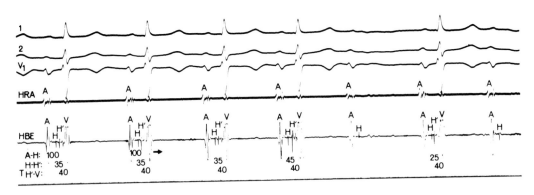

Fig. 7–4. Wenckebach type of conduction within the His bundle. Conducted beats demonstrate two His bundle deflections (H-H'). First three complexes are conducted with H-H' intervals of 35 msec; however, prior to nonconducted atrial impulse, H-H' interval increases to 45 msec. Note that fifth atrial impulse is blocked distal to proximal His bundle deflection as suggested by presence of a single H deflection. Note also, that following the blocked atrial impulse, next conducted beat demonstrates shorter H-H' interval of 25 msec. A-H intervals (100 msec) and H-V intervals (40 msec) of conducted beats remain constant.

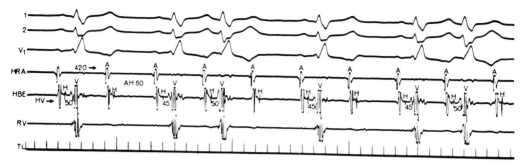

Fig. 7–5. Type I second degree and 2:1 A-V block within HPS in presence of RBBB and LAHB. Patient demonstrated alternating 2:1 and 3:2 AV conduction ratio. During 3:2 AV conduction, there is prolongation of H-V interval (45 to 50 msec) before nonconducted atrial impulse which is blocked below bundle of His.

conduction abnormalities requires HBE studies. Wenckebach type of conduction within the HB is uncommon. It is associated with split HB potentials on the HBE. There is progressively increasing delay between the two recorded HB potentials with ultimate failure in transmission in the distal HB (Fig. 7–4). This form of block in the main bundle may occur in the presence of normal or wide QRS complexes.

Type I second degree AV block within the bundle branch Purkinje system may begin as (1) progressive changes in QRS configuration from normal to a complete BBB configuration, with progressive increase in H-V interval and progressive changes in QRS configuration; (2) fixed

BBB with progressive prolongation of H-V intervals with resultant block within the bundle branch Purkinje system as denoted by the observation of a HB deflection that is not followed by a QRS complex (Fig. 7–5). The latter variety will ultimately progress to complete heart block. Permanent pacemaker implantation is justified in this form of block.

TYPE II SECOND DEGREE AV BLOCK (MOBITZ II). Type II second degree AV block is electrocardiographically characterized by a sudden unexpected blocked P wave.[75] The P-R interval of conducted beats remains constant, and the nonconducted P wave is not preceded by P-R prolongation. It is usually associated with a

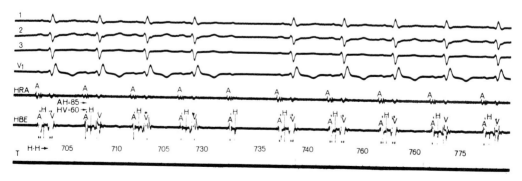

Fig. 7–6. Type II second degree A-V block (Mobitz II) in a patient with RBBB and LAHB. Conducted beats demonstrate normal A-H interval of 85 msec and prolonged H-V interval of 60 msec. Both A-H and H-V intervals stay constant until sudden unexpected block of fifth atrial impulse below bundle of His.

BBB or bifascicular block pattern. The AV conduction ratio may be 3:2 or greater. His bundle recordings in patients with type II second degree AV block have demonstrated that the site of block is below the bundle of His (Fig. 7–6).[15–18,22,24,30] Occasionally the ECG pattern of type II second degree AV block may be confused for a subtle form of AV nodal Wenckebach block. The presence of a normal QRS complex and the findings on the HBE will clarify the issue. In the absence of an HBE, the intravenous administration of atropine can considerably help in establishing the diagnosis. If the block is below the HB, atropine will increase atrial rate with a greater number of nonconducted atrial beats. Thus, a 5:4 conduction ratio may be converted to a 4:3 or a 3:2 AV ratio. If the block is at the level of the AV node, atropine will shorten the P-R interval and decrease the number of nonconducted P waves; thus a 3:2 AV conduction ratio may be converted to a 4:3 or 5:4 or 1:1 AV conduction. Type II second degree AV block usually progresses to complete heart block. A permanent pacemaker should be implanted in these patients.

High Degree AV Block

High degree AV block is generally manifested with a fixed 2:1, 3:1 AV conduction ratio. It may result from block within the AV node, the HB and the bundle branch Purkinje system. Localization of the site of block can be precisely accomplished by HBE.[15,32,77,80] Figure 7–7 is an example of 2:1 AV block within the HB in a patient with a normal QRS complex. The conducted beats are associated with split HB deflections (H-H' = 25 msec). The nonconducted beat has a single HB deflection indicating that the block is within the HB but distal to the proximal HB potential. Figure 7–8A is an example of 2:1 AV block below the HB in a patient with RBBB and left axis deviation. A single HB deflection is noted in the conducted beats with an H-V interval of 55 msec. In the nonconducted beat the A wave is blocked below the HB, indicating block in the bundle branch Purkinje system.

Although an HBE is essential for localization of the site of block, a careful examination of the surface ECG and clinical circumstances can lead to the appropriate diagnosis. The following are ECG and clinical features suggesting AV nodal block: (1) normal QRS complex in conducted beats (rarely, however, a normal QRS complex is associated with intra-Hisian block) (Fig. 7–7); (2) Wenckebach phenomenon in tracings prior to the development of high degree AV block; (3) inferior wall myocardial infarction, digitalis toxicity, and

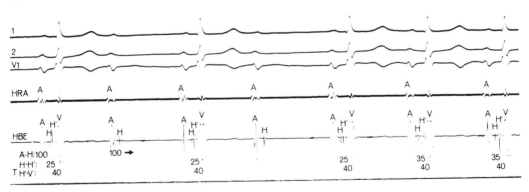

Fig. 7–7. 2:1 A-V block within His bundle in patient with normal QRS complex. Conducted beats demonstrate split His bundle deflections (H-H' = 25 msec). The nonconducted atrial impulse has a single His bundle deflection denoting that block is within His bundle but distal to proximal His bundle deflection. A-H and H-V intervals remain constant.

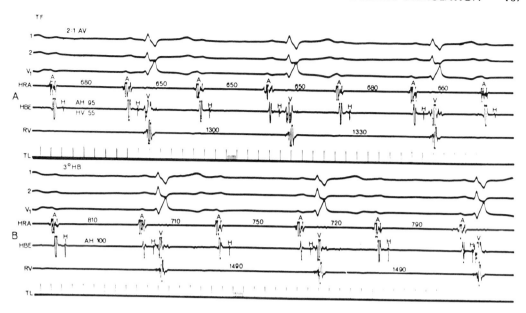

Fig. 7–8. A, 2:1 A-V block below His bundle in patient with RBBB and LAHB. A-H intervals measure 95 msec and H-V intervals of conducted beats measure 55 msec. In nonconducted beat atrial impulse is blocked below bundle of His, indicating block within bundle branch Purkinje system. B, Complete heart block in same patient. Atrial impulses are dissociated from ventricles. Nonconducted atrial impulses are followed by His bundle deflections indicating that block is below bundle of His.

drug therapy with propranolol; and (4) reversion to 1:1 AV conduction following atropine. The following are ECG features that suggest block below the HB: (1) BBB or bifascicular block in conducted beats, but it should be noted that block within the AV node may also be present in patients with BBB; (2) either no change in the conduction ratio or an increase with acceleration of the atrial rate after patients have taken atropine.

When 2:1 AV block is due to a lesion within the AV node, a pacemaker is not indicated if the patient is asymptomatic, the block is drug related, and the ventricular response increases during exercise and/or after the administration of atropine or isoproterenol. However, if the patient is symptomatic, in congestive heart failure, and the ventricular rate is < 40 beats/minute without appreciable acceleration after atropine,

then a permanent pacemaker is justified. In contrast, patients with 2:1 AV block within the HPS should have a permanent pacemaker. These patients are generally symptomatic. Acceleration of the atrial rate during exercise or after atropine usually results in higher AV conduction ratios. Importantly, 2:1 His-Purkinje block is a forerunner of complete heart block.

Complete Heart Block

In complete heart block, the atria beat regularly in response to the sinus pacemaker; the ventricles beat regularly but independently at rates ranging from 20 to 45 beats/minute in response to their pacemaker situated in the lower portion of the AV junction, the bundle of His, or the bundle branch Purkinje system. Complete

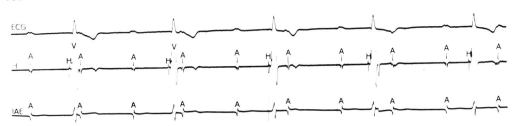

Fig. 7–9. Complete heart block in patient with a normal QRS complex. Atrial impulses are dissociated from ventricles. Nonconducted atrial impulses are not followed by His bundle deflections indicating block within AV node. His bundle deflection precedes each QRS complex suggesting junctional location of escape pacemaker. Abbreviations; H = His bundle electrogram; IAE = intra-atrial recording.

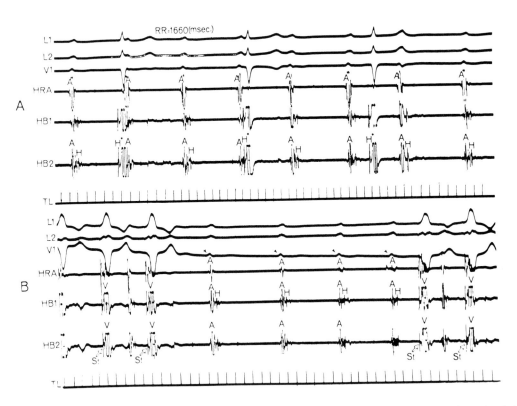

Fig. 7–10. A, Complete heart block in patient with a normal QRS complex. Each nonconducted atrial impulse is followed by His bundle deflection (H) and each QRS complex is preceded by His bundle deflection (H*) with abbreviated H-V interval suggesting that escape pacemaker is located in distal His bundle. (HBE₁ and HBE₂ refer to two separate recordings of His bundle activity.) B, Recovery time of subjunctional pacemaker in same patient following ventricular pacing. First three beats demonstrate right ventricular apical pacing. Note that following abrupt termination of pacing there is overdrive suppression of subjunctional pacemaker. All atrial impulses are followed by His bundle deflections indicating that block is below proximal His bundle.

heart block may be due to a lesion within the AV node (Fig. 7–9), the HB (Fig. 7–10A), or the bundle branch Purkinje system (Fig. 7–8B). When complete heart block is associated with a normal QRS complex, it generally indicates block within the AV node.

The ventricles are driven by a junctional pacemaker, the rate of discharge of such pacemakers being generally in the range of 40 to 60 beats/minute. These pacemakers are relatively stable and respond to exercise, atropine, and isoproterenol by increasing the rate of discharge. Rarely, lesions within the HB itself may produce complete heart block with normal QRS complexes. Such an example is demonstrated in Figure 7–10A. The nonconducted atrial impulses are followed by His bundle deflections (suggesting block distal to the HB), and each normal QRS complex is also preceded by an HB deflection with an abbreviated H-V interval suggesting that the pacemaker is located in the distal portion of the common bundle. The functional integrity of these pacemakers should be tested by exercise, atropine, or isoproterenol. The recovery time of these pacemakers can be tested by ventricular pacing. Often these pacemakers are unstable and have long recovery times. After cessation of ventricular pacing, the pacemaker is completely suppressed (Fig. 7–10B), and the occurrence of premature ventricular contractions can suppress subjunctional pacemakers.

A pacemaker is not absolutely indicated for an asymptomatic patient with complete heart block within the AV node if the junctional pacemaker is found to accelerate with exercise. Indication for pacemaker implantation in these patients include (1) symptoms of dizziness and/or syncope, (2) congestive heart failure, (3) inappropriate acceleration of junctional pacemaker on exercise, and (4) ventricular arrhythmias. A permanent pacemaker is indicated in patients with complete heart block due to lesions within the HB or bundle branch Purkinje system.

BIFASCICULAR AND TRIFASCICULAR BLOCKS

Block in two of three fascicles of the infranodal specialized conducting system is commonly referred to as bifascicular block. The ECG patterns include RBBB and LAHB, RBBB and LPHB, and LBBB. If conduction through the remaining fascicle is also partially or totally impaired, then an incomplete or a complete trifascicular block will result. Complete block within the trifascicular system will obviously result in complete heart block. It has been observed frequently that patients with bifascicular and/or incomplete trifascicular disease run a definite risk of developing complete heart block. Lasser, Haft, and Friedberg observed that 59% of patients with complete heart block had a pattern of RBBB and marked left axis deviation during periods of intact AV conduction.[81] However, the progression to AV block in patients with RBBB and LAHB is estimated to be less than 10%/year.[81,82] The causes of bilateral BBBs include sclerodegenerative disease involving the cardiac conducting system, arteriosclerotic heart disease, hypertensive heart disease, calcific aortic stenosis, cardiomyopathy, and other organic heart disease.

Right BBB and LAHB is the most common pattern of bifascicular block. This ECG pattern is estimated to occur in about 1% of patients in a large New York Hospital. Left anterior hemiblock in the presence of RBBB is diagnosed on the ECG by the presence of left axis deviation ($> -30°$) in the frontal plane. Rosenbaum and his colleagues suggest that left axis deviation be greater than $-45°$ but concede this to be an arbitrary number.[83]

The combination of RBBB and LPHB is much less frequent but potentially more dangerous. Left posterior hemiblock in the presence of RBBB is diagnosed on the basis of abnormal right axis deviation (RAD) ($+ 120°$) in the frontal plane.[68,83] The diagnosis of LPHB is fraught with error in the presence of anterolateral myocardial infarction, right ventricular hypertrophy, pulmonary disease, and extreme vertical hearts. Of the infranodal conducting system, the left posterior fascicle, in contrast to the left anterior fascicle and the right bundle, is the least vulnerable and most stable. When LPHB is associated with RBBB, the abnormality is diffuse and widespread; conduction is maintained over the more vulnerable anterior fascicle and increases the risk of complete heart block.

The pattern of LBBB implies conduction defect in the main left bundle and/or in both fascicles of the left bundle and perhaps less often in the His bundle. The exact frequency with which patients with LBBB develop complete heart block is currently unclear, although it is believed that the incidence is less than with either of the two bifascicular patterns. Abnormalities in cardiac function are frequent in patients with LBBB.[84]

His Bundle Electrocardiographic Findings in Bifascicular Blocks

His bundle studies have revealed that more than 17% of patients with RBBB and LAHB,[29,33,36,38,40] more than 50% of patients with RBBB and LPHB,[37,78] and more than 36% of patients with LBBB[29,33,78,85,86] have a prolonged H-V interval. However, markedly prolonged H-V intervals are less frequent. In one study only 4.6% of 388 patients had H-V intervals > 80 msec,[87] whereas in another study, 35% of 121 patients had H-V intervals of > 70 msec and 65% of patients had H-V intervals < 70 msec.[88] A prolonged H-V interval in patients with bifascicular block suggests some degree of impairment in the remaining fascicle (incomplete trifascicular block), although it is unclear what degree of H-V interval prolongation and over how long a time complete failure in the remaining fascicle will result. It has been suggested that a prolonged P-R interval in patients with one or the other pattern of bifascicular block implies impairment in conduction through the third fascicle. However, HB studies in patients with first degree heart block and bifascicular block have revealed that 44% of patients with LBBB, 50% of patients with RBBB and LAHB, and 14% of patients with RBBB and LPHB have normal H-V intervals.[78] In these patients, the prolonged P-R interval is due to A-V nodal conduction delay.

Clinical Approach to the Patient with Bifascicular Blocks

Often in clinical practice elderly patients with an ECG pattern of bifascicular block

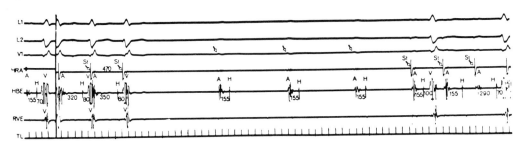

Fig. 7–11. Atrial pacing induced His-Purkinje block in patient with first degree heart block and RBBB and LAHB. Sinus beat is demonstrated on extreme left; note that the P-R prolongation is due to both AV nodal (A-H = 155 msec) and His-Purkinje (H-V interval = 70 msec) delay. During atrial pacing (cycle length = 470 msec), there is AV nodal Wenckebach block and also H-V prolongation (80 msec). Following sudden interruption of pacing, spontaneous atrial impulses are all blocked below bundle of His as noted by observation of His bundle deflection following each atrial electrogram. On resumption of atrial pacing (extreme right) 2:1 His-Purkinje block ensues.

have symptoms of lightheadedness, dizziness, and/or syncope. Causes of syncope may well be other than intermittent AV block and include central nervous system disease, postural hypotension, hypoglycemia, idiopathic vasovagal attacks, sick sinus syndrome and supraventricular and ventricular arrhythmias. These patients should have a complete neurologic, medical, and noninvasive cardiac evaluation to determine the cause of symptoms. If no cause is apparently discernible, then electrophysiologic studies (see study methods) to stress the AV conducting system are indicated. Occasionally it is possible to induce block within the HPS during atrial pacing (Fig. 7–11). Nonetheless, the inability to induce block in the laboratory does not imply the absence of intermittent AV block. Below is an outline of the clinical approach to the patient with bifascicular block.

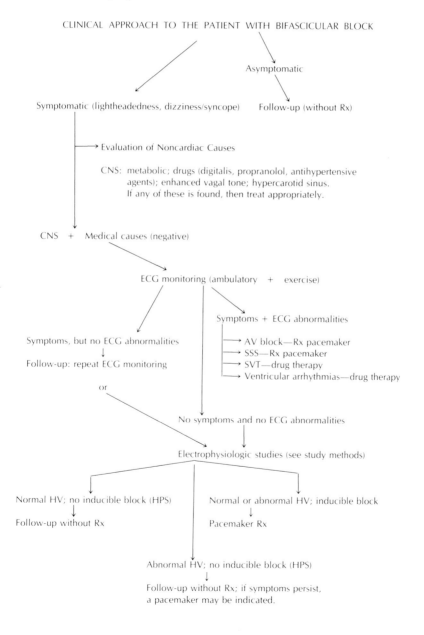

CLINICAL APPROACH TO THE PATIENT WITH BIFASCICULAR BLOCK

Asymptomatic

Symptomatic (lightheadedness, dizziness/syncope)   Follow-up (without Rx)

→ Evaluation of Noncardiac Causes

CNS: metabolic; drugs (digitalis, propranolol, antihypertensive
agents); enhanced vagal tone; hypercarotid sinus.
If any of these is found, then treat appropriately.

CNS + Medical causes (negative)

ECG monitoring (ambulatory + exercise)

Symptoms + ECG abnormalities

Symptoms, but no ECG abnormalities   → AV block—Rx pacemaker
↓   → SSS—Rx pacemaker
Follow-up: repeat ECG monitoring   → SVT—drug therapy
                                            → Ventricular arrhythmias—drug therapy

or

No symptoms and no ECG abnormalities

Electrophysiologic studies (see study methods)

Normal HV; no inducible block (HPS)   Normal or abnormal HV; inducible block
↓   ↓
Follow-up without Rx   Pacemaker Rx

Abnormal HV; no inducible block (HPS)
↓
Follow-up without Rx; if symptoms persist,
a pacemaker may be indicated.

Prognostic and Therapeutic Implications of the H-V Interval

It has been suggested that patients with bifascicular block and a prolonged H-V interval have a higher mortality and run a greater risk of developing complete heart block. Scheinman and co-workers reported 7 patients with chronic BBB with H-V intervals of 80 msec or greater and transient neurologic symptoms.[42] Six of these patients had complete heart block on admission. Narula and co-workers reported on 10 patients with RBBB and LAD and H-V intervals > 65 msec who were followed for 1 to 6 years.[41] Of these 10 patients, 8 died over a period of 1.32 years, for a yearly mortality of 61%. It should be noted, however, that the cause of death in these patients was unclear. Vera and co-workers reported a prolonged H-Q interval of 65 msec or greater in 47 of 50 patients with Mobitz II or transient complete heart block.[89] Both Vera and Narula suggested that patients with a prolonged H-V interval and bilateral BBB should be considered for prophylactic pacemaker insertion.

More recently Scheinman and co-workers reported their experience in a total of 121 patients followed up to 18 months.[88] They observed a significantly greater incidence of progression to second degree or third degree A-V block (21% of patients) and severe congestive heart failure (38% of patients) with H-Q interval > 70 msec compared to those with H-Q intervals of < 70 msec (1.3% and 16%, respectively). The risk of sudden death was also greater in patients with H-Q intervals of > 70 msec and severe congestive heart failure. They suggested prophylactic insertion of a pacemaker in patients with marked H-Q prolongation (> 70 msec) and no other cause of neurologic symptoms. In contrast, Dhinghra and associates reported on 18 of 388 patients with H-V intervals of 80 msec or greater followed prospectively for 103 to 1919 days.[87] They observed a high morbid-

ity and mortality in patients with marked H-V prolongation and symptomatic heart disease. They concluded that prophylactic pacing did not appreciably modify the clinical course of patients with symptomatic heart disease and is not indicated in asymptomatic people.

Our own follow-up studies (11 to 57 months) suggest that H-V intervals and refractory periods of the HPS are unreliable indices in predicting the imminence of complete heart block.[90] It is apparent from these studies that (1) patients with bifascicular block and a prolonged H-V interval have a higher morbidity and mortality and a greater incidence of organic heart disease and congestive heart failure; (2) the modus of sudden death is currently unclear and in all likelihood may be related to new coronary events, congestive heart failure, ventricular arrhythmias, and to a lesser extent from the development of complete heart block; (3) although the majority of patients with Mobitz II and/or periods of intermittent complete heart block have markedly prolonged H-V intervals (> 70 msec), the incidence of marked H-V prolongation in patients with bifascicular block is low (4.6 to 38%).

Considering the cost of pacemaker insertion and the inherent complications of pacemakers, it is unclear whether prophylactic pacemaker insertion will significantly alter the long-term prognosis and the modus of sudden death in these patients. Clearly, long-term prospective studies with larger numbers of patients and subsets of patients are required before these questions are answered. Until then we believe that prophylactic pacemakers are not indicated in asymptomatic individuals, irrespective of the H-V interval. We believe that patients with symptoms and a prolonged H-V interval should be closely followed with repeated ECG monitoring. If symptoms are still persistent, then a pacemaker may be considered. Temporary prophylactic pacemakers are not recommended in asymptomatic patients with bifascicular block who are undergoing surgery and general anesthesia.[91]

Bifascicular Block in Acute Myocardial Infarction

Intraventricular conduction abnormalities are not uncommon in acute myocardial infarction, the most commonly encountered patterns being RBBB and LAHB and LBBB whereas RBBB and LPHB are much less frequent. Anteroseptal, anterior, or anterolateral sites of infarction are the most common location of infarction that result in bifascicular block. However, patients with myocardial infarction of the inferior wall in whom collaterals from the posterior descending coronary artery are the major supply to the interventricular septum may also develop RBBB with or without LAHB. The mechanism of development of bundle branch blocks in association with acute myocardial infarction has been found to be ischemic injury to the interventricular conducting system.

It has been repeatedly demonstrated that patients who develop bifascicular block in the acute phase of myocardial infarction are at a high risk of developing complete heart block. The incidence of complete heart block is estimated to be 11 to 14% for RBBB without axis deviation,[92,93] 27 to 64% for RBBB and LAHB,[92,94] 29 to 43% for RBBB and LPHB,[93,95-97] and 8 to 30% for LBBB.[92,98] It is believed that the presence of first degree heart block in association with one of the bifascicular patterns increases the risk of complete heart block. Scanlon et al. reported episodes of complete heart block in 5 of 7 patients with RBBB and LAHB and first degree heart block.[94] Similarly Saltups et al. observed that 7 of 11 patients with RBBB and first degree heart block developed complete heart block.[93] In contrast, Lie et al. found that the P-R interval was of no use in predicting prolongation of H-V interval, the development of complete heart block, and mortality.[99]

His bundle recordings seem to be of some value in predicting the short-term prognosis in patients with bifascicular block. Leichstein and co-workers reported 8 deaths in 12 patients with bifascicular block and prolonged H-V interval; in contrast there was one death in 4 patients with bifascicular block and a normal H-V interval.[100] Similarly, Lie et al. observed a significantly higher mortality in patients with bifascicular block and prolonged H-V intervals (81%) in comparison to those with normal H-V interval (47%).[99] Of interest also were their findings that 11 of 15 patients with bifascicular block and prolonged H-V intervals progressed to complete heart block as compared to 1 of 10 patients with a normal H-V interval. In all likelihood a prolonged H-V interval reflects the amount of myocardial damage.

Temporary pacemaker therapy is recommended in patients who during the acute phase of infarction develop (1) RBBB and LAHB or LPHB with or without first degree heart block,[99,101] (2) LBBB with or without first degree heart block, and (3) alternating BBB. Temporary insertion of a pacemaker does not appear to be necessary if (1) the block is of short duration (< 6 hours), (2) only RBBB develops, and (3) the block appears 24 hours after the infarction. It should be pointed out, however, that the mortality in these patients is not significantly altered by temporary implantation of pacemakers, since the cause of death in the majority is pump failure rather than complete heart block. The disappointing results despite pacemaker implantation in these patients have been amply emphasized by Norris and co-workers[102] and Lie and co-workers.[99]

It remains unclear whether patients with persistent bifascicular block following recovery from myocardial infarction and those with temporary second or third degree His-Purkinje block are candidates for permanent pacemakers. Based on the short-term follow-up studies of Waugh and co-workers and Atkins and co-workers who demonstrated a higher incidence of syncope and/or sudden death in non-paced patients in contrast to those with AV block who received pacemakers,[101,103] it would seem wise to consider permanent pacemaker insertion in patients with transient second or third degree His-Purkinje block in the presence of bifascicular block.

SICK SINUS SYNDROME (SSS)

Normal sinus node function is dependent on a close and complex interaction between intrinsic sinus node automaticity, sinoatrial conduction and extrinsic autonomic regulatory mechanisms. Disturbances in sinus node automaticity and sinoatrial conduction, perhaps in association with alteration in autonomic mechanisms, result in dysfunction of the sinus node clinically referred to as the sick sinus syndrome.[104,105,106]

The sick sinus syndrome is a constellation of electrocardiographic abnormalities that may manifest as (1) nondrug-induced sinus bradycardia, (2) sinus arrest, (3) sinoatrial block, and (4) bradycardia-tachycardia syndrome.[104] The hallmark of these electrocardiographic abnormalities is symptoms of cerebral dysfunction, namely, lightheadedness, dizzy spells, or syncope. Often patients with the sick sinus syndrome have disorders of AV nodal and intraventricular conduction. In these patients the symptoms need not relate to malfunction of the sinus node but to intermittent AV block. In patients with the bradycardia-tachycardia syndrome, the tachycardia component is most often atrial fibrillation, but atrial flutter or paroxysmal atrial tachycardia is also known to occur. The bradycardia component consists of braydycardia with or without periods of sinus arrest and/or sinoatrial block.

Symptoms of palpitations are followed by symptoms of dizziness or syncope during transition from rapid to slow heart rates.[107,108] The inability to resume normal sinus rhythm following cardioversion for paroxysmal atrial fibrillation, atrial flutter, or atrial tachycardia should also alert the clinician to the diagnosis of sick sinus syndrome.

Electrophysiologic Assessment of Sinus Node Function

Symptomatic sinus bradycardia can often be the only apparent manifestation of the SSS. However, nondrug-induced sinus bradycardia alone is not uncommon and is frequently seen in the young, the old, and the athlete. Often these subjects do not have abnormalities of sinus node function, and the sinus bradycardia is a reflection of enhanced vagal tone. Ferrer and Narula have suggested that persistent asymptomatic sinus bradycardia may be a precursor of SSS.[104,109] Nonetheless, it remains unclear whether asymptomatic sinus bradycardia is a separate entity of itself or over how long a time these patients will ultimately demonstrate other abnormalities of sinus function if at all.

Over the years several clinical tests and electrophysiologic methods have been developed to assess sinus node function. To date there are no available means to reliably record sinus node potentials in the intact human heart, although techniques to that effect are being developed by Hoffman and his associates.[71] However, indirect means of assessing sinus node function have been the subject of considerable investigation. The electrophysiologic evaluation of sinus node function consists of measurement of (1) sinus node recovery time (SNRT) by overdrive suppression, which reflects the automaticity of the sinus node, and (2) sinoatrial conduction time by premature atrial stimulation studies.

Sinus Node Recovery Time

Sinus node recovery time (SNRT) is assessed by interrupted atrial pacing starting at rates slightly in excess of sinus rhythm. The atria are paced consistently at a preset rate for a period of 1 to 2 minutes after which pacing is abruptly stopped and spontaneous sinus rhythm is allowed to return. The patient is kept in spontaneous sinus rhythm for at least 30 seconds before the next paced rate is begun, which is generally 10 beats above the original rate. Overdrive suppression is assessed up to rates of 150 to 160 beats/minute. Sinus node recovery time is defined as the interval from the last paced P wave or high atrial electrogram (if one is recorded) to the following spontaneous P wave or A wave. Sinus node recovery time is best expressed after correction for the spontaneous sinus rate prior to pacing. The corrected sinus node recovery time (CSNRT) is obtained by subtracting the average spontaneous P-P or A-A interval from the SRT. Thus,

$$CSNRT \ (msec) = P\text{-}P \ (or \ A\text{-}A) \ interval - SNRT.$$

While assessing SNRT it is of importance to record at least two or more ECG leads and note the polarity of the P wave and the sequence of atrial activation (i.e., high to low) if two or more atrial electrograms are recorded.

Overdrive suppression of the sinus node is seen in normal patients as well as in those with sinus node dysfunction (Fig. 7–12). The separation of the latter group, however, depends upon the degree of suppression. Although various laboratories have somewhat differed in characterizing normal from abnormal, CSNRT values above 525 msec are generally considered as abnormal.[44] Sinus node recovery time can also be expressed as a percentage of the basic sinus cycle. In our laboratory, a value equal to or greater than 150% of the basic sinus cycle is considered abnormal. The measurement of SNRT in patients with the SSS has yielded variable results. Mandel and co-workers found that 93% of 31 patients with the SSS had an abnormal SNRT.[43] Rosen and co-workers and Narula and co-workers reported abnormal suppression in 40% of 10 patients and 57% of 28 patients, respectively.[44,110] In contrast, Gupta and co-workers reported abnormal values in only 35% of 17 patients with the SSS.[111] In a more recent study, Breithardt and associates reported abnormal CSNRT in 75% of 41 patients with sinus node dysfunction.[112]

The wide variability of the SNRT in patients with SSS, although unclear, may

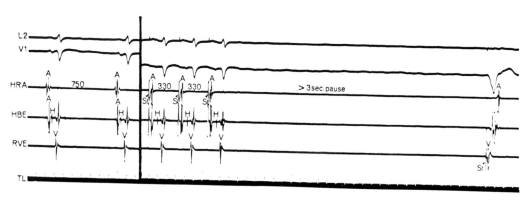

Fig. 7–12. Overdrive suppression of sinus node in patient with sick sinus syndrome. Spontaneous sinus rhythm with A-A interval of 750 msec is demonstrated on extreme left. Note that following termination of atrial pacing (cycle length = 330 msec), there is prolonged pause of > 3 seconds without any escape pacemaker. Pause was terminated by right ventricular pacing (extreme right).

be related to several factors: (1) variability in selection of patients and in the definition of what really constitutes the clinical SSS, (2) shift of the origin of the recovery pacemaker to a low atrial or junctional focus, (3) induction of sinus node reentry, (4) variability in the site of atrial stimulation, and (5) incomplete suppression due to entrance block into the sinus node during rapid atrial pacing particularly at rates above 140 beats/minute.[113] At times repeat atrial pacing after the administration of atropine may result in an abnormal response. Abolition of entrance block and/or enhancement of atriosinus conduction following atropine may allow consistent penetration of the sinus node resulting in enhanced suppression and a longer recovery time.[114] At times analysis of secondary pauses when the first postpacing pause is normal may uncover sinus node dysfunction.[115]

Sinoatrial Conduction Time (SACT)

Langendorf and co-workers originally estimated SACT by analyzing sinus cycles during spontaneous atrial ectopic beats.[116] In 1973, Strauss and co-workers measured SACT by the technique of programmed premature atrial stimulation.[45] According to this method, programmed premature atrial stimuli (A_2) are introduced after every eighth spontaneous sinus beat (A_1). Stimuli are introduced late in atrial diastole and progressively moved earlier by 10 msec intervals until atrial muscle refractoriness. The $A_1 A_1$ interval is the spontaneous sinus cycle preceding the premature atrial depolarization; $A_1 A_2$ is the coupling interval of the premature atrial response, and $A_2 A_3$ interval is the return cycle or the postextrasystolic pause. On plotting the normalized test cycle ($A_1 A_2/A_1 A_1$) against the return cycle ($A_2 A_3/A_1 A_1$), Strauss and co-workers observed two types of responses:

1. A fully compensatory pause followed premature atrial depolarizations (PADs)

elicited late in atrial diastole. As the $A_1 A_2$ intervals decreased, the $A_2 A_3$ intervals increased. They postulated that PADs falling late in atrial diastole fail to penetrate the SA node and therefore fail to discharge it prematurely. The range of $A_1 A_2$ interval over which a fully compensatory pause occurred, defined the "non-reset zone."

2. When PADs fell earlier in diastole, the $A_2 A_3$ interval was no longer fully compensatory but greater than the spontaneous $A_1 A_1$ cycle. Progressive shortening of the $A_1 A_2$ test cycle did not result in reciprocal lengthening of the return cycle ($A_2 A_3$), but the returned cycle remained constant. It was postulated that in this zone, the sinus node was reset by the PAD (zone of reset). The range over which the return cycles ($A_2 A_3$) exceed spontaneous cycles ($A_1 A_1$) in the zone of reset reflects conduction time of the atrial impulse into the atriosinus and sinoatrial direction. Half the difference between return and spontaneous sinus cycles reflect SACT. Thus,

$$SACT \ (msec) = \frac{A_2 A_3 - A_1 A_1}{2}$$

It is to be pointed out that this is an indirect method of measuring SACT requiring several assumptions: (1) no change in sinus node automaticity as a result of premature atrial stimulation; (2) atriosinus and sinoatrial conduction is equal, and (3) all premature impulses are capable of resetting the sinus node in the "zone of reset." However, the validity of the technique has been questioned because of (1) a poor correlation between direct and indirect measurements of SACT in rabbit hearts,[117] (2) the occasional presence of chaotic pattern of return cycles and of sinus node reentrant beats at close coupling intervals,[112,118] and (3) the occasional absence of a zone of reset.[45,119]

Narula has introduced a new method of estimating SACT.[119] According to this method the atria are paced at a rate slightly faster (< 5 to 10 beats/minute) than sinus rate for 8 to 16 consecutive beats after which pacing is terminated and recordings are continued for a subsequent 8 or more spontaneous sinus beats. SACT by this method is calculated by deducting the mean sinus cycle length from the interval between the last paced atrial electrogram and the first escape sinus cycle and represents the sum total of the conduction time into and out of the sinus node. This method seems to be simpler and quicker than the Strauss method. However, whether the new method will be of greater clinical value than the Strauss method is currently unclear.

Recently several laboratories have reported normal values of SACT. Steinbeck et al. reported value of 40 to 70 msec (mean = 56 ± 22 msec) in 5 patients.[120] Massini et al. reported values of 39.5 to 97.5 msec (mean = 70 ± 30 msec) in 18 patients,[121] whereas Engel et al. reported values of 28.5 to 115.5 msec (mean = 84.5 ± 26 msec).[122] Dhinghra and associates reported values of 40 to 153 msec (mean = 92 ± 60 msec) in 36 patients.[123] Although upper limits of normal have somewhat varied between different laboratories, values greater than 120 msec are considered as abnormal.[112,118] The measurement of SACT as a means of differentiating normal from abnormal sinus node function have also shown considerable variation. Strauss and co-workers reported values of 68 to 156 msec in 4 patients with sinus node disease.[45] Narula and co-workers observed normal values of SACT in patients with sinus bradycardia, SA block, and a prolonged SNRT.[109] Steinbeck and co-workers reported values of 105 to 150 msec (mean = 133 msec) in 3 patients with sinus node dysfunction.[120] Massini and co-workers reported values of 75.5 to 148.5 msec (mean = 126 msec) in 7 patients with sinus node dysfunction.[121] Dhinghra and co-workers reported abnormal values in only 29% of patients with suspected sinus node disease.[123] Of interest were the findings of Breithardt and co-workers who reported prolongation of SACT more often in patients with spontaneous SA block and the bradycardia-tachycardia syndrome; in contrast, patients with asymptomatic and symptomatic sinus bradycardia had abnormal prolonged SACT less often.[112]

Value of Electrophysiologic Parameters

The SSS is a clinical diagnosis based primarily on symptoms, signs, and electrocardiographic findings. We believe that the presence of a prolonged SNRT and/or SACT in patients with symptomatic sinus bradycardia, sinus arrest, SA block, and the bradycardia-tachycardia syndrome is confirmatory of the diagnosis. The presence of a normal SNRT and/or SACT in these patients is of no significant clinical or therapeutic value. A careful analysis of the electrocardiogram and particularly 24-hour ambulatory Holter monitoring are of greatest value in establishing the diagnosis. Pacemaker therapy is recommended in patients in whom a cause-and-effect relationship has been demonstrated between ECG abnormalities and symptoms, regardless of electrophysiologic studies. A preliminary report on long-term follow-up of patients with sinus node dysfunction indicates that clinical signs, symptoms, and ECG findings are the best guides in predicting response to pacemaker implantation and eventual outcome; in contrast the determination of SNRT and/or SACT is of little value.[124]

The demonstration of abnormal SNRT and/or SACT in asymptomatic patients with nondrug-induced sinus bradycardia, sinus arrest, and/or SA block, although helpful, should not appreciably influence the choice of therapy. Close and careful follow-up is indicated in asymptomatic patients with evidence of sinus node dysfunction and abnormal SNRT and/or SACT in regard to the future need of pacemaker therapy. Additionally, we advocate cautious use of quinidine in such patients, since a recent study in our laboratory demonstrated that

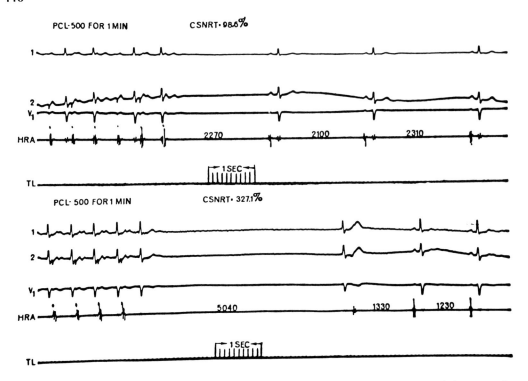

Fig. 7–13. Quinidine and CSNRT in patient with sinus node dysfunction. Top panel shows tracings during control study. Following termination of atrial pacing (for 1 minute) at pacing cycle length of 500 msec the CSNRT is 98.6%. Bottom panel shows tracings following quinidine. CSNRT is prolonged (327.1%) following 1 minute of atrial pacing at similar cycle length.

quinidine exaggerated sinus node dysfunction and recovery times were greatly prolonged (> 5 sec) in patients with SSS (Fig. 7–13).[125]

REFERENCES

1. Damato, A.N., et al.: Study of atrioventricular conduction in man using electrode catheter recordings of His bundle activity. Circulation, 39:287, 1969.
2. Damato, A.N., et al.: Recording of specialized conducting fibers (A-V nodal, His bundle and right bundle branch) in man using an electrode catheter technique. Circulation, 39:435, 1969.
3. Damato, A.N., et al.: A study of atrioventricular conduction in man using premature atrial stimulation and His bundle recordings. Circulation, 40:61, 1969.
4. Wit, A.L., et al.: Patterns of atrioventricular conduction in the human heart. Circ. Res., 27:345, 1970.
5. Wit, A.L., et al.: Phenomenon of the gap in atrioventricular conduction in the human heart. Circ. Res., 27:79, 1970.
6. Damato, A.N., and Lau, S.H.: Concealed and supernormal atrioventricular conduction. Circulation, 49:967, 1971.
7. Damato, A.N., et al.: Functional 2:1 A-V block within the His-Purkinje system. Simulation of type II second degree A-V block. Circulation, 47:534, 1973.
8. Castellanos, A., et al.: Functional properties of the human atrioventricular and intraventricular conduction during premature atrial stimulation. Cardiovasc. Res., 6:716, 1972.
9. Agha, A.S., et al.: Type I, type II and type III gap in bundle branch conduction. Circulation, 47:325, 1973.
10. Denes, P., et al.: The effect of cycle length on cardiac refractory periods in man. Circulation, 49:32, 1974.
11. Akhtar, M., et al.: Unmasking and conversion of gap phenomenon in the human heart. Circulation, 49:624, 1974.
12. Akhtar, M., et al.: The gap phenomenon during retrograde conduction in man. Circulation, 49:624, 1974.

13. Damato, A.N., et al.: A study of heart block in man using His bundle recordings. Circulation, 39:297, 1969.

14. Damato, A.N., and Lau, S.H.: Clinical value of the electrogram of the conducting system. Progr. Cardiovasc. Dis., 13:119, 1970.

15. Lau, S.H., and Damato, A.N.: Mechanisms of A-V block. Cardiovasc. Clin., 2:50, 1970.

16. Narula, O.S., et al.: Analysis of the A-V conduction defect in complete heart block utilizing His bundle electrograms. Circulation, 41:437, 1970.

17. Narula, O.S., and Samet, P.: Wenckebach and Mobitz II A-V block due to block within the His bundle and bundle branches. Circulation, 41:947, 1970.

18. Narula, O.S., et al.: Localization of A-V conduction defects in man by recording of the His bundle electrogram. Am. J. Cardiol., 25:228, 1970.

19. Puech, P., et al.: Leurigistrement de L'activite electrique du faisceau de His dans les blocs AV spontanes. Arch. Mal. Coeur, 63:784, 1970.

20. Rosen, K.M., et al.: Site of heart block in acute myocardial infarction. Circulation, 42:925, 1970.

21. Damato, A.N., et al.: Use of His bundle recordings in diagnosing conduction disturbances. Bull. N.Y. Acad. Med., 47:905, 1971.

22. Haft, J.I., Weinstock, M., and De Guia, R.: Electrophysiologic studies in Mobitz type II second degree heart block. Am. J. Cardiol., 27:682, 1971.

23. Castellanos, A., et al.: Contribution of His bundle recordings in the understanding of clinical arrhythmias. Am. J. Cardiol., 28:499, 1971.

24. Rosen, K.M., et al.: Electrophysiological significance of first degree atrioventricular block with intraventricular conduction disturbance. Circulation, 43:941, 1971.

25. Narula, O.S., et al.: Atrioventricular block. Localization and classification by His bundle recordings. Am. J. Med., 50:146, 1971.

26. Rosen, K.M., et al.: Site of heart block as defined by His bundle recordings: Pathologic correlation in three cases. Circulation, 45:965, 1972.

27. Steiner, C., et al.: Electrophysiologic documentation of trifascicular block as a common cause of complete heart block. Am. J. Cardiol., 28:436, 1971.

28. Schuillenberg, R.M., and Durrer, D.: Conduction disturbances located within the His bundle. Circulation, 45:612, 1972.

29. Raganathan, N., et al.: His bundle electrogram in bundle branch block. Circulation, 44:282, 1972.

30. Damato, A.N., Gallagher, J.J., and Lau, S.H.: Application of His bundle recordings in diagnosing conduction disorders. Prog. Cardiovasc. Dis., 14:601, 1972.

31. Kelly, D.T., et al.: Bundle of His recordings in congenital complete heart block. Circulation, 45:277, 1972.

32. Rosen, K.M.: Catheter recording of His bundle electrogram. Mod. Concepts Cardiovasc. Dis., 42:23, 1973.

33. Berkowitz, W.D., et al.: The use of His bundle recordings in the analysis of unilateral and bilateral bundle branch block. Am. Heart J., 81:340, 1973.

34. Hecht, H.H., et al.: Atrioventricular and intraventricular conduction: Revised nomenclature and concepts. Am. J. Cardiol., 31:232, 1973.

35. Dhinghra, R.C., et al.: The significance of second degree AV block and bundle branch block. Circulation, 49:638, 1974.

36. Haft, J.I., et al.: Assessment of atrioventricular conduction in left and right bundle branch block using His bundle electrograms and atrial pacing. Am. J. Cardiol., 27:474, 1971.

37. Castellanos, A. Jr., et al.: Significance of complete right bundle branch block with right axis deviation in absence of right ventricular hypertrophy. Br. Heart J., 32:85, 1970.

38. Narula, O.S., and Samet, P.: Right bundle branch block with normal left or right axis deviation; analysis by His bundle recordings. Am. J. Med., 51:432, 1971.

39. Narula, O.S.: Intraventricular conduction defects. In His Bundle Electrocardiography and Clinical Electrophysiology. Edited by O.S. Narula. Philadelphia, F.A. Davis Co., 1975, p. 177.

40. Denes, P., et al.: H-V interval in patients with bifascicular block (right bundle branch block and left anterior hemiblock). Clinical, electrocardiographic and electrophysiologic correlations. Am. J. Cardiol., 35:23, 1975.

41. Narula, O.S., Gann, D., and Samet, P.: Prognostic value of H-V intervals. In His Bundle Electrocardiography and Clinical Electrophysiology. Edited by O.S. Narula. Philadelphia, F.A. Davis Co., 1975, p. 437.

42. Scheinman, M., Weiss, A., and Kunkel, F.: His bundle recordings in patients with bundle branch block and transient neurologic symptoms. Circulation, 48:322, 1973.

43. Mandel, W.J., et al.: Evaluation of sino-atrial node function in man by overdrive suppression. Circulation, 44:59, 1971.

44. Narula, O.S., Samet, P., and Javier, R.P.: Significance of sinus node recovery time. Circulation, 45:140, 1972.

45. Strauss, H.C., et al.: Premature atrial stimulation as a key to the understanding of sino-atrial conduction in man. Presentation of data and critical review of the literature. Circulation, 47:86, 1973.

46. Castellanos, A., et al.: His bundle electrograms in two cases of Wolff-Parkinson-White (pre-excitation) syndrome. Circulation, 41:399, 1970.

47. Durrer, D., et al.: The role of premature beats in the initiation and termination of supraventricular tachycardia in the Wolff-Parkinson-White syndrome. Circulation, 36:644, 1967.

48. Narula, O.S.: Wolff-Parkinson-White syndrome—a review. Circulation, 47:872, 1973.

49. Wellens, H.J.J., and Durrer, D.: Patterns of ventriculo-atrial conduction in the Wolff-Parkinson-White syndrome. Circulation, 49:22, 1974.

50. Goldreyer, B.N., and Bigger, J.T. Jr.: Site of reentry in paroxysmal supraventricular tachycardia in man. Circulation, 43:15, 1971.

51. Goldreyer, B.N., and Damato, A.N.: Essential role of atrioventricular conduction delay in the initiation of paroxysmal supraventricular tachycardia. Circulation, *43*:679, 1971.

52. Denes, P., et al.: Demonstration of dual A-V nodal pathways in patients with supraventricular tachycardia. Circulation, *48*:549, 1974.

53. Akhtar, M., et al.: Antegrade and retrograde conduction characteristics in three patterns of paroxysmal atrioventricular junctional reentrant tachycardia. Am. Heart J., *95*:22, 1978.

54. Akhtar, M., et al.: Electrophysiological effects of atropine on atrioventricular conduction studied by His bundle electrocardiogram. Am. J. Cardiol., *33*:327, 1974.

55. Caracta, A.R., et al.: Electrophysiological properties of diphenylhydantoin. Circulation, *47*:1234, 1973.

56. Josephson, M.E., et al.: Effects of lidocaine on refractory periods in man. Am. Heart J., *84*:778, 1972.

57. Josephson, M.E., et al.: Electrophysiological evaluation of disopyramide in man. Am. Heart J., *86*:771, 1973.

58. Josephson, M.E., et al.: The electrophysiological effects of intramuscular quinidine on the atrioventricular conduction system in man. Am. Heart J., *87*:55, 1974.

59. Josephson, M.E., et al.: Electrophysiologic properties of procaine amide in man. Am. J. Cardiol., *33*:596, 1974.

60. Damato, A.N., et al.: The effects of commonly used cardiovascular drugs on AV conduction and refractoriness. *In* His Bundle Electrocardiography and Clinical Electrophysiology. Edited by O.S. Narula. Philadelphia, F.A. Davis Co., 1975, p. 105.

61. Gomes, J.A., et al.: The effects of digitalis on refractoriness and reentry within the His-Purkinje system in man. Am. J. Cardiol., *41*:442, 1978.

62. James, T.N.: Anatomy of the human sinus node. Anat. Rec., *141*:109, 1961.

63. James, T.N., et al.: Comparative ultrastructure of the sinus node in man and dog. Circulation, *34*:139, 1966.

64. James, T.N.: Morphology of the human atrioventricular node, with remarks pertinent to its electrophysiology. Am. Heart J., *62*:756, 1961.

65. Lev, M.: The conduction system. *In* Pathology of the Heart and Blood Vessels. Edited by S.E. Gould. Springfield, Ill., Charles C Thomas, 1968, p. 180.

66. Hoffman, B.F., and Cranefield, P.F.: The physiologic basis of cardiac arrhythmias. Am. J. Med., *37*:670, 1964.

67. Massing, G.K., and James, T.N.: Anatomical configuration of the His bundle and bundle branches in the human heart. Circulation, *53*:609, 1976.

68. Rosenbaum, M.B., Elizari, M.V., and Lazzari, J.O.: Las Hemibloqueos. Buenos Aires, Ed., Pardos, 1968.

69. Demontin, J.C., and Kulbertus, H.E.: His-topathological examination of concept of left hemiblock. Br. Heart J., *34*:807, 1972.

70. Davies, M.J.: Pathology of Conducting Tissue of the Heart. New York, Appleton-Century-Crofts, 1971.

71. Hoffman, B.F., et al.: Electrical activity during the P-R interval. Circ. Res., *13*:1200, 1960.

72. Scherlag, B.J., et al.: Catheter technique for recording His bundle activity in man. Circulation, *39*:13, 1969.

73. Gallagher, J.J., et al.: Antecubital vein approach for recording His bundle activity in man. Am. Heart J., *85*: 199, 1973.

74. Meister, S.G., et al.: A balloon tipped catheter for obtaining His bundle electrograms without fluoroscopy. Circulation, *49*:42, 1974.

75. Katz, L.N., and Pick, A.: Clinical electrocardiography. *In* The Arrhythmias. Philadelphia, Lea & Febiger, 1956.

76. Bellett, S.: Clinical disorders of the heart beat, Third Edition. Philadelphia, Lea & Febiger, 1971.

77. Narula, O.S.: Conduction disorders in the AV transmission system. *In* Cardiac Arrhythmias. Edited by L.S. Dreifus and W. Likoff, New York, Grune & Stratton, 1973, p. 259.

78. Levites, R., and Haft, J.I.: Significance of first degree heart block (prolonged P-R interval) in bifascicular block. Am. J. Cardiol., *34*:259, 1974.

79. Friedman, H.S., Gomes, J.A.C., and Haft, J.I.: An analysis of Wenckebach periodicity. J. Electrocardiol., *8*:307, 1975.

80. Damato, A.N., Schnitzler, R.N., and Lau, S.H.: Recent advances in the bundle of His electrogram. *In* Progress in Cardiology. Edited by P.N. Yu and J.F. Goodwin. Philadelphia, Lea & Febiger, 1973, p. 181.

81. Lasser, R.P., Haft, J.I., and Friedberg, C.K.: Relationship of right bundle branch block and marked left axis deviation (with left parietal or peri-infarction block) to complete heart block and syncope. Circulation, *37*:429, 1968.

82. Kulbertus, H.E.: The magnitude of risk of developing complete heart block in patients with LAD-RBBB. Am. Heart J., *86*:278, 1973.

83. Rosenbaum, M.B., Elizari, M.V., and Lazzari, J.O.: The hemiblocks. Oldsmar, Florida, Tampa tracings, 1970.

84. Haft, J.I., Herman, M.V., and Gorlin, R.: Left bundle branch block. Etiologic hemodynamic and ventriculographic considerations. Circulation, *43*:279, 1971.

85. Cannom, D.S., Goldreyer, B.N., and Damato, A.N.: Atrioventricular conduction system in left bundle branch block with normal QRS axis. Circulation, *46*:129, 1972.

86. Spurell, R.A.J., Krikler, D.M., and Sowton, E.: Study of intraventricular conduction times in patients with left bundle branch block and left axis deviation and in patients with left bundle branch block and normal QRS axis using His bundle electrograms. Br. Heart J., *34*:1244, 1972.

87. Dhinghra, R.C., et al.: Prospective observations in patients with chronic bundle branch block and

marked H-V prolongation. Circulation, *53*:600, 1976.

88. Scheinman, M.M., et al.: Prognostic value of infranodal conduction time in patients with chronic bundle branch block. Circulation, *56*:240, 1977.

89. Vera, Z., et al.: Prolonged His-Q interval in chronic bifascicular block. Relation to impending complete heart block. Circulation, *53*:46, 1976.

90. Foster, J.R., et al.: Prognostic value of His bundle recordings in right bundle branch block and left anterior hemiblock. One-to-five year follow-up. Circulation, *51*:II, 1975.

91. Pastore, J.O., et al.: The risk of advanced heart block in surgical patients with right bundle branch block and left axis deviation. Circulation, *57*:677, 1978.

92. Goodman, M.J., Lasser, B.W., and Julian, D.G.: Complete bundle branch block complicating acute myocardial infarction. N. Engl. J. Med., *282*:237, 1970.

93. Saltups, A., Bett, N., and McLean, K.H.: Prognostic factors in right bundle branch block complicating acute myocardial infarction. J. Med., *1*:25, 1973.

94. Scanlon, P.J., Pryor, R., and Blount, G.S.: Right bundle branch block associated with left superior or inferior intraventricular block: Associated with acute myocardial infarction. Circulation, *42*:1135, 1970.

95. Waugh, R.A., et al.: Immediate and remote prognostic significance of fascicular block during acute myocardial infarction. Circulation, *47*:765, 1973.

96. Gann, D., et al.: Prognostic significance of chronic versus bundle branch block in acute myocardial infarction. Chest, *67*:298, 1975.

97. Gould, L., et al.: Prognosis of right bundle branch block in acute myocardial infarction. J.A.M.A., *219*:502, 1972.

98. Norris, R.M., and Croxson, M.S.: Bundle branch block in acute myocardial infarction. Am. Heart J., *79*:728, 1970.

99. Lie, K.I., et al.: Factors influencing prognosis of bundle branch block complicating acute anteroseptal infarction. The value of His bundle recordings. Circulation, *50*:935, 1974.

100. Lichtstein, E., et al.: Findings of prognostic value in patients with incomplete bilateral bundle branch block complicating acute myocardial infarction. Am. J. Cardiol., *32*:913, 1973.

101. Atkins, J.M., et al.: Ventricular conduction blocks and sudden death in acute myocardial infarction. Circulation, *47*:765, 1973.

102. Norris, R.M., Mercer, C.J., and Croxson, M.S.: Conduction disturbances due to antero-septal infarction and their treatment by endocardial pacing. Am. Heart J., *84*:560, 1972.

103. Waugh, R.A., et al.: Immediate and remote prognostic significance of fascicular block during acute myocardial infarction. Circulation, *47*:765, 1973.

104. Ferrer, M.I.: The sick sinus syndrome. Circulation, *47*:635, 1973.

105. Rubenstein, J.J., et al.: Clinical spectrum of the sick sinus syndrome. Circulation, *46*:5, 1972.

106. Jordan, J.L., Yamaguchi, I., and Mandel, W.J.: Studies on the mechanism of sinus node dysfunction in the sick sinus syndrome. Circulation, *57*:217, 1978.

107. Short, D.S.: The syndrome of alternating bradycardia and tachycardia. Br. Heart J., *16*:208, 1954.

108. Kaplan, B.N., et al.: Tachycardia-bradycardia syndrome (so-called 'sick sinus syndrome'). Pathology, mechanism and treatment. Am. J. Cardiol., *31*:497, 1973.

109. Narula, O.S.: Disorders of sinus node function: Electrophysiologic evaluation. *In* His Bundle Electrocardiography and Clinical Electrophysiology. Edited by O.S. Narula. Philadelphia, F.A. Davis Co., 1975, p. 275.

110. Rosen, K.M., et al.: Cardiac conduction in patients with symptomatic sinus node disease. Circulation, *43*:836, 1971.

111. Gupta, P.K., et al.: Appraisal of sinus nodal recovery time in patients with sick sinus syndrome. Am. J. Cardiol., *34*:265, 1974.

112. Breithardt, G., Seipel, L., and Loogen, F.: Sinus node recovery time and calculated sino-atrial conduction time in normal subjects and patients with sinus node dysfunction. Circulation, *56*:43, 1977.

113. Goldreyer, B.N., and Damato, A.N.: Sino-atrial node entrance block. Circulation, *44*:789, 1971.

114. Reiffel, J.A., Bigger, J.T., and Giardina, V.E.G.: Paradoxical prolongation of sinus nodal recovery time after atropine in the sick sinus syndrome. Am. J. Cardiol., *36*:98, 1975.

115. Benditt, D.G., et al.: Analysis of secondary pauses following termination of rapid atrial pacing in man. Circulation, *54*:436, 1976.

116. Langendorf, R., et al.: Atrial parasystole with interpretation. Observations on prolonged sino-atrial conduction time and sinus cycle length. Circulation, *50*(supp III): 79, 1974.

117. Miller, H.C., and Strauss, H.C.: Measurement of sino-atrial conduction time by premature atrial stimulation in the rabbit. Circ. Res., *35*:935, 1974.

118. Talano, V., et al.: Sinus node dysfunction. An overview with emphasis on anatomic and pharmacologic consideration. Am. J. Med., *64*:773, 1978.

119. Narula, O.S.: A new technique for measurement of sino-atrial conduction time. *In* The Sinus Node: Structure, Function and Clinical Relevance. Edited by C.I. Bonke. The Hague, Martinus Nijhoff Med. Div., 1978, p. 65.

120. Steinbeck, G., and Luderitz, B.: Comparative study of sino-atrial conduction time and sinus node recovery time. Br. Heart J., *37*:956, 1975.

121. Massini, G., Dianda, R., and Graziina, A.: Analysis of sino-atrial conduction in man using premature atrial stimulation. Cardiovasc. Res., *9*:498, 1975.

122. Engel, T.R., Bond, R.C., and Schall, S.F.: First

degree sino-atrial block. Sino-atrial block in the sick sinus syndrome. Am. Heart J., *37*:956, 1975.

123. Dhinghra, R.C., et al.: Sino-atrial conduction time. Circulation, *55*:8, 1977.

124. Abbott, J.A., et al.: Prognostic indicators in patients with sinus node disease. Clin. Res., *26*(2):88A, 1978.

125. Calon, A.H. et al.: Quinidine in sinus node dysfunction. Circulation, *54*(II):907, 1976.

8

Hemodynamic Effects of Cardiac Pacing

RICHARD A. WALSH
ROBERT A. O'ROURKE

Since Zoll first employed transthoracic pacing in 1952, there has been a rapid and continuous expansion in pacemaker technology. As a result, the clinician is faced with a wide variety of pacing modalities. A major consideration in the choice of the proper type of pacing device is its ultimate hemodynamic effect in a given patient. The purpose of this chapter is to review variables that are important determinants of cardiac output during pacing in order to provide rational guidelines for patient management (Fig. 8–1). Because of the tremendous variation in ventricular function between patients, it is highly desirable to document an important hemodynamic advantage of atrial or AV sequential pacemaker therapy prior to chronic implantation.

EFFECT OF CHANGE IN HEART RATE ON CARDIAC OUTPUT

The extent to which cardiac output is dependent upon changes in heart rate is contingent on the physiologic setting. Atrial pacing in either the anesthetized or conscious animal results in a linear decrease in stroke volume as heart rate increases. This decline in stroke volume is due to a decrease in the length of end-diastolic muscle fiber. The usual explanation evoked to explain this observation is a mechanical limitation in ventricular filling owing to the shortening of diastole which occurs during tachycardia. However, the greatest portion of ventricular filling occurs in the first third of diastole, and other factors, such as alterations in the timing of atrial systole or rate-induced changes in diastolic compliance, may be equally important.

Because of the reciprocal relationship between heart rate and stroke volume, the ability to utilize the Starling mechanism will be compromised at low heart rates. In the setting of profound bradycardia, end-diastolic fiber length and hence stroke volume approach a maximum, and other reserve mechanisms must be utilized to increase cardiac output in response to physiologic needs. On the other hand, myocardial oxy-

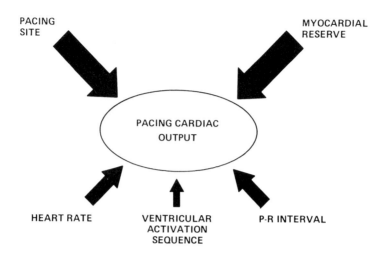

Fig. 8–1. Schematic representation illustrating relative effects of five factors influencing cardiac output during pacing.

gen consumption, a factor of critical importance in patients with ischemic heart disease, is greater when cardiac output is increased through changes in heart rate rather than by an increment in stroke volume.

The net effect of heart rate on cardiac output in three different situations is illustrated in Figure 8–2. In the conscious animal with normal left ventricular performance, there is a modest but definite increase in cardiac output with increasing heart rate, despite the decline in stroke volume. However, in human subjects with

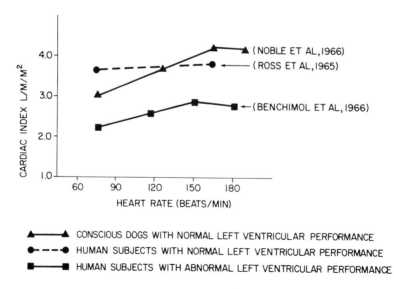

Fig. 8–2. This graph uses data points obtained from literature to compare effects of increase in heart rate on cardiac index in the awake dog and in patients with normal and impaired left ventricular function.

normal ventricular function, a significant rate-induced increase in cardiac output has not been observed at physiologic heart rates. Finally, in patients with abnormal left ventricular performance, a variable rate-related increment in cardiac output occurs.

The available data indicate that cardiac output is not dependent upon the pacing rate but is adjusted largely by alterations in stroke volume in normal subjects and in pacemaker patients with otherwise normal cardiovascular function. Yet, in the presence of impaired left ventricular performance, the stroke volume is relatively fixed, and the cardiac output is more heart rate-dependent.

Thus far we have considered only heart rate-induced modifications of cardiac output within the physiologic range of 60 to 150 beats/min. Numerous investigators have documented a rate-related increase in cardiac output in patients with complete heart block during incremental ventricular pacing up to 70 or 80 beats/min. The magnitude of the cardiac output increase is directly related to the degree of underlying myocardial dysfunction, with greater increments being noted in those with more severely impaired function. Although linear increases in cardiac output have been noted with pacing rates up to 110 per minute in individual patients, meaningful increases are uncommon beyond pacing rates of 70 to 80 beats/min in most patients. This observation explains the frequently used pacing heart rate of 72 beats/min in patients with pronounced bradyarrhythmias requiring permanent pacemakers. In patients with normal myocardial function, the resting cardiac output is largely independent of heart rate above a minimum of 45 to 50 beats/min. Under these circumstances the *theoretical* "optimum" pacing rate would be the slowest ventricular rate at which an adequate cardiac output and systemic arterial pressure can be maintained. This lower limit might be an important practical consideration in patients with severe ischemic heart disease who have associated conduc-

tion abnormalities, in whom heart rate-induced increases in myocardial oxygen demand must be minimized.

EFFECT OF ATRIAL CONTRACTION ON CARDIAC OUTPUT

The hemodynamic importance of atrial systole is well-documented. A properly timed atrial contraction at end-diastole serves to abruptly increase ventricular pressure and volume. This increase permits a relatively lower mean right or left atrial pressure during most of diastole than would occur if effective atrial contraction were absent (e.g., atrial fibrillation) or improperly timed (e.g., A-V dissociation). The atrial contribution to end-diastolic left ventricular volume is of particular importance in patients with diminished ventricular compliance as occurs in conditions causing left ventricular hypertrophy. It is of considerably less importance in the setting of normal left ventricular function. Although atrial systole contributes to ventricular filling and stroke volume in all situations, the normal left ventricle utilizes compensatory mechanisms such as enhancement of inotropic state and chamber dilatation to maintain cardiac output. These compensatory reserves are less readily available in the setting of reduced left ventricular performance, and therefore the loss of atrial systole may be less readily tolerated. The adverse effects of an improperly timed atrial contraction are illustrated in Figure 8–3. In this patient right ventricular pacing produced retrograde atrial activation with 30 mmHg "cannon A waves" on the pulmonary capillary wedge tracing. Atrial pacing at the same rate produced a 25% increase in cardiac output at a greatly reduced left ventricular filling pressure.

It seems clear, therefore, that the desirability of maintaining a properly timed atrial contraction in the pacemaker-dependent patient is greatest in patients with severely reduced left ventricular compliance (e.g.,

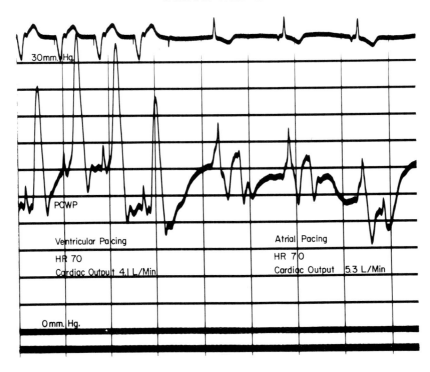

Fig. 8–3. Deleterious effect of ventricular pacemaker induced retrograde atrial activation on pulmonary capillary wedge pressure (PCWP) and cardiac output. PCWP decreases and cardiac output increases during atrial pacing (see text).

aortic stenosis, hypertrophic cardiomyopathy), in patients with severely compromised left ventricular performance, and in those in whom ventricular pacing produces hemodynamically significant retrograde atrial activation.

ACQUIRED COMPLETE HEART BLOCK

The following comments describe the circulatory aberrations that occur in patients with chronic complete heart block caused by fibrodegenerative disease of the conduction system or ischemic heart disease. Since congenital complete heart block differs in terms of pathophysiology and functional significance, it will be discussed separately.

The hemodynamic alterations in adult patients with complete heart block have been well characterized, and individual differences reflect variations in myocardial impairment related to age and underlying heart disease (Fig. 8–4). The cause in the majority of patients is abnormal *distal* conduction, and the ventricular rate is abnormally low, ranging between 10 and 40 beats/min. Since the subsidiary pacemaker is idioventricular in origin, there is little, if any, autonomic influence on heart rate. The resting cardiac index is reduced, and ranges between 1.5 and 2.5 $l/min/m^2$ despite an increase in stroke volume index averaging 65 ml/m^2. The impaired cardiac output is a reflection of profound bradycardia and a variable degree of impaired left ventricular performance. Thus, pacing at physiologic rates may normalize resting output, but an abnormally high ventricular filling pressure often persists. The difference in arteriovenous oxygen is greatly increased, with total

HEMODYNAMICS OF COMPLETE HEART BLOCK

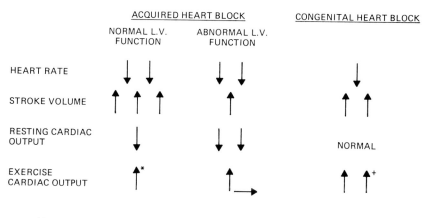

*Slight increase in stroke volume
+Normal increase in cardiac output with exercise

Fig. 8–4. Effects of acquired and congenital heart block on resting and exercise hemodynamics. In addition, hemodynamic consequences of acquired heart block in presence of normal and abnormal left ventricular (LV) function are compared (see text).

oxygen consumption being in the normal to slightly reduced range, particularly in patients with extremely slow heart rates. The primary effect on the systemic circulation is an increase in the arterial systolic, mean, and pulse pressures, as well as in the peripheral vascular resistance. Mild pulmonary hypertension may be present if the left ventricular filling pressure is elevated, and a mild increase in pulmonary vascular resistance often occurs in elderly patients. Atrioventricular asynchrony results in beat-to-beat variations in systemic pressures with increases being noted when atrial systole occurs fortuitously near end-diastole. Likewise, when atrial systole occurs during ventricular systole, cannon A waves may be noted in right atrial or pulmonary capillary wedge pressure tracings. The distribution of regional blood flow to the cerebral, renal, splanchnic, and coronary circulations is uniformly reduced. Underperfusion of these vascular beds leads to various functional and metabolic derangements which may be corrected by pacing. The

severity of these alterations is dependent upon the resting cardiac output and the integrity of the regional vasculature.

The response of patients with acquired complete heart block to exercise is severely compromised. Resting stroke volume is already increased, thus limiting further use of the Frank-Starling mechanism, and the idioventricular rate remains essentially unaltered because the relative lack of innervation prevents the reflex increase in heart rate mediated by the autonomic nervous system. The modest increase in cardiac output usually observed during exercise is accomplished by a slight increase in stroke volume due to an increased inotropic state and a decrease in systemic arterial resistance.

CONGENITAL COMPLETE HEART BLOCK

The etiology, electrophysiology, and natural history of congenital heart block differs from those of the acquired form.

Therefore, it is not surprising that the circulatory disturbances differ as well (Fig. 8-4). Most patients are asymptomatic, and the diagnosis is made because of an abnormally low resting heart rate. However, examples of presyncope, syncope, and sudden death are well recorded, particularly in infants and young children. The electrocardiogram characteristically reveals AV dissociation with narrow QRS complexes. For this reason, it has been assumed that the escape pacemaker focus is located in the *proximal* conduction system. This observation has recently been confirmed by His bundle electrocardiography. Because of the junctional nature of the escape focus, the resting heart rate is faster than in the acquired form and averages between 40 and 80 beats/min. The cardiac output in the resting state is normal to slightly reduced. In contrast to acquired complete heart block, the stroke volume is sufficiently increased to maintain a normal cardiac output despite a low ventricular rate. This difference probably reflects the absence of underlying myocardial disease in most of these patients. The resting end-diastolic pressures are usually normal but may be slightly elevated. During exercise the heart rate increases almost normally, since the junctional pacemaker responds to sympathetic stimulation and the response of cardiac output to exercise is normal to slightly decreased. Because these patients have a more benign natural history than those with acquired complete heart block, syncope is the most commonly used indication for permanent pacemaker placement.

PACING MODALITIES AND CARDIAC FUNCTION

Thus far we have reviewed heart rate and atrial systole as they relate to pacing-induced changes in cardiac function. In addition, the hemodynamic alterations that occur during acquired or congenital complete heart block have been discussed. It is our purpose now to apply these principles to the commonly employed forms of pacemaker therapy.

Fixed Rate Ventricular Pacing

Ventricular pacing in complete heart block is analogous to an accelerated idioventricular rhythm. It does not restore the normal temporal relationship between atrial and ventricular depolarization. Consequently, only a portion of atrial contractions occur at an appropriate interval before a subsequent ventricular systole, and the advantages of coordinated AV activity are not present. The heart rate is fixed in the most commonly employed units at 840 msec (heart rate 72 beats/min), and the ventricular activation sequence is abnormal, since the pacing electrode is positioned at the right ventricular apex with transvenous pacemakers and on the surface of the right or left ventricles with epicardial pacing systems. However, several animal and human studies have indicated that the abnormal ventricular activation sequence per se is hemodynamically unimportant. The major disadvantages of this form of pacemaker therapy are the loss of synchronized atrial contraction and the fixed rate.

Tachycardia is a normal cardiovascular accompaniment of exercise. Whether the heart rate is limited spontaneously (because of complete heart block) or by a fixed rate pacemaker, the usual response of the cardiac output to exercise is suboptimal. The level of cardiac output observed at a given exercise load will be entirely a function of stroke volume, which in turn is largely dependent upon the underlying contractile state. Several clinical studies have documented improved peak exercise capacity at pacing heart rates up to 110 beats/min when compared to idioventricular rates in patients with complete heart block. This occurs because resting stroke volume is smaller at faster heart rates and the ability

TABLE 8–1

Hemodynamic Indications for Atrial Pacing

1. Patients with moderately to severely depressed left ventricular performance
2. Patients with severely reduced left ventricular compliance such as those with aortic stenosis and hypertrophic cardiomyopathy
3. Retrograde activation of the atria with ventricular pacing
4. Complete heart block in physically active patients with normal atrial activity

to utilize the Frank-Starling mechanism is correspondingly greater.

Despite these potential hemodynamic disadvantages, ventricular pacing remains the most frequently employed form of permanent pacemaker therapy. The reasons for this wide usage include economy and simplicity of operation, as well as long-term experience. Most patients requiring long-term pacing are elderly (average age 72) and are relatively sedentary. Therefore, the potential benefits derived from variable rate

units are less applicable. Except for selected subsets of patients (Table 8–1), properly timed atrial systole provides measurable but clinically unimportant increases in cardiac output. The continued use of fixed-rate noncompetitive pacemakers in elderly patients with chronic complete heart block but otherwise reasonably normal ventricular function seems justified.

Atrial Pacing

Cardiac output increases when atrial pacing and ventricular pacing at identical heart rates are compared in patients with normal or abnormal left ventricular function (Fig. 8–5). The magnitude of the greater increase with atrial pacing will be highest in those subgroups listed in Table 8–1.

Two general types of atrial pacemakers are available for clinical use. The first is widely used in patients with isolated sinus node dysfunction and consists of an electrode positioned in the right atrial appendage or, more commonly, in the coronary sinus. This form of pacemaker maintains properly timed atrial systole at a noncom-

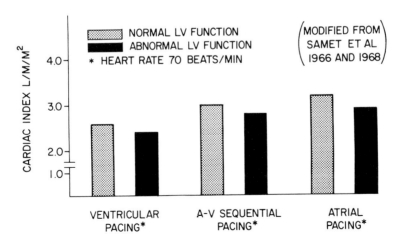

Fig. 8–5. Effect of three modes of pacing on cardiac index in patients with normal and abnormal LV function at identical rates (see text). (Modified from Samet, P., Castillo, C., and Bernstein, W.H.: Hemodynamic sequelae of atrial ventricular, and sequential atrioventricular pacing in cardiac patients. Am. Heart J., 72:725, 1966; Hemodynamic consequences of sequential atrioventricular pacing. Am. J. Cardiol., 21:207, 1968.)

TABLE 8–2

Contraindications to Atrial-triggered Pacing

1. Atrial flutter and fibrillation
2. Sick sinus syndrome
3. Ischemic heart disease with normal left ventricular function (relative)
4. Frequent occupational exposure to electromagnetic fields (relative)

petitive fixed rate in patients with chronic or intermittent bradyarrhythmias originating from the sinus node. The only disadvantage of this type of unit is the limitation of a fixed heart rate during exercise, which may be important in young, physically active patients with chronic or intermittent complete heart block. This problem is eliminated with the second type of atrial pacemaker referred to as an atrial-triggered unit. This device relies on an electrode positioned at the atrial level to sense intrinsic atrial activity and, after a preset delay, to stimulate an electrode placed at the right ventricular apex. The advantages of properly timed atrial systole and exercise-induced increments in heart rate are thus restored in patients with complete heart block *unassociated with atrial dysrhythmias* (Table 8–2). As compared to fixed-rate ventricular pacing at identical exercise levels, substantial increases in cardiac output are noted and range from 15 to 25%. However, it should be reemphasized that rate-related increases in cardiac output are less desirable in patients with symptomatic ischemic heart disease. In this subgroup, comparable increases in cardiac output may be achieved by increases in stroke volume when the heart rate is fixed, resulting in a smaller increment in myocardial oxygen demand.

AV Sequential Pacing

The AV sequential pacemaker has been reported to improve hemodynamics in a variety of clinical circumstances when compared with ventricular pacing. These situations include chronic complete heart block in the setting of normal or impaired left ventricular function (Fig. 8–5) and heart block complicating myocardial infarction or cardiac surgery. Pacing electrodes are positioned at both the atrial and the ventricular levels. The atrium is paced at a fixed noncompetitive rate followed by ventricular pacing after a preset delay. A major difference from other pacing devices is the ability to vary the interval between atrial and ventricular depolarization.

The hemodynamic importance of the duration of atrioventricular delay may be understood by considering the results of two extremes. Inappropriately reduced AV delay may not provide adequate time for an effective atrial contraction before ventricular systole resulting in cannon A waves and a reduction in cardiac output. Unusually prolonged AV delay, as occurs with extreme first degree heart block, may diminish stroke volume by causing premature mitral valve closure. The hemodynamic importance of small differences in the P-R interval has been demonstrated most convincingly in clinical situations resulting in *acutely* depressed myocardial function such as immediately after cardiac surgery or early after myocardial infarction. In this setting, deviation from the optimal P-R interval by less than 50 msec has been shown to decrease cardiac output by as much as 33% in individual patients with similar hemodynamics. This may reflect differences between the electrical and mechanical AV delay owing to varying positions of the pacing electrodes and intra-atrial or intraventricular conduction disturbances.

SELECTED READINGS

Benchimol, A., and Liggett, M.S.: Cardiac hemodynamics during stimulation of the right atrium, right ventricle, and left ventricle in normal and abnormal hearts. Circulation, *33*:933, 1966.

Hartzler, G. O., et al.: Hemodynamic benefits of atrioventricular sequential pacing after cardiac surgery. Am. J. Cardiol., 40:232, 1977.

Karlof, I.: Haemodynamic studies at rest and during exercise in patient treated with artificial pacemaker. Acta Med. Scand. (Suppl.) 565:1, 1974.

Noble, M.J.M., Trenchard, D., and Guz, A.: Effect of changing heart rate on cardiovascular function in the conscious dog. Circ. Res., 19:206, 1966.

Rosenquist, A.N., et al.: Hemodynamic changes during ventricular pacing in patients with complete heart block and aortic and mitral valvular heart disease. Am. Heart J., 89:144, 1975.

Ross, J., Jr., Linhart, J.W., and Braunwald, E.: Effects of changing heart rate in man by electrical stimulation of the right atrium. Circulation, 32:549, 1965.

Samet, P.: Physiologic aspects of cardiac pacing. In Cardiac Pacing. Edited by N. Segel and P. Samet. Grune & Stratton, 1973.

Samet, P., Castillo, C., and Bernstein, W. H.: Hemodynamic sequelae of atrial ventricular, and sequential atrioventricular pacing in cardiac patients. Am. Heart J., 72:725, 1966.

Samet, P., Castillo, C., and Bernstein, W. H.: Hemodynamic consequences of sequential atrioventricular pacing. Am. J. Cardiol., 21:207, 1968.

9

Temporary and Emergency Cardiac Pacing

LEONARD S. DREIFUS
KHALID R. CHAUDRY
SATOSHI OGAWA

The indications for artificial pacing of the heart have expanded since its first application in 1952 by Zoll for cardiac standstill. Today, artificial cardiac pacing is used in a variety of conduction and rhythm disturbances both as a temporary life-saving procedure and as a long-term means of life support. In this chapter the subject of artificial temporary cardiac pacing will be specifically discussed.

Controversy still exists regarding the indications for cardiac pacing, and precise criteria vary in accordance to the institution. Temporary cardiac pacing is used to increase the heart rate in the presence of acute or chronic AV heart block. Furthermore, it can be used as a diagnostic tool to uncover or confirm the existence of preexcitation, atrioventricular heart block, or sinus node dysfunction or to reproduce and identify the mechanism of an arrhythmia. Temporary cardiac pacing can be beneficial to identify hemodynamic abnormalities. A trial of temporary cardiac pacing is often indicated before a permanent cardiac pacemaker is implanted. Table 9–1 summarizes the indications for temporary cardiac pacing.

TABLE 9–1

Indications for Temporary Pacing

DIAGNOSTIC
Preexcitation
Sinus nodal dysfunctions
AV heart block
Induction of reentry dysrhythmias
Hemodynamic assessment of the heart
Anti-arrhythmic drug testing
PROPHYLACTIC
Acute myocardial infarction
Acute and chronic AV block
Overdrive suppression of dysrhythmia
THERAPEUTIC
Adams-Stokes attack due to SA, AV block, bradycardia, and tachycardias

DIAGNOSTIC INDICATIONS

Preexcitation

Atrial and ventricular pacing studies, in conjunction with His bundle electrocardiography, are being utilized to localize various pathways and map ventricular activation in the presence of preexcitation syndromes. The QRS complexes during preexcitation sometimes cause diagnostic problems by simulating myocardial infarction and bundle branch block patterns. Precise diagnosis of preexcitation is required to prevent or treat potentially fatal dysrhythmias.

In some patients with recurrent tachyarrhythmias, AV bypass tracts capable only of retrograde conduction (ventriculoatrial) can be identified (concealed Wolff-Parkinson-White syndrome). These patients usually do not show evidence of preexcitation on the surface electrocardiogram (ECG), and the diagnosis will be missed unless ventricular pacing studies and atrial activation patterns are studied.

AV Block

AV block is relatively easy to diagnose on the surface ECG. Atrial pacing studies may be required to evaluate AV nodal function when intermittent AV block is clinically suspected, but the ECG is not diagnostic of advanced or second degree AV block.

Evaluation of AV nodal function by atrial pacing is also required before an atrial pacemaker is implanted. As a general rule, it is safe to implant an atrial pacemaker if AV conduction is not interrupted (Wenckebach point) at pacing rates 20 to 30 beats above the desired pacing rate.

Sinus Nodal Dysfunction

Sinus and AV nodal function must be evaluated when no cause can be found for episodes of syncope or lightheadedness and long term ECG monitoring fails to demonstrate sinus node disease or second degree AV block. Syncope due to sinus node disorders may be associated with AV nodal disease, and subsidiary pacemakers may fail to prevent symptoms. Sinus node recovery time (SNRT) and sinoatrial conduction time (SACT) can be measured from surface ECGs during spontaneous termination of supraventricular tachycardia or by a return cycle following an atrial premature systole.

Sinus node recovery time and sinoatrial conduction time can be determined by atrial

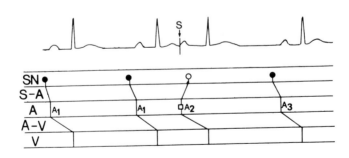

$$SACT = \frac{A_2 A_3 - A_1 A_1}{2}$$

Fig. 9–1. Sinoatrial conduction time (SACT), as measured by extrastimulus technique. Calculation should be done only when reset of the sinus node occurs, which can be assumed to occur if A_2A_3 is longer than A_1A_1 and A_2A_3 is shorter than $A_1A_1 \times 2$. SACT above 120 msec is abnormal.

overdrive pacing or by the extrastimulus method of atrial excitation. Overdrive pacing or spontaneous tachycardia results in suppression of the sinus node. When pacing ceases or tachycardia terminates abruptly, a sinus pause is observed, which is called SNRT. Normal SNRT should not exceed 150% of the basic sinus cycle length. SNRT can be corrected for sinus rate by subtracting the basic cycle length from the observed SNRT. The corrected SNRT should not exceed 525 msec. Measurement of SA conduction time is described in Figure 9–1.

Arrhythmias

Atrial and ventricular pacing can be used to (1) differentiate between supraventricular and ventricular tachycardia, (2) identify the pathogenesis of an arrhythmia and to determine optimal therapy, (3) overdrive supraventricular or ventricular tachycardias (overdrive suppression), and (4) identify concealed retrograde bypass tracts.

THERAPEUTIC INDICATIONS

Temporary and emergency cardiac pacing is used mainly to sustain life in the presence of heart rates too slow to maintain adequate cardiac output. The term *Adams-Stokes attack* was originally used to describe attacks of syncope and convulsions incident to extreme slowing of the arterial pulse. This definition can now be more generalized as "dizziness or syncope produced by a dysrhythmia." These syncopal attacks can be attributed to cerebral ischemia resulting from bradycardia or tachycardia associated with a decreased stroke or minute volume. An artificial cardiac pacemaker is indicated in symptomatic patients with either slow or rapid ventricular rates.

Slow Ventricular Rates

The major rhythm disturbances in this subgroup are the following:

1. Sick sinus syndrome.
2. Nonconducted premature atrial complexes with long return cycle.
3. AV block.
4. Exit block from a subsidiary pacemaker.
5. Downward displacement of the pacemaker.

Symptomatic sinus node dysfunction can be associated with AV nodal disease as well as failure of subsidiary pacemakers. Sinus bradycardia is generally not associated with symptoms, but if the ventricular rate is slower than 35 to 40 beats/min and does not increase with exercise, syncope may occur. Extreme sinus bradycardia may also precipitate ventricular tachycardia or fibrillation, and prophylactic pacing may be necessary. SA arrest, on the other hand, can cause syncope, depending on its duration and emergence of a subsidiary pacemaker. Syncope associated with carotid sinus stimulation or sensitivity is one such example.

Sinus arrest following sudden cessation of an ectopic tachycardia, as in paroxysmal atrial tachycardia or paroxysmal atrial fibrillation, may cause syncope. Persistent nonconducted premature atrial systoles can decrease the ventricular rate to almost half and may be associated with syncope, since the return cycle after premature atrial complex is usually longer than the sinus cycle. If antiarrhythmic agents fail to control the premature atrial systoles, electrical pacing will be indicated. Figure 9–2 demonstrates persistent nonconducted premature atrial systoles causing extreme bradycardia and recurrent syncope.

Second degree and third degree AV blocks are the commonest cause of Adams-Stokes attacks. Two-to-one (2:1) AV block may not have any significant hemodynamic effect, but sudden dropping of two or three ventricular complexes may cause syncope. This most commonly occurs with AV block associated with QRS complexes greater than 120 msec, and the AV block is considered to be below the His

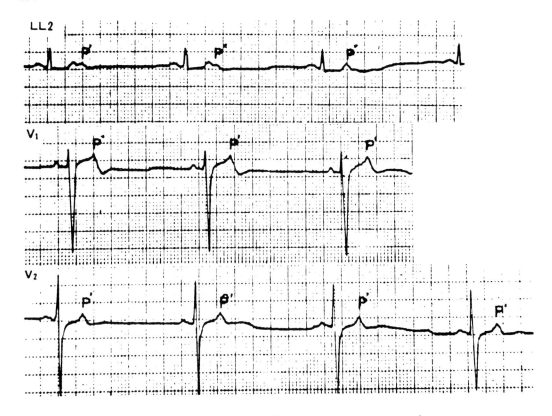

Fig. 9–2. Syncope caused by persistent nonconducted atrial premature systoles.

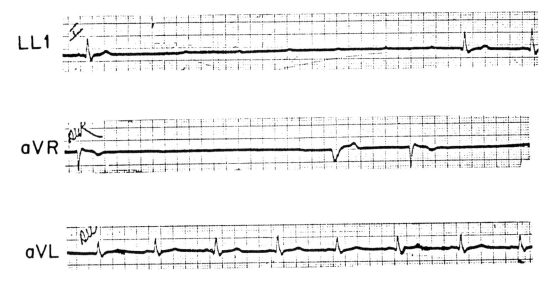

Fig. 9–3. Advanced second-degree AV block, Type II, with great variation in conduction ratio.

bundle. The rate of the subsidiary pacemaker is usually slow (30 to 40/min) and insufficient to prevent symptoms. On the other hand, AV block associated with narrow QRS complexes indicates that the level of block is in the AV node. Subsidiary junctional pacemakers are usually rapid enough to prevent symptoms. An example of syncope associated with the Type II AV block (wide QRS) is seen in Figure 9–3. Marked variation in the AV conduction ratio can easily cause syncope. Exit block from the subsidiary pacemaker may further slow the ventricular rate and adversely influence hemodynamic response.

Medication or intrinsic disease may depress automaticity in all potential pacemaker sites, so-called downward displacement of the pacemaker. In this situation, a rescuing pacemaker either fails to emerge, or the rate is too slow to sustain life. This occurs more often in Type II AV block with a wide QRS (Fig. 9–4). These patients usually do not respond to pacing, and the outlook is rather poor.

Third degree AV block is not always an indication for placement of an artificial pacemaker, and the need for pacing depends upon the rate and stability of the subsidiary pacemaker. A pacemaker is not mandatory when the rate is rapid enough to maintain an adequate cardiac output and the patient is free of symptoms, as commonly occurs with narrow QRS complexes. On the other hand, third degree AV block with wide QRS complexes is generally associated with a slow ventricular rate and symptoms of syncope. A pacemaker is indicated in almost all of these instances.

Rapid Ventricular Rates

Syncope or Adams-Stokes attacks may occur with rapid ventricular rates, and pacing may be required to control these arrhythmias. Sophisticated pacemakers may be required to control resistant or complex arrhythmias on a permanent basis, and temporary pacing wires are required in the

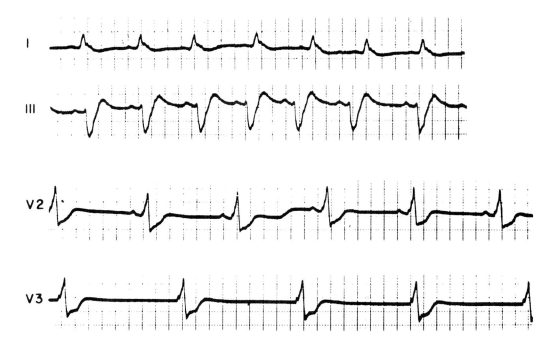

Fig. 9–4. So-called downward displacement of pacemaker.

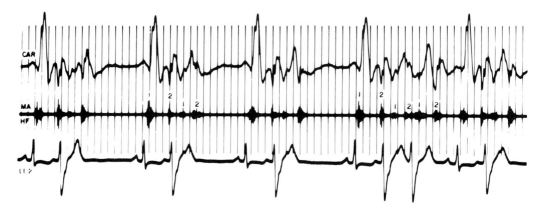

Fig. 9–5. Syncope caused by persistent ventricular bigeminy or trigeminy. Carotid and phonocardiographic recordings (upper tracing); Lead II (lower tracing).

ventricle or atria (coronary sinus) to identify the precise electrophysiologic mechanisms and types of stimulation sequence to control the tachycardia. Atrial or ventricular overdrive suppression and AV sequential timed, orthorhythmic pacing are some examples of the use of the new so-called smart pacemakers.

Frequent premature ventricular complexes, ventricular tachycardia, or ventricular fibrillation can be prevented with overdrive suppression by appropriately designed electronic pacemakers. Supraventricular reentrant tachycardias can be terminated by timed atrial or ventricular premature depolarizations or AV sequential pacing to interrupt reentry circuits. Control of supraventricular or ventricular premature systoles becomes essential when these beats are hemodynamically significant as in

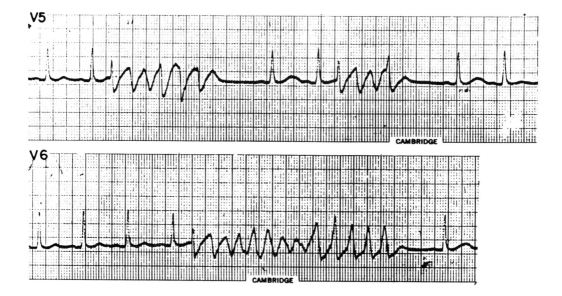

Fig. 9–6. Recurrent ventricular tachycardia associated with prolonged QT. Ventricular premature systoles falling on T wave.

bigeminal rhythm (Fig. 9–5). Electronic pacing may abolish the PVCs by overdrive suppression or shorten the QT interval and shorten an abnormally prolonged spread of repolarization to enhance the electrical safety factors of the heart. Figure 9–6 is an example of a prolonged QT interval and PVC in which recurrent ventricular tachycardia could be controlled only with overdrive suppression pacing. The following tachyarrhythmias may need temporary or permanent electrical pacing for their control:

1. Premature atrial or ventricular complexes.
2. Prolonged QT with premature ventricular complexes.
3. Reentrant supraventricular arrhythmias.
4. Ventricular tachycardia and ventricular fibrillation.

PROPHYLACTIC INDICATIONS

The most controversial issue in the subject of artificial pacemakers is prophylactic use. Current opinions generally held by most authorities will be summarized. For a better understanding, the subject is subdivided into acute myocardial infarction, chronic AV block, and tachycardia.

Acute Myocardial Infarction

Indications for temporary cardiac pacing in acute myocardial infarction are generally accepted. Table 9–2 summarizes the mandatory and possible indications for temporary pacing.

The site of AV block associated with an acute inferior wall infarction is generally located proximal to the His bundle. The QRS complexes are usually narrow, and the rate of the subsidiary pacemaker is rapid enough to maintain an adequate cardiac output. A pacemaker is indicated when

TABLE 9–2

Indications for Pacing in Acute Myocardial Infarction with Newly Acquired Subjunctional Block

	TEMPORARY	PERMANENT
LAH	0	0
LBBB	0	0
RBBB	+*	0
RBBB + 1°	+	0
RBBB + LAD	+	+
RBBB + LPH	+	+
LPH	+	+

*Placement of a temporary pacemaker must be judged on the clinical course of the patient. If only transitory RBBB, observation alone may be sufficient.
0 = not indicated; + = indicated. LAH = left anterior hemiblock; LBBB = left bundle branch block; RBBB = right bundle branch block; LAD = left axis deviation; LPH = left posterior hemiblock; 1° = first degree AV block.

cardiac output is inadequate, blood pressure falls, and there are symptoms of cerebral ischemia. Other indications are sinus bradycardia, second degree AV block, or any other situation causing a slow ventricular rate associated with an inferior myocardial infarction.

As AV block usually occurs below the His bundle and the rate of the subsidiary pacemaker is often slow in the presence of an anteroseptal myocardial infarction, a temporary pacemaker is indicated. The necessity for long-term pacing should be evaluated before the patient leaves the hospital. First degree AV block in acute anterior wall infarction should be considered an ominous sign, whereas in inferior wall infarction it is generally benign. We do not recommend temporary pacing for patients with an acute anterior wall infarction and left bundle branch block (with or without left axis deviation) because it does not seem to affect the prognosis. On the other hand, newly acquired right bundle branch block with or without left axis deviation ($-45°$) may be an indication for temporary cardiac pacing.

The use of a temporary pacemaker in tachyarrhythmia or bradytachycardia syndrome in acute myocardial infarction is infrequent, but mortality seems to remain high, as these arrhythmias are generally associated with cardiogenic shock or congestive heart failure. The major cause of death in anterior myocardial infarction is pump failure, and artificial pacing cannot improve myocardial contractility beyond what can be expected by changing the preload.

Chronic AV Block

Asymptomatic fascicular block with or without first degree AV block is not an indication for the implantation of a temporary pacemaker.

Tachycardia

The use of temporary cardiac pacing in the treatment or prevention of cardiac dysrhythmia has been discussed under therapeutic indications.

IMPLANTATION

Temporary cardiac pacing should be started as soon as the suspicion of its need arises. Decision for electrical pacing should be made promptly and before an emergency situation arises. In expert hands, cardiac pacing is a safe procedure and can be performed with or without fluoroscopic control as the situation dictates. Fluoroscopic control makes the procedure much simpler, and effective pacing can be rapidly initiated.

In emergency situations, external cardiac pacing can be used while the operator is putting in the endocardial lead. External cardiac pacing is rarely effective and when used requires high energy for effective control of the heart.

Routes of Access

For temporary transvenous cardiac pacing the electrode is placed in the apical endocardium of the right ventricle. The selected route of access depends upon the immediate need for pacing. Transthoracic temporary pacing can be attempted when rapid electrical control of the heart is required. It is a dangerous procedure and should be used only in emergency situations. Pneumothorax, cardiac tamponade, or laceration of a coronary artery may occur following insertion of a transthoracic needle into the heart. The subclavian, femoral, brachial, or jugular vein constitute the usual routes for temporary transvenous pacing. Selection of the venous route is dependent upon the physician's experience and the type of electrode catheter. Floating and semifloating electrode catheters may be introduced into the brachial vein, but the subclavian approach is preferable.

Several practical points should be mentioned. Balloon-tipped electrode catheters can be placed with relative ease into the femoral vein even during cardiovascular collapse. The likelihood of contamination in the femoral area increases the chance of infection when the percutaneous transfemoral approach is used. Access to the subclavian or jugular vein during cardiopulmonary resuscitation may be difficult.

Electrode position is relatively more stable with the subclavian approach than with the brachial vein. The latter approach may easily produce lead displacement incident to arm movements. The time required for temporary pacing will therefore influence selection of the site of venous entry.

Electrode Type

Bipolar electrodes obviate the need for attaching the positive or anodal electrode to the skin. Unipolar leads may be more sensitive to extraneous signals. Highly sensitive unipolar electrode systems may detect intercostal myopotentials or external signals and inappropriately inhibit demand pacing function. Special temporary endocardial leads with a longer distance between the positive and negative electrodes are designed to increase sensitivity to the available cardiac signal at the electrode site. Fibrillation threshold for bipolar leads is also slightly lower than for unipolar leads. This difference in fibrillation threshold may become clinically important when temporary endocardial pacing is indicated in acute myocardial infarction.

A Zucker semirigid catheter is preferred for coronary sinus (atrial) pacing. This catheter usually retains its position in the proximal coronary sinus. Position of the catheter can also be appraised by injection of a radiopaque bolus into the catheter lumen. The lumen is then sealed subsequent to catheter installation.

Tripolar and hexapolar catheters are available for electrophysiologic studies of the heart. Hexapolar catheters may be used for temporary AV sequential pacing, although two separate electrodes are preferred—one in the coronary sinus and the other at the right ventricular apex. Special catheters can be designed to secure stable pacing from different regions of the heart by modifying the electrode site on the catheter.

Technique

A venous cutdown is usually indicated when the jugular or brachial vein is used for catheter entry. Subclavian and femoral veins may be entered percutaneously. A needle is inserted into the vein and a guide wire is introduced into the vein through the needle. The needle is then removed and a vein dilator and introducer are guided over the guide wire. The dilator and guide wire are then replaced by the pacing electrode catheter.

Floating and semifloating catheters can be passed through a large bore needle without an introducer and a dilator. The pacing catheter is then advanced to the right ventricular apex under fluoroscopic control or electrocardiographic guidance (see Chapter 18). The pacing electrode is positioned into the apex of the ventricle, preferably under fluoroscopic control.

It is essential to select an endocardial site that offers a low pacing threshold, a high sensing measurement, and ECG evidence of ventricular capture. A 4 mV QRS signal should be obtained from the electrographic bipolar signal to ensure satisfactory electrode position. Good electrode placement is also evaluated by the presence of the current of injury on the electrographic signal and the maintenance of intact pacing and sensing function after deep respiration, Valsalva maneuver, or coughing.

Occasionally a RBBB complex can be seen in the V_1 ECG lead. This finding may indicate electrode malposition or placement into the coronary sinus or cardiac vein or may also represent a physiologic pattern. The transition of a left bundle to right bundle branch block pattern may suggest septal perforation. A RBBB pattern may be physiologic on occasion when activation of the septal Purkinje system depolarizes the left ventricle earlier than the right ventricle.

Pacemaker Design

Various types of pacemakers have been developed over the past several years. In most instances, a simple ventricular demand type pacemaker may suffice for temporary pacing. An atrial or ventricular sequential pacemaker may be used. Fixed rate pacemakers may produce competition between the intrinsic QRS activity and pacer rhythm. This will often dispose to discomforting clinical symptoms such as syncope, vascular pulsations of the neck, and palpitatory sensations. In the presence of acute myocardial infarction, fixed rate pacing may engender serious ventricular arrhythmias. Asynchronous pacing can be used in patients with high degree AV block where competition is not a consideration.

The pacing rate is usually established at about 70 beats/min and the current pulse amplitude at twice the stimulation threshold. The pacing system is maintained in accordance with the clinical situation and the assessed need. The pacemaker is turned off and maintained for approximately one day before it is removed.

COMPLICATIONS

Emergency cardiac pacing and temporary cardiac pacing are associated with certain complications that must be acknowledged. The untoward sequelae are principally related to the physician's technique and experience, venous entry point, and type of catheter used.

Semifloating and floating catheters may knot within the heart and occasionally require open heart surgery for their removal. Rigid catheters may perforate the ventricular wall and produce hemopericardium or, rarely, cardiac tamponade. Infection and thrombophlebitis can be avoided by using meticulous sterile techniques. Endocarditis can result from electrode trauma.

A subclavian vein approach may be complicated by pneumothorax or hemothorax and should be utilized only by an experienced physician. The antecubital cutdown site may result in injury to the median nerve. Vena caval thrombosis and obstruction have been reported, and thromboem-

bolism and cardiac arrhythmia resistant to medical therapy may necessitate removal of the pacing electrode.

Hemodynamic Consequences

Competition from sensing failure or the use of a fixed rate pacemaker may result in palpitations. Life-threatening ventricular arrhythmias may result when the R on T phenomenon is manifest. Syncope may be associated with periods of rapid heart action caused by interpolation of paced beats with sinus rhythm. Ventricular pacing in patients with borderline cardiac output may vitiate the hemodynamic response and cause symptomatic hypotension. Retrograde VA conduction and inappropriate atrial contraction may be responsible for untoward effects on cardiovascular dynamics. Atrial flutter or fibrillation may arise when a retrograde P wave occurs within the atrial vulnerable period (Fig. 9–7). It is important to select the optimal AV interval when using the AV sequential pacemaker. Small adjustments in the AV interval may account for considerable differences in the cardiac output. Figure 9–8 shows the effect of varying AV interval on left ventricular systolic pressure and left atrial pressure.

Reciprocal beating or ventricular premature systoles with a fixed rate ventricular pacemaker may cause an apparent tachycardia and decrease peripheral perfusion. Bigeminal rhythm with demand pacemakers may decrease the effective rate of the pacemaker and may even cause syn-

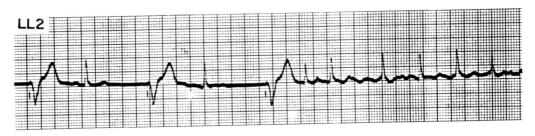

Fig. 9–7.   Retrograde conduction to atrium causing atrial fibrillation.

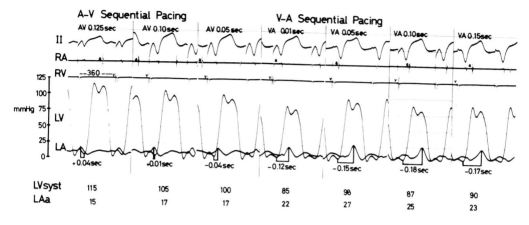

Fig. 9–8. Effect of varying AV interval on left ventricular systolic pressure.

cope. It is quite obvious that pacemakers should be implanted only when indicated and undue delay should be avoided. The procedure should be performed under fluoroscopic control to avoid complications.

The rhythm should be monitored carefully to detect pacemaker malfunction, reciprocal beating, or a multiple reset phenomenon. Patients should be questioned about their symptoms, and their blood pressures and hemodynamic status should be checked regularly. Pacing time should be kept to a minimum, and the pacer should be turned off for at least 24 hours before the electrode is removed.

SELECTED READINGS

Advances in cardiac pacemakers. Ann. N.Y. Acad. Sci., *267*:505, 1969.

Cardiac Pacing. Proceedings of the Vth International Symposium Tokyo, March 14–18, 1976. Amsterdam, Excerpta Medica, 1977.

Dreifus, L.S.: Clinical judgement is sufficient for the management of conduction defects. *In* Cardiovascular Clinics. Edited by E. Corday. Philadelphia, F.A. Davis, 1977, p. 195.

Furman, S., and Escher, D.J.W.: Modern Cardiac Pacing: A Clinical Overview. Bowie, Md., The Charles Press Publishers, Inc. 1974, pp. 3–74.

Lie, K.I., et al.: Factors influencing prognosis of bundle branch block complicating acute myocardial infarction. Circulation, *50*:935, 1974.

Samet, P.: Cardiac Pacing. New York, Grune & Stratton, Inc., 1973, pp. 143–167.

Siddons, H., and Sowton, E.: Cardiac Pacemakers. Springfield, Ill., Charles C Thomas Publisher, 1974, pp. 51–64.

Watanabe, Y., and Dreifus, L.S.: Cardiac Arrhythmias. Electrophysiological Basis for Clinical Interpretation. New York, Grune & Stratton, Inc., 1977, pp. 320–338.

Zoll, P.M.: Resuscitation of the heart in ventricular standstill by external electric stimulation. N. Engl. J. Med., *247*:768, 1952.

10

Surgical Techniques for Permanent Ventricular Pacing

EMIL A. NACLERIO
PHILIP VARRIALE

The treatment of complete heart block and a variety of other cardiac arrhythmias with an implanted pacemaker has evolved spectacularly and rapidly in the past two decades. In 1958, Lillehei first applied direct electrical stimulation to the ventricle to treat surgically induced heart block. In his procedure a wire with a small diameter was sutured to the ventricle and attached to an external pacemaker. In 1959, Furman established the feasibility of right ventricular endocardial stimulation with a transvenously introduced endocardial electrode, also attached to an external pacemaker device.

Untoward effects associated with an external pacemaker system include infection, accidental disconnection, and the inconvenience of an externally worn appliance. Such disadvantages prompted the development of a fully implantable lead and pulse generator system. The first successful totally implanted pacemaker system was installed by Chardack in 1960 using a thoracotomy approach. Other implantable pacing systems developed by Zoll and Frank and Kantrowitz followed in rapid succession.

The first successfully implanted transvenous endocardial lead system was reported in 1963 by Siddons and Davies. In a few years, this pacing method gained popularity and readily replaced the transthoracic method. In 1963, Nathan and his associates clinically applied an implantable atrial synchronous pacemaker system with a sensing electrode to the atrium. An implantable pulse generator programmed by spontaneous ventricular activity or demand function was introduced by Parsonnet et al. in 1966. This demand or noncompetitive pacing system provided the first valuable alternative to fixed rate competitive pacing.

Today the transvenous method of endocardial stimulation is used in over 80% of all pacemaker implantations. Indeed, many pacemaker physicians and surgeons prefer this method almost exclusively. However,

145

interest in the thoracotomy approach for direct myocardial stimulation as an alternate method has prevailed, since the transvenous method has, on occasion, proved unsuccessful or, for a number of reasons, impossible.

The introduction of the Medtronic sutureless myocardial lead in 1973 by Hunter provided an entirely novel technique to affix the electrode directly to the myocardium without sutures via a limited thoracotomy. The relative simplicity of this technique reawakened interest in the transthoracic approach, and currently approximately 10 to 15% of all primary lead implantations are of the direct myocardial variety.

The once prohibitive complications of thoracotomy and direct myocardial pacing have been considerably reduced, and complications now compare favorably with those associated with transvenous endocardial pacing. Better selection of patients, improved instrumentation, easier lead installation, less extensive surgery, advances in anesthetic techniques, and improved methods in preoperative and postoperative care are responsible for the reduced complications.

TRANSTHORACIC VERSUS TRANSVENOUS TECHNIQUES

The merits of direct transthoracic myocardial electrode implantation include the following:

1. An optimal pacing site can be precisely selected with preliminary electrophysiologic testing using a myocardial test probe (see Chapter 19).
2. Secure electrode fixation is provided and the incidence of electrode dislodgment reduced.
3. Ventricular perforation by the electrode is minimized.
4. The fluoroscopic hazard is eliminated.

Although direct transthoracic electrode implantation is used less frequently, it is preferred in the following circumstances: (1) for installing a pacemaker if one is needed during open-heart corrective surgery, (2) in infants and children requiring pacing therapy, and (3) after repeated electrode complications following transvenous installation. Unlike the transvenous method, direct myocardial electrode implantation has notable limitations. It should not be used in patients with serious underlying cardiac disease, such as congestive heart failure, advanced coronary artery disease, and recent acute myocardial infarction, in elderly debilitated patients, and in patients with pulmonary disease and/or renal dysfunction. The transvenous endocardial pacing method, on the other hand, can be applied to most patients; age and underlying disease states are not contraindications.

The ease of transvenous electrode placement requires only local anesthesia and limits the surgical risk. This approach is also associated with a lower mortality, ranging from 0 to 2%. Additionally, complications of this procedure may often be successfully reversed by a second procedure with little risk to the patient.

Nonetheless, the complications of electrode dislodgment and perforation are frequent sequelae to this method. Loss of intimate contact between the electrode and the endocardial surface usually leads to loss of pacing. The reported incidence of malposition varies between 2 and 20%. This complication is deemed an inherent feature of the transvenous approach rather than a function of the skill of the operator. Other infrequent problems of transvenous pacing include difficulty in endocardial electrode placement, axillary or subclavian venous thrombosis with or without consequent embolic phenomena, and bacterial endocarditis.

PREOPERATIVE REQUISITES

Before describing the surgical techniques used for implantation of cardiac pacemak-

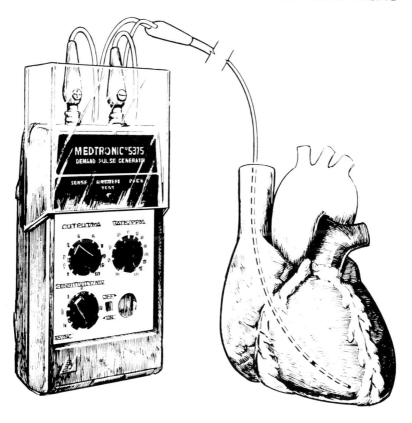

Fig. 10–1. Externally battery operated pulse generator connected to temporary transvenous lead with electrode tip wedged into trabeculations of right ventricular apex. This provides precise electrical control.

ers a number of important preoperative requisites will be briefly considered. Psychologic preparation is indeed a major preoperative consideration often ignored by both the attending cardiologist and the operating surgeon. Such preparation is important because the procedure involves the implantation of an electrical device in the patient's body and an electrode attachment to the heart. The patient's acceptance of this procedure therefore requires a far greater understanding of the underlying concepts than is necessary with more conventional surgical procedures. An intelligent explanation of what is to be done surgically, how the pacemaker operates, and what is to be expected after the operation will considerably lessen the patient's apprehension.

Temporary transvenous endocardial pacing prior to permanent electrode implantation is recommended for most patients for more precise control of cardiac rate and rhythm (Fig. 10–1). A solution of 2% lidocaine should be available for use in the suppression of premature ventricular contractions or bursts of ventricular tachycardia that may emerge during the procedure.

A cardiac catheterization laboratory, an x-ray special procedures room, or an operating room equipped with a fluoroscopic unit with an image intensifier and viewing screen is required. Equipment for cardiac monitoring, defibrillation, and cardiorespiratory resuscitation must be available throughout the procedure. A pacing system analyzer such as the Medtronic Model 5300, Cordis Model 209A, CPI

Model 2200, or Telectronics Model PMA 200 should also be available for determining stimulation thresholds and sensing measurements appropriate for permanent pacing.

PERMANENT TRANSVENOUS IMPLANTATION

Patients are premedicated with a sedative, a narcotic agent, or a tranquilizing drug in doses appropriate to the patient's age, weight, and general health. Diazepam (Valium) may be administered intravenously in increments of 2.5 to 5.0 mg every few minutes until the desired degree of sedation and tranquilization is achieved. Narcotic agents are usually avoided in elderly or high risk patients.

Local anesthesia is generally used during the procedure, with a 1% solution of lidocaine being the anesthetic agent of choice. If necessary, small doses of diazepam may be administered intravenously during the operation. In the anxious or uncooperative patient, general anesthesia may be indicated. An anesthetist or anesthesiologist should be available on standby.

The cephalic vein (right or left) is preferred for insertion of an endocardial lead (Fig. 10–2). Selection of a cephalic vein requires only one incision for insertion of a permanent transvenous electrode and the development of a pocket for the pulse generator. If approach through the cephalic vein is not feasible or the vein is not found (these circumstances occur in about 8% of our patients), entrance through either the external or the internal jugular vein is recommended. When these veins are used, two separate incisions are required, a cervical incision for insertion of the electrode and a subclavicular incision for the development of a pocket for the pulse generator.

An incision, approximately 10 cm long, is made through the skin and subcutaneous

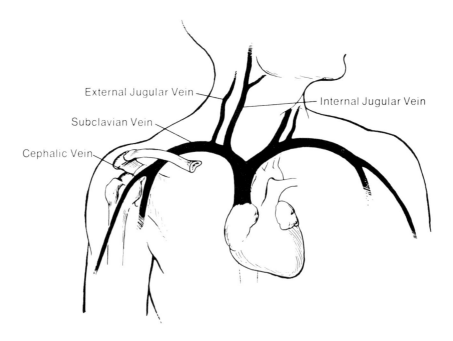

Fig. 10–2. The cephalic vein (right or left) is used for lead entry for permanent transvenous electrode implantation. The external jugular or internal jugular vein in that order is used when the cephalic vein is not available.

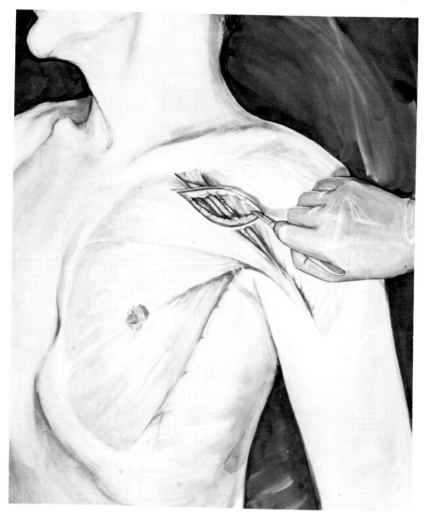

Fig. 10–3. An incision through the skin and subcutaneous tissue into deltopectoral groove permits access to the cephalic vein and development of the pulse generator pocket.

tissues about 2 cm below the medial portion of the clavicle and is extended laterally into the deltopectoral groove for the cephalic vein approach. An incision into the deltopectoral groove provides easy access to the cephalic vein and simple creation of a pocket for the pulse generator (Fig. 10–3).

The cephalic vein is readily located, since it lies deep in the deltopectoral groove and is embedeed in fat. A polyester ligature (3–0 Mersilene) is doubly looped loosely around the central end of the cephalic vein after it is dissected free for a distance of about 5 cm. The peripheral end is ligated. In the segment between the two ligatures, a small transverse incision is made for insertion of the electrode.

The endocardial lead is then prepared for insertion into the vein (Fig. 10–4). A stylet guide wire is gently bent with the thumb and the index finger about 15 cm from its distal end to create an approximate 80-degree angle; a smooth-surfaced sterile instrument may also be used. The stylet wire

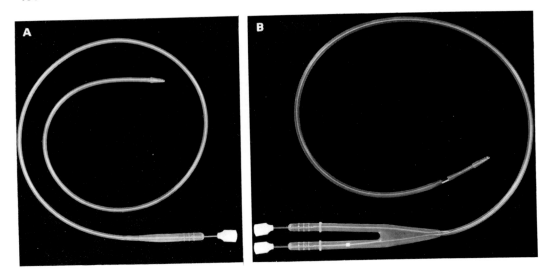

Fig. 10–4.   Electrodes. A, Unipolar. B, Bipolar with stylet wires in position to facilitate insertion into vein.

is inserted into the lead lumen so that the lead can be maneuvered during insertion with the necessary curvature.

The endocardial lead is then inserted into the cephalic vein and advanced toward the subclavian vein. Advancement of the catheter may be impeded because of fragility or small size of the cephalic vein or sharp angles at venous junctions. Impedance may occur despite manipulation of the patient's arm, shoulder, or head. The external jugular vein is selected when the lead cannot be passed beyond the cephalic vein. In a few patients the cephalic vein cannot be found.

Access to the external jugular vein will be provided by a 2 to 3 cm skin incision over its visible superficial course in the neck. If not seen, it may be located by extending the skin incision about 5 cm in length approximately two finger-breadths above the clavicle and slightly lateral to the sternocleidomastoid. A segment of the vein is exposed and encircled with two silk ligatures. The upper end of the vein is tied, and an incision is made in its wall. If brisk back bleeding occurs, it is controlled by exerting traction on the proximal ligature.

The internal jugular vein is chosen when

the external jugular vein proves unsuitable. This vein is selected in approximately 5% of our patients. The sternocleidomastoid muscle is divided between its medial and lateral clavicular insertions, and the internal jugular vein is exposed and ligated distally and a tourniquet ligature is positioned proximally, using 2–0 black silk. An incision is made in the vein between the ligatures for catheter electrode insertion. Untoward effects from interruption of the internal jugular vein have not resulted in our experience.

Lead insertion may also be accomplished by lateral venotomy using a pursestring suture of 3–0 black silk placed around the electrode point of entry. The electrode is advanced into the right ventricle under fluoroscopic control. The endocardial lead with its contained stylet slightly curved near the tip is passed into the right atrium and placed against the lateral wall of the right atrium to form a loop. This loop is then advanced backwards across the tricuspid valve while the lead is rotated until the tip falls into the right ventricle. Loop passage across the tricuspid valve avoids entry into the coronary sinus or the cardiac veins (Fig. 10–5).

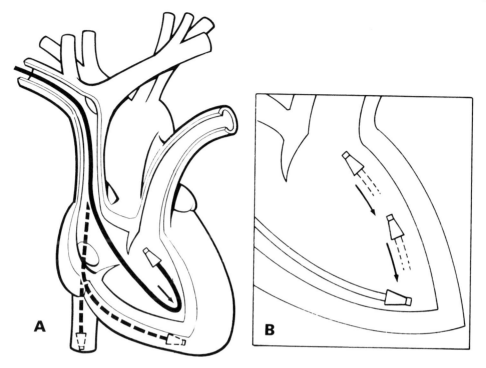

Fig. 10–5. A, Endocardial lead with contained wire stylet passed across tricuspid valve as a loop into right ventricle. This maneuver avoids entry into inferior cava and coronary sinus (dotted lines). B, Distal endocardial lead in pulmonary outflow tract. As catheter is withdrawn, it falls into apex of right ventricle.

The endocardial lead is then withdrawn slowly until the electrode tip lies about three quarters of the way down the ventricular septum, where the tip will usually suddenly fall into the apex of the right ventricle. Next, the stylet is withdrawn 1 or 2 inches, and the lead is gently advanced to wedge its tip firmly into the ventricular apex (Fig. 10–6). This maneuver will avoid perforation of the relatively thin right ventricular myocardium.

With the catheter tip finally lodged at its appropriate ventricular site, the wire stylet is withdrawn to a point corresponding to the upper region of the superior vena cava. The catheter electrode position and course are again noted. The segment in the right atrium should form a gentle curve in order to transmit slight tension to the electrode tip wedged in the apex of the right ventricle.

The section of the catheter traversing the tricuspid valve should buckle only slightly during each cardiac systole. The segment of the catheter within the right ventricle should be smooth and buckle upward slightly proximal to the tip electrode during each cardiac systole.

The patient is instructed to cough and breathe deeply while the anatomic position and stability of the apically located electrode are observed. A fluoroscopic examination with the patient in the lateral position and an electrogram may be necessary to determine that the lead is not lodged in the coronary sinus or cardiac vein.

At this juncture, stimulation and sensing measurements and intracavitary electrograms are taken to ascertain a satisfactory position of the electrode. A low stimulation threshold and an adequate sensing mea-

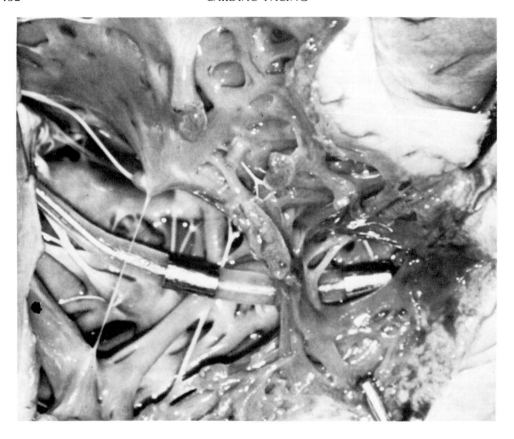

Fig. 10–6. Endocardial lead with electrode tip wedged into trabeculations of right ventricular apex. Autopsy photograph for demonstration.

surement are requisites for good electrode-endocardial contact. Stimulation and sensing measurements should be taken with an external pacing system analyzer (PSA), whose operational characteristics conform to the specifications of the pulse generator being implanted. The QRS signal for pacemaker sensing may also be determined from a properly recorded cardiac electrogram (Chapter 18).

When a unipolar endocardial lead is used, the negative connector of the extension cable should be attached to the terminal pin of the endocardial electrode and the positive connector to a large indifferent electrode plate in contact with moist subcutaneous tissue (Chapter 17). When a bipolar lead system is used, polarity should be carefully observed with electrode connections.

An acute stimulation threshold measurement for an implantable endocardial lead should not exceed 1.0 volt using a constant voltage device or 1.0 mA when measured with a constant current external generator. An initially low stimulation threshold value provides a desirable safety margin and minimizes postoperative pacing problems. An acute sensing measurement for endocardial leads should be greater than 5 millivolts when measured with a PSA testing device. If the electrical testing determinations prove unsatisfactory, it is essential to reposition the catheter electrode, several times if necessary, until all electrical requirements are satisfactorily met. The operational parameters of the pulse generator that include pulse amplitude, width, and interval are also tested using an appropriately calibrated PSA device. On rare occasion, a pulse generator proves defective under such preliminary testing.

Diaphragmatic stimulation should be ruled out by application of a momentary deliberate high amplitude pulse of 10 mA or 5 V. If the hemidiaphragm contracts, the endocardial lead requires repositioning. The remaining length of the wire stylet is then slowly removed from the catheter, and the lead is fixed in position in the vein with four to six 2–0 polyester (Mersilene) sutures. The sutures are tied around the vein and also around the bare lead. A relatively fixed position of the lead is dependent upon proper placement of sutures. The ligatures should be tightened sufficiently for fixation, yet avoid severance of the vein or over-constriction of the lead insulation.

The infraclavicular pulse generator pocket is developed by sharp and blunt dissection in the plane between the subcutaneous tissue and the underlying pectoralis major muscle. When the pocket is created precisely in the correct plane and made large enough to accept the pulse generator without tension, impairment of blood supply of the subcutaneous tissues is avoided even in very thin patients. Placement is particularly important in patients in whom a tight pocket may cause the unit to erode through the skin. When tissue vascularity is sparse, the pulse generator should be placed behind the pectoralis major. In our experience, however, infrapectoral placement of the pulse generator has not been deemed necessary.

If there is fear of excessive migration of the pacemaker, it can be enclosed in a synthetic (Dacron) pouch as advocated by Parsonnet, sutured to the pectoral fascia with 1–0 black silk placed around the boot of the battery or sutured to the fascia by using the suture hole in the pulse generator. The latter may prove hazardous, since the nonabsorbable suture may become a ful-

crum about which the lead electrode may become twisted and result in lead disruption.

When the external or internal jugular vein is used for lead insertion, a subcutaneous tunnel is created anterior to the medial end of the clavicle between the cervical venotomy and infraclavicular pocket incisions using a long, curved Kelly forceps. The Kelly instrument is then passed upward through the infraclavicular incision via the subcutaneous tunnel to the cervical incision where the lead connector pin is placed and fixed inside a Penrose drain with a heavy ligature. The ligature and lead are then pulled through the subcutaneous tunnel to the infraclavicular pulse generator pocket without incurring damage to the lead terminal pin. The pulse generator is then connected to the lead terminal pin using the manufacturer's recommended technique and is placed in the carefully fashioned generator pocket.

The wounds are thoroughly irrigated with saline solution, and the incisions are closed without drainage. Closure is accomplished with three layers of sutures, two in the subcutaneous tissues and one in the skin, using interrupted 3–0 black silk. Posteroanterior and lateral x-ray views of the chest are taken to ascertain good anatomic location of the lead system (Fig. 10–7).

The patient is monitored postoperatively with continuous electrocardiography for 1 or 2 days until reliable permanent cardiac pacing has been ensured. Antibiotics are administered orally for 5 days.

MYOCARDIAL LEAD IMPLANTATION

The surgical approaches generally employed for direct permanent myocardial electrode implantation include (1) left anterolateral transpleural thoracotomy, (2) left parasternal extrapleural mediastinotomy, and (3) inferior extrapleural mediastinotomy, consisting of subxiphoid, transxiphoid, transxiphisternal, or subcostal extrapleural techniques.

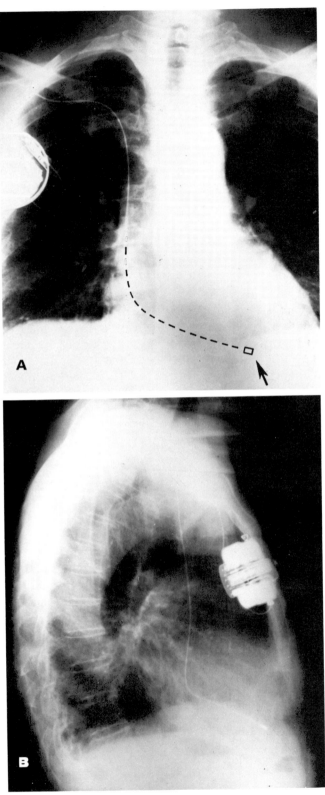

Fig. 10–7. Roentgenograms of patient with a permanent endocardial pacemaker. A, Posteroanterior view. Note position of pulse generator and electrode tip at apex of right ventricle. B, Lateral view. Catheter tip is anteriorly placed, the correct position.

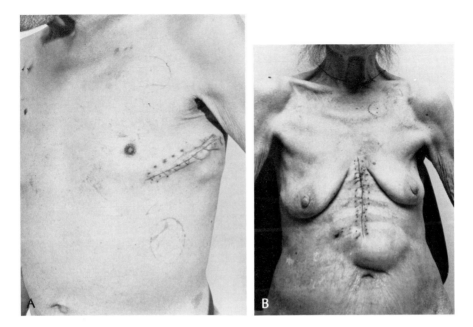

Fig. 10–8. A, Patient with permanent left ventricular implant installed via an anterior transaxillary minithoracotomy. Pulse generator bulge is seen in midaxillary area. B, Patient with right ventricular implant inserted via transxiphisternal extrapleural approach. Pulse generator bulge is seen in left subcostal area. Both 7 days postoperative.

We use two basic approaches, depending upon whether the right ventricle or the left ventricle is selected for permanent lead implantation (Fig. 10–8). An anterior axillary minithoracotomy is used when the left ventricle is chosen. A transxiphisternal (extrapleural) procedure using an incision that overlies the lower midright ventricular wall is utilized when the right ventricle is selected.

The optimal site for electrode insertion, a prerequisite for myocardial lead installation, is determined for either ventricle by precise electrophysiologic studies using a specially designed myocardial test electrode (MTE). The pacing site selected should offer the most satisfactory stimulatory and sensing measurements.

Left Ventricular Electrode Implantation

The left ventricle is the chamber of choice for permanent cardiac pacing. A left anterior transaxillary minithoracotomy approach is used (Fig. 10–9).

Preoperative insertion of a temporary transvenous pacemaker is recommended for most patients for control of cardiac rate and rhythm. This procedure may prove necessary for operative success because it prevents severe bradyarrhythmias, transient asystole, or even ventricular fibrillation provoked during anesthetic induction or thereafter.

Topical anesthesia is applied to the larynx to facilitate endotracheal intubation. General anesthesia is administered, and local anesthesia is applied to the surgical field to reduce the amount of general anesthesia.

The patient is placed supine on the operating table with the left chest slightly elevated and the padded forearm secured to the crossbar of the anesthetic screen (Fig. 10–9A). Skin preparation should include a large area to facilitate the counting of ribs and insertion of a chest tube.

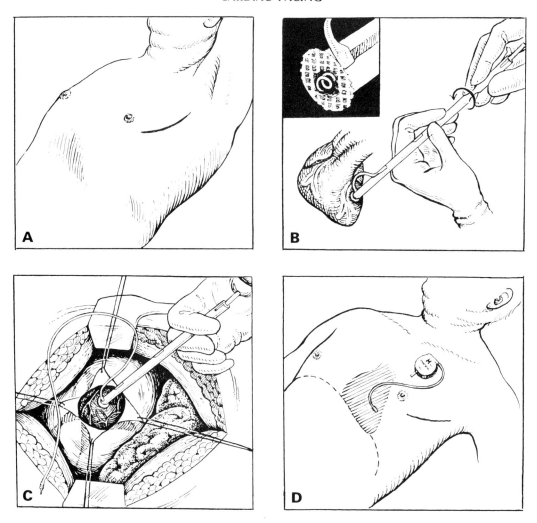

Fig. 10–9. Anterior axillary minithoracotomy for left ventricular lead implantation. A, Operative position and anterior axillary incision. B, Insertion of sutureless electrode. C, Release of electrode with finger-grip syringe-like action. D, Final positions of lead and pulse generator.

→

Fig. 10–10. A, Implanted sutureless lead, lead loop in pericardial sac, and lead loosely sutured to pericardial edge. Peanut sponge on forceps retracting left atrium. B, Second retractor creates window exposure. Note size of thoracotomy incision and its relation to axilla and nipple. Proximal lead pin and expanded lung are demonstrated.

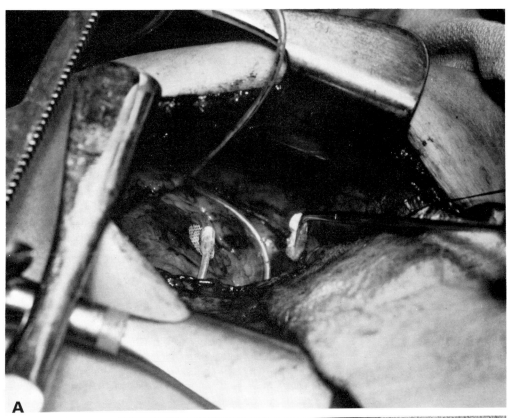

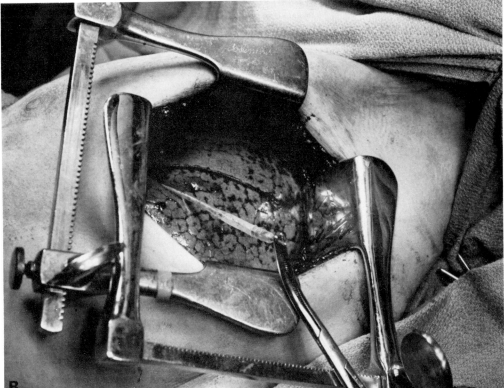

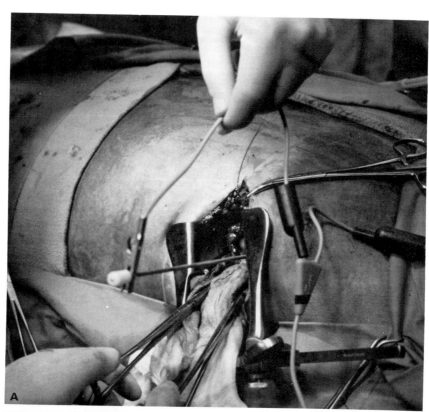

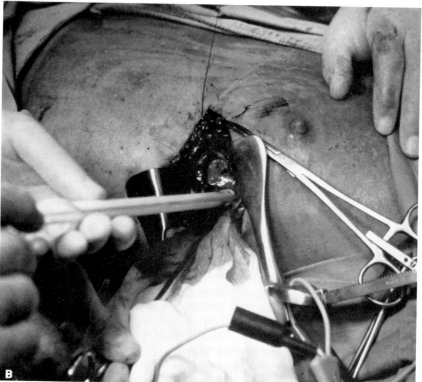

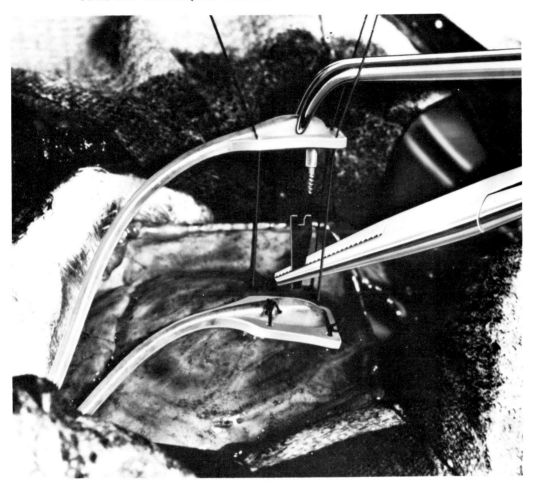

Fig. 10–12. Suture-electrode technique. Note placement of sutures, stab wound into myocardium, and fixation of electrode leads to ventricular myocardial wall.

←

Fig. 10–11. **A,** Selection of optimal myocardial lead implantation site using myocardial test electrode. **B,** Sutureless lead being rotated into myocardium. The precise depth that yields best stimulation threshold is determined sequentially during rotation of lead.

An anterior transaxillary skin incision is made along the course of the fifth rib and is extended from the pectoralis major anteriorly to the latissimus dorsi posteriorly. The subcutaneous tissues are then loosely and rapidly divided along the line of incision and dissected down to the rib cage. The incision can be carried forward in women to conform to the inframammary fold.

The surgeon may choose to enter the fourth or fifth interspace or remove a section of the fifth rib; the latter is preferred. Subperiosteal resection of a portion of rib provides a window exposure.

The posterior periosteal bed of the rib and the underlying pleura are incised, and the pleural cavity is entered. The subjacent intercostal artery, vein, and nerve at each end of the thoracotomy incision are ligated and divided, and the periosteal bed is retracted with stay sutures. A medium-sized self-retaining retractor is inserted into the pleural cavity and is opened slowly to minimize vagovagal stimulation and sufficiently to allow exposure of the anterolateral surface of the left ventricle. A second retractor in the opposite direction often maintains an improved exposure (Fig. 10–10).

The pericardium is incised 3 to 5 cm anterior and parallel to the phrenic nerve. Sutures of 3–0 black silk, attached to Kelly forceps, are used to retract the pericardial edges to expose the anterolateral aspect of the left ventricle. The pacing site is selected by preliminary electrophysiologic measurements obtained with a myocardial test electrode (Fig. 10–11). This site should be relatively free of epicardial fat, coronary vessels, or fibrosis.

A sutureless or suture electrode can then be affixed to the ventricular myocardium. Since the introduction of the sutureless myocardial lead (Medtronic Model 6917) in 1973, the suture electrode technique has been used less and less, and today this method has been practically abandoned (Fig. 10–12). Implantation of the suture electrode poses a number of problems. At the electrode insertion site it requires a myocardial stab wound which often engenders hemorrhage. Suturing of the electrode lead to the myocardium may produce an undesirable angulation and unstable electrode position. Also, a more extensive surgical incision is required for adequate exposure of the heart.

The sutureless myocardial lead has reawakened interest in the thoracotomy approach. Because of the "corkscrew" electrode design (Fig. 10–13), the lead can be inserted into the myocardium quickly and securely under direct vision through a small extrapleural or transpleural approach. Secure electrode placement is achieved without sutures (Fig. 10–14). The specially designed electrode coil is coated with silicone rubber except for its distal area which is the stimulating portion of the electrode. Sutureless leads are now being developed and tested by other manufacturers.

When a suitable pacing site has been selected, the Medtronic Model 6917 three-turn sutureless lead should be examined to be sure it is properly mounted on the handle. The handle is then held perpendicular to the selected site above the heart, and the electrode tip is gently thrust into the myocardium, minimally rotated, and slightly pulled back to ascertain whether the electrode tip has become attached to the myocardial wall. This maneuver is important, since an initial good grasp of the heart by the electrode tip is essential for proper electrode insertion. The electrode is then slowly torqued into the myocardial wall with clockwise turns, preferably during systole (Figs. 10–9B, 10–11). Little pressure is required during its insertion by virtue of the corkscrew configuration of the electrode.

Sutureless leads are provided with spiral electrodes that have varying depths of penetration. Depending on lead specifications, manufacturers recommend two or three complete clockwise turns for satisfactory lead implantation (Fig. 10–13). The final degree of rotation and depth of elec-

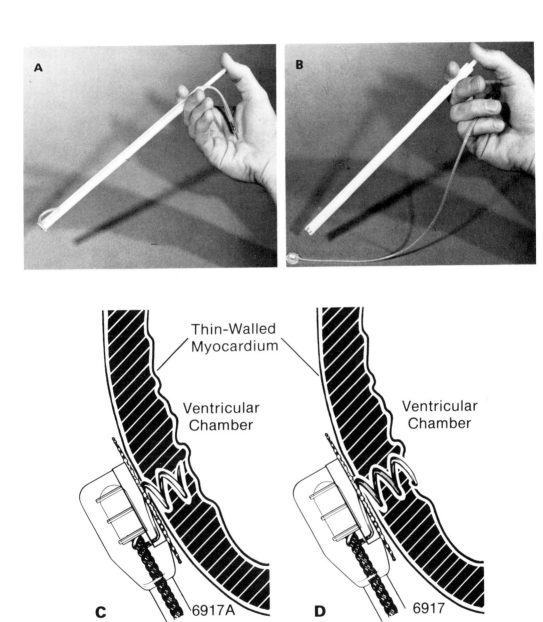

Fig. 10–13. Medtronic sutureless myocardial leads. A, Lead is preloaded on specially designed handle for rotating spiral electrode into myocardium. B, Release of electrode and conductor is accomplished by gripping handle between two fingers in finger grip depressions and applying pressure on protruding rod in syringe-like action. C, Model 6917A, two-turn electrode with penetration depth of 3.5 mm is suited to right ventricular implantation. D, Model 6917, three-turn electrode with penetration depth of 6.0 mm tends to perforate the thin-walled right ventricle; for left ventricular installations, the 6917 is preferred.

trode penetration should correspond to the precise position that yields the best stimulation threshold, which is determined sequentially during rotation of the lead. Hence, for any sutureless lead the ultimate rotation of the electrode into the myocardium may be slightly more or less than the recommended specifications of the manufacturer.

We have used both the Medtronic 6917 three-turn and 6917A two-turn lead for left

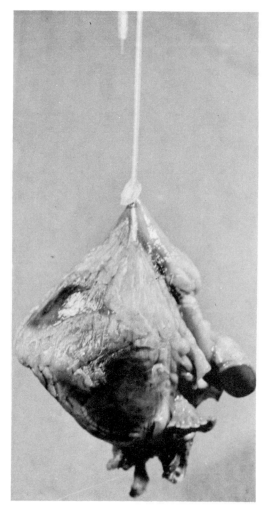

Fig. 10–14. Cadaver heart showing excellent retentive properties (ability to withstand pull) of spiral electrode when implanted in myocardium. This was observed by one of us (E.A.N.) in 25 consecutive necropsy hearts.

ventricular implantation (Fig. 10–13). It has been observed on a number of occasions that there is significantly more effective electrode anchorage and fixation in myocardial tissue with little or no tendency for electrode derotation or angulation with the Model 6917 three-turn electrode.

A second lead is installed in the ventricular wall approximately 2.5 cm away from the first lead if bipolar pacing is desired. Unipolar pacing is usually satisfactory provided the sutureless lead has been properly implanted in a site that offers appropriate stimulatory and sensing properties. To circumvent the potential complication of exit block, some surgeons prefer a unipolar pacing system and leave a second capped implanted lead in reserve.

Following electrode insertion, stimulation threshold and sensing measurements are again tested after several minutes, and if still satisfactory, the lead conductor and electrode are released from the handle (Figs. 10–9C, 10–13B). If these measurements are not satisfactory, another implantation site is sought (Chapter 17).

A loop of the lead is then placed in the pericardial sac and is loosely sutured to the pericardial edge. The lead connecting terminal pin is brought out of the chest cavity through the thoracotomy wound or an appropriate interspace (Fig. 10–10). The pericardium is left open. If the edges of the incised pericardium impinge upon the electrode plate with each cardiac systolic contraction, the edges are then loosely brought together with several sutures so that an intact pericardium extends over the implanted electrodes.

A chest drainage tube is inserted in a lower intercostal space in the posterior axillary area, the lung is expanded, and the connector pin of the myocardial lead is connected to the pulse generator. The generator is placed subcutaneously in the midaxillary or subclavicular region of the chest; the latter site is preferred. The conductor lead should not be unduly angulated or kinked at any point.

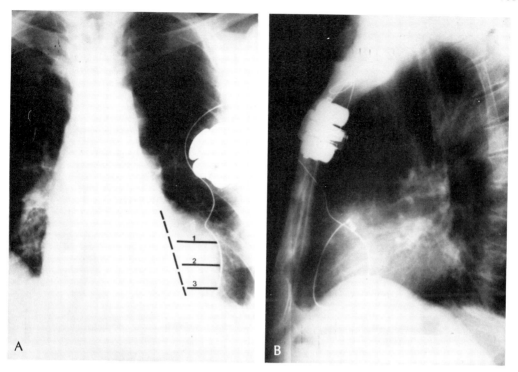

Fig. 10–15. A, Posteroanterior and B, lateral roentgenograms of patient treated by left anterior transaxillary minithoracotomy. Electrode tip is seen in area 1 of anterolateral wall of left ventricle. Pulse generator is often placed in subcutaneous infraclavicular pocket. Pulse generator in this area is more comfortable than in axillary region.

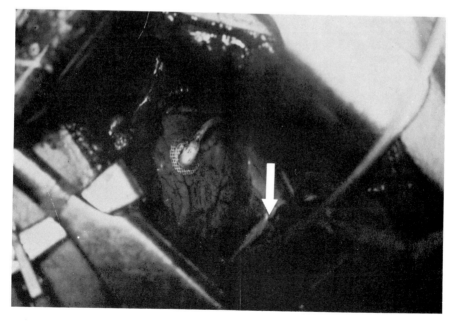

Fig. 10–16. Portion of fourth rib is resected for independent electrode installation to both left atrium and left ventricle. Note pinch-on atrial lead attachment to atrium.

The periosteal bed, muscular layers, subcutaneous tissues of the chest wall, and skin are approximated and sutured with interrupted 3–0 silk. Antibiotics are administered, and the postoperative management is similar to that of any thoracotomy procedure (Fig. 10–15). The patient is monitored electrocardiographically for several days.

Resection of a segment of the fifth rib is recommended for left ventricular implantations. However, for atrioventricular synchronous or sequential pacing to provide independent electrode installation to both left atrium and left ventricle, a portion of the fourth rib should be resected for appropriate exposure (Fig. 10–16).

Right Ventricular Electrode Implantation

We prefer the left ventricle for permanent electrode implantation and rarely resort to right ventricular implant. The latter method is used only for the rare patient in whom the transvenous technique has repeatedly failed and the transpleural procedure poses too great a risk.

The right ventricular procedure utilizes a transxiphisternal extrapleural approach (Fig. 10–17). The operation is performed under general inhalation anesthesia or field infiltration with lidocaine (Xylocaine) and an intercostal nerve block, supplemented with small increments of intravenous analgesics and tranquilizers. A vertical midline incision, approximately 15 cm long, is made through skin and subcutaneous tissues (Fig. 10–17B). The incision is begun at the level of the fourth costal cartilage and extended over the lower sternum and xiphoid and through the linea alba, exposing preperitoneal fat. The right and left costal arches are retracted laterally.

The xiphoid is freed from surrounding tissues sufficiently to permit introduction of the index finger into the anterior mediastinum. The xiphoid is then grasped with Kocher's forceps and removed with Mayo scissors. Excision of the xiphoid is a key point in the operation. Its removal provides optimal right ventricular exposure because its elimination combined with the release of the many muscles attached to this structure results in a relatively large free anatomic space. The operation is therefore facilitated. Only if further exposure is necessary, a 1 cm segment of adjacent sternum is then removed with a large double-action bone rongeur.

The fixed sternum is brought forward; the costal segments are retracted laterally and the diaphragm, inferiorly. Proper retraction of these structures provide excellent exposure of the pericardium and the heart. The pericardial fat is grasped at the midline and is separated from the pericardium by blunt dissection. The pericardium is then incised close to its diaphragmatic attachment using an inverted Y incision to expose the anterior wall of the right ventricle (Fig. 10–17C).

Following pericardiotomy, a retractor is inserted into the pericardial sac and the necessary traction is applied. This maneuver permits visualization of the lower right ventricular anterior surface extending to the interventricular groove. The myocardial test electrode is utilized to select an optimal electrode insertion site in the lower region of the anterior wall of the right ventricle. The site that offers the lowest stimulation threshold and a high sensing measurement threshold is selected as the pacing site for permanent electrode insertion and the Medtronic Model 6917A two-turn sutureless electrode is inserted there. This lead is more suitable for right ventricular implantation. Intraoperative electrical studies and the method of electrode insertion are similar to those used for left ventricular implantation (Fig. 10–9).

Far greater care is required during right ventricular insertion, since this chamber, unlike the left ventricle, swings significantly during each cardiac systole and has a muscle wall only 2 to 3 mm in thickness (Fig. 10–17D). A moderately thick layer of

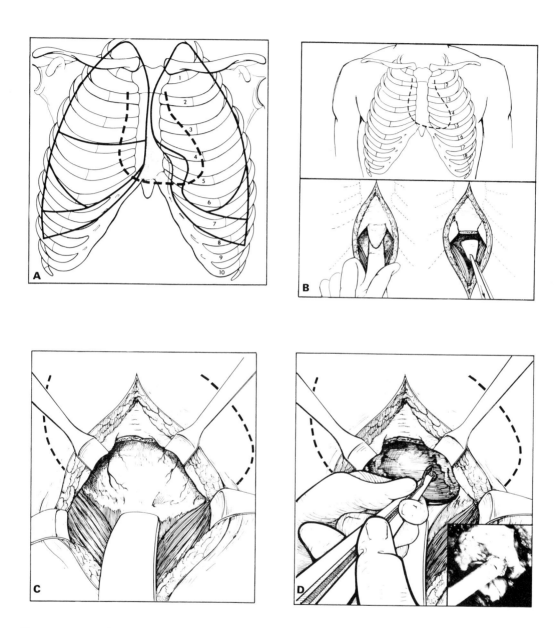

Fig. 10–17. Right ventricular lead implantation using a transxiphisternal extrapleural approach. A, Projection of extrapleural space (dotted) to anterior wall of thorax. B, Site of operative incision and excision of xiphoid. C, Pericardiotomy using inverted Y incision. D, Insertion of sutureless lead.

epicardial fat on the anterior surface of the right ventricle does not preclude electrode insertion.

The diaphragmatic surface that characteristically bears an area free of epicardial fat and coronary vessels is used by some surgeons for electrode insertion. It must be emphasized that several surgical pitfalls are associated with electrode placement into this area of the heart. The heart must be retracted, lifted, rotated, and held in a relatively fixed position for varying periods of time. Disturbing ventricular arrhythmias and hypotension may occur. A life-threatening situation and the need for prompt major thoracotomy may also ensue if excessive bleeding occurs. We therefore prefer the anterior wall of the right ventricle for pacemaker implantation.

Following implantation, stimulation threshold and sensing measurements are again obtained prior to releasing the myocardial lead from its handle. The myocardial lead connector pin is then connected to the pulse generator. The left subcostal area is usually selected for the subcutaneous pocket for pacemaker implantation.

The pericardium is left open and a multifenestrated catheter is placed inferiorly in the lower anterior mediastinum. Suction drainage is applied for 24 to 48 hours. The drainage catheter is brought out through a separate stab wound, and the subcutaneous tissues and skin are approximated. Antibiotics are administered. The postoperative care is similar to that following any thoracic intervention (Fig. 10–18).

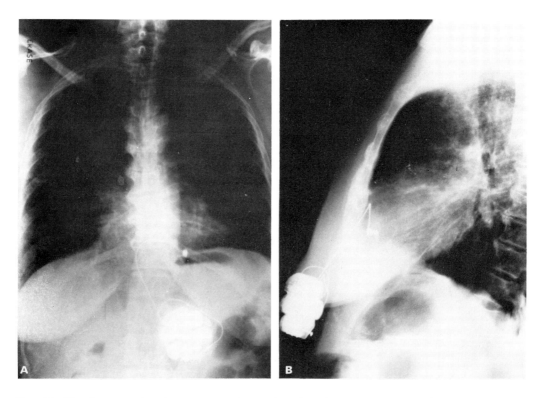

Fig. 10–18. Postoperative A, posteroanterior and B, lateral roentgenograms of patient treated by transxiphisternal extrapleural approach. Electrode is clearly seen in anterior wall of right ventricle. Myocardial lead courses inferiorly to pulse generator placed in subcutaneous pocket in left subcostal region.

PULSE GENERATOR REPLACEMENT

Pulse generator replacement is necessary for a variety of reasons at some interval of time following initial implantation. Newer and more reliable power sources and improved electronic circuitry obviously will make the need for this reoperation less frequent. It is recommended that the pulse generator at initial implantation be placed in a subcutaneous tissue plane where it can be readily and easily approached when replacement is required. Other locations such as retroperitoneal or submuscular entail a more complicated surgical procedure that may be associated with increased morbidity.

Electrocardiographic monitoring, cardiorespiratory resuscitative equipment, drugs for cardiac support, and a pacing system analyzer are required during pulse generator replacement. Knowledge of the pacing lead system previously implanted is necessary if a proper connection is to be established with the new pulse generator. It is essential to have a full range of pacing accessories and kits (splicing and nonsplicing types) for adapting different types of electrode leads to a specific pulse generator when this need arises. A second pulse generator should be available when the new pulse generator is unacceptable or has become contaminated.

Pulse generator replacement is relatively simple and is performed under local anesthesia and mild sedation. A skin incision is made along the periphery of the pulse generator which is almost always apparent and palpable (Fig. 10–8). The sac that has formed around the generator is fibrous, tough, smooth, and glistening. The sac abuts the subcutaneous tissues and closely conforms to the shape of the pacemaker. This sac should be carefully incised in order to avoid damage to the insulator and/or conductor wire.

Once the lead is detached from the pulse generator, stimulation and sensing measurements should be tested with an appropriate PSA. The stimulation threshold in most instances will be two to three times that obtained at initial electrode implantation. Occasionally, a high stimulation threshold is found and the cause established by properly performed electrical testing. Causes include increased perielectrode fibrosis, lead malposition, or increased lead resistance incident to partial lead fracture. In these circumstances, the surgeon should anticipate and be prepared for revision of the lead system when indicated.

The lead connector to the pulse generator is not secured until an acceptable stimulation threshold and an appropriate sensing measurement are obtained. The generator is then placed in the fibrous sac. A relaxing incision of the sac capsule is often necessary to facilitate placement of the generator into the sac. Hemostasis is obtained, and the wound is irrigated with saline solution. Wound closure is accomplished with 3-0 interrupted silk sutures. The electrode lead should not be unduly angulated or positioned in a manner that will result in lead stress or fracture.

The patient is discharged from the hospital one to three days following surgery when there are no contraindications. Prophylactic antibiotics are administered. The sutures are removed at the first postoperative office visit four to five days later.

SELECTED READINGS

Bernstein, V., Rotem, C.E., and Peretz, D.I.: Permanent pacemakers, 8-year follow-up study. Incidence and management of congestive heart failure and perforations. Ann. Intern. Med., 74:361, 1971.

Brenner, A.S., et al.: Transvenous, transmediastinal and transthoracic ventricular pacing. Circulation, 49:407, 1974.

Brenner, A.S., et al.: Transvenous, transmediastinal and transthoracic ventricular pacing: A comparison after complete two-year follow-up. Circulation, 49:407, 1974.

Buffle, P.J.: Ventricular pacing with epigastric transdiaphragmatic electrodes. J. Thorac. Cardiovasc. Surg., 72:226, 1976.

Calvin, J.W., et al.: Clinical application of parasternal mediastinotomy. Arch. Surg., 102:322, 1971.

Chardack, W.M.: Cardiac pacemakers and heart block. Gibbon's Surgery of the Chest, 3rd Ed.

Edited by D.C. Sabiston and F.C. Spencer. Philadelphia, W.B. Saunders Co., 1976, p. 1252.

Chardack, W.M., Gage, A.A., and Greatbatch, W.: Correction of complete heart block by self-contained and subcutaneously implanted pacemaker. J. Thorac. Cardiovasc. Surg., *42*:814, 1961.

Conklin, E.F., Giannelli, S., Jr., and Nealon, T.F., Jr.: Four hundred consecutive patients with permanent transvenous pacemaker. J. Thorac. Cardiovasc. Surg., *69*:1, 1975.

Dixon, S.H., Jr., et al.: Transmediastinal permanent ventricular pacing: A comparison with the transvenous method. Ann. Thorac. Surg., *14*:206, 1972.

Furman, S., and Escher, D.J.W.: Principles and Techniques of Cardiac Pacing. New York, Harper and Row, 1970.

Furman, S., and Norman, J.C.: Cardiac Pacing and Pacemakers. Cardiac Surgery, 2nd Ed. New York, Appleton-Century-Crofts, 1972, p. 495.

Furman, S., and Robinson, G.: Use of intracardiac pacemaker in correction of total heart block. Surg. Forum, 9:245, 1958.

Goldstein, S., Moss, A., and Ribers, R., Jr.: Transthoracic and transvenous pacemakers—a comparative clinical experience with 131 implantable units. Br. Heart J., *32*:35, 1970.

Goldstein, S., et al.: Comparative clinical experience with implantable transthoracic and transvenous pacemakers. Am. J. Cardiol., *19*:131, 1967.

Green, G.E., et al.: A four year review of cardiac pacing in Glasgow. 181 Medtronic generators implanted in 127 patients. Am. Heart J., *83*:265, 1972.

Hunter, S.W., et al.: A new myocardial pacemaker lead (sutureless). Chest, *63*:430, 1973.

Kantrowitz, A., et al.: The treatment of complete heart block with an implanted controllable pacemaker. Surg. Gynec. Obstet., *115*:415, 1962.

Lawrie, G.M., et al.: Left subcostal insertion of the sutureless myocardial electrode. Ann. Thorac. Surg., *21*:350, 1976.

Mansour, K.A., et al.: Cardiac pacemakers: Comparing epicardial and pervenous pacing. Geriatrics, *28*:151, 1973.

Mansour, K. A., Fleming, W.H., and Hatcher, C.R., Jr.: Initial experience with a sutureless, screw-in electrode for cardiac pacing. Ann. Thorac. Surg., *16*:127, 1973.

Medtronic News.7:7, 1977.

Morris, J.J., Jr., et al.: Permanent ventricular pacemakers. A comparison of transthoracic and transvenous implantation. Circulation, *36*:587, 1967.

Naclerio, E.A., and Varriale, P.: A Comparison of Left and Right Ventricular Pacing Using Medtronic Sutureless Lead. Presented American College Cardiology, 1977 Annual Meeting, Las Vegas, March 7–10, 1977.

Naclerio, E. A., and Varriale, P.: Screw-in electrode: New method for permanent ventricular pacing. N.Y. State J. Med., *74*:2391, 1974.

Nathan, D.A., et al.: An implantable synchronous pacemaker for the long-term correction of complete heart block. Am. J. Cardiol., *11*:362, 1963.

Parsonnet, V., et al.: Clinical use of an implantable standby pacemaker. J.A.M.A., *196*:104, 1966.

Siddons, H., and Davies, J.G.: A new technique for internal cardiac pacing. Lancet, 2:1204, 1963.

Sowton, F., Hendrix, G., and Roy, P.: Ten year survey of treatment with implanted cardiac pacemaker. Br. Med. J., *3*:155, 1974.

Stewart, S.: Placement of the sutureless epicardial pacemaker lead by the subxiphoid approach. Ann. Thorac. Surg., *18*:308, 1974.

Varriale, P., Naclerio, E.A., and Niznik, J.: Selection of site for permanent epicardial pacing using myocardial testing electrode. N.Y. State J. Med., 77:1272, 1977.

Weirich, W.L., Gott, V.L., and Lillehei, C.W.: The treatment of complete heart block by the combined use of a myocardial electrode and an artificial pacemaker. Surg. Forum, 8:360, 1957.

Zoll, P.M., et al.: Long-term electrical stimulation of the heart for Stokes-Adams disease. Ann. Surg., *154*:330, 1961.

11

Atrial Programmed Pacing

NICHOLAS P. D. SMYTH

Patients with symptomatic bradycardia usually are managed by ventricular demand pacing. For most of them this pacing mode is adequate, but for some, especially those with myocardial disease in addition to conduction disturbance, the contribution of the atrial "kick" is important, and in a few cases essential.[1-4]

The advantage of the atrial transport mechanism may be maintained by pacing the atrium in patients with disease of the sinus node alone (AOO, AAI, or AAT).* There must be no evidence of disease of the AV node or conduction system and preferably no history of atrial fibrillation.

In patients with disease of the AV node or conduction system alone, the mechanism is preserved by atrial sensing and synchronized ventricular pacing (VAT).[5] The sinus mechanism must be normal for the success of this system. When both systems are diseased, AV sequential pacing of both chambers must be used (DVI or DDT).[6,7]

All of these systems, with one exception, may be grouped under the heading "Atrial Programmed Pacing" used frequently in Europe. The exception is the bifocal (DVI) AV sequential system which is ventricular programmed. All systems, however, depend for their function on the availability of a good atrial lead. The difficulty in providing this without thoracotomy has slowed the development of these more complex pacing systems, as well as systems designed to control tachyarrhythmias by atrial overdrive pacing.

The placement of an atrial lead adjacent to the left atrium by mediastinoscopy was first described by Carlens et al.[8] This method has been widely used in Sweden and in Germany but has been largely abandoned because of instability of the lead and inadequate P wave sensing.[9]

Transvenous placement of an atrial lead has generally followed two courses. In one, the lead is lodged in the coronary sinus adjacent to the left atrium,[10] and in the other a J-shaped lead is hooked in the right atrial appendage.[11]

The coronary sinus approach has been

*Generic Pulse Generator Identification System described in Parsonnet, V., Furman, S., and Smyth, N.: Implantable cardiac pacemakers: Status report and resource guideline. Circulation, 50:A 21, 1974.

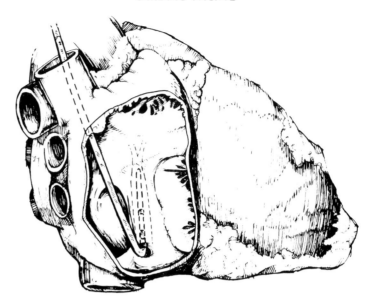

Fig. 11–1.   Lead shown in position in coronary sinus.

successful for some surgeons.[12] The coronary sinus is particularly suitable for pacing because the musculature of the vein wall is cardiac and not smooth muscle as in other veins (Fig. 11–1). We have paced one patient's atrium successfully for ten years by this method, but our subsequent experience showed an unacceptable instability of the lead, poor P wave sensing, and high pacing thresholds. We have therefore concentrated on the J lead approach.

ATRIAL LEADS

The first lead was a simple J (Fig. 11–2).* The mechanism of insertion is illustrated in Figure 11–3. With this lead, 31 patients were successfully paced (20 AAT, 1 AOO, 4 VAT, and 6 DDT).

Experimental work in dogs showed that atrial fixation of the lead was unlikely and that stimulating or pacing thresholds would be higher than in the ventricle—usually by a factor of three times.[11] Both findings were

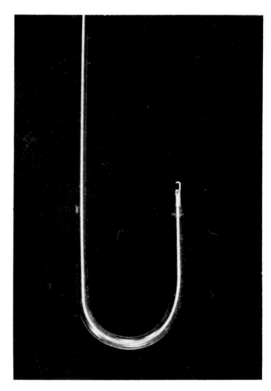

Fig. 11–2.   J lead with stylet withdrawn to allow lead to assume its preformed J configuration.

---

* Cordis Corporation, Miami, Florida.

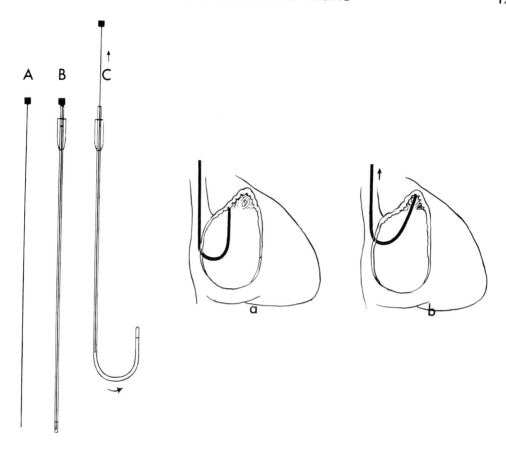

Fig. 11–3. Diagram illustrating use of stylet to straighten J lead during insertion. The lead is shown pulled up into the atrial appendage on the right (a, b). A, Stylet. B, Stylet inserted into lead. C, Stylet being withdrawn.

confirmed in trials in patients.[13] The reason for the higher stimulating thresholds in the atrium are not clear, although the difference in ultrastructure of atrial and ventricular myocardium is an intriguing possibility.[14]

PULSE GENERATOR

For atrial pacing, the Cordis R wave triggered pulse generator, the Cordis Ectocor (VVT) has been modified to function as a P wave triggered unit by increasing the sensitivity from 2.0 millivolts to 1.0 millivolt to sense the smaller P wave (AAT).

TECHNIQUE

In the atrial group, preliminary temporary atrial pacing is carried out to determine whether atrioventricular conduction will be maintained at faster rates, because of the known association of atrioventricular conduction defects in many of these patients. His bundle recordings are useful but not essential in the preoperative evaluation of these patients.

The operation is performed with local anesthesia. The lead is positioned in the right atrial appendage under fluoroscopic control. An intra-atrial unipolar electrogram is obtained to determine the magnitude of the P wave, and a complete series of unipolar stimulating thresholds is measured in volts and milliamperes at pulse durations ranging in the first series, from 0.5 msec to 2.5 msec. The P wave values in the first series ranged from 1.0 millivolts to 5.0 millivolts with a mean value of 2.5 millivolts. The stimulating thresholds are shown in Figures 11–4 (current) and 11–5 (voltage). The typical x-ray appearance of the lead is shown in Figure 11–6. The pulse generator is connected to the lead in the usual way and buried subcutaneously in the right pectoral area.

In the VAT group, P wave values are similar. No stimulating thresholds are recorded, since the lead performs a sensing function only. The "sensitive" (0.5 mv) Cordis Atricor is used in all cases.

We have used bifocal AV sequential pacing (DVI) infrequently and prefer an atrial

programmed system (DDT). The latter is not a standard system and is still under development. However, it is an atrial programmed system and for this reason will be briefly described.

In the DDT AV sequential system the sensitive Cordis Ectocor pulse generator is used with the atrial lead to pace the atrium. A standard ventricular lead is connected to a modified sensitive Atricor generator usually placed on the opposite side of the chest. This unit is modified to sense and stimulate through a single lead. The electrode detects the atrial pacing signal in the ventricle and relays it to the pulse generator. After a 120-millisecond delay, the modified Cordis Atricor paces the ventricle sequentially. The Atricor plug contains a 20,000 ohm resistor across the sensing and stimulating terminals in order to prevent damage to the sensing circuit by the large output signal. The atrial pacer thus

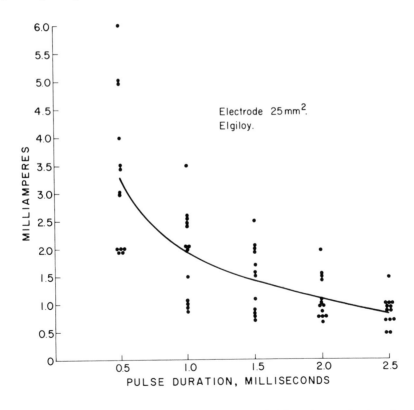

Fig. 11–4. Average strength duration curve for current thresholds with actual values for 13 patients.

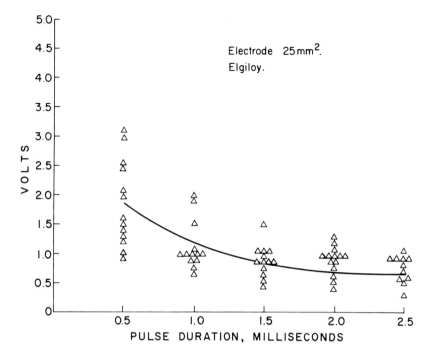

Fig. 11–5. Average strength duration curve for voltage thresholds with actual values for 13 patients.

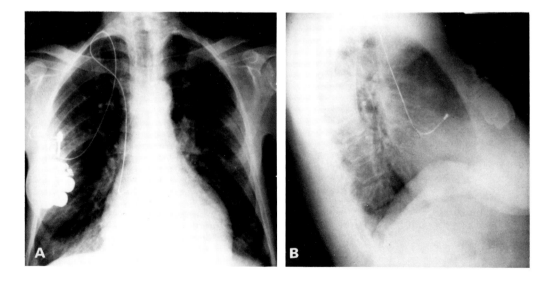

Fig. 11–6. A, Posteroanterior and B, lateral chest radiographs showing typical appearance of J lead in right atrial appendage. J configuration opens out to reverse "check mark" configuration when properly positioned in atrial appendage.

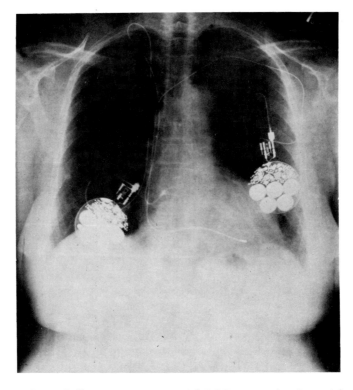

Fig. 11–7. Chest radiograph illustrating AV sequential (DDT) system showing atrial system on patient's right and ventricular "slave" system on patient's left side.

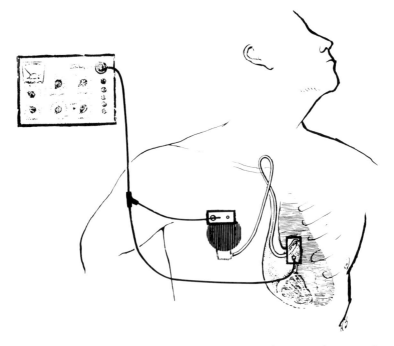

Fig. 11–8. External (indirect) overdrive system used in checking function of an AAT (P wave triggered) atrial pacing system.

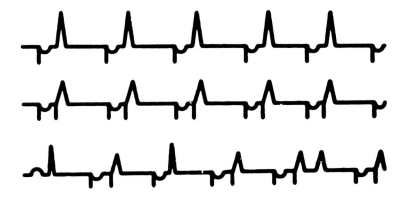

Fig. 11–9. Diagrammatic ECG tracings. DVI pacer functioning as an atrial pacer (top). AV sequential mode (middle). All three modes: sinus rhythm, atrial and AV sequential pacing (bottom).

operates on the P wave triggered principle and the ventricle is paced sequentially by a unit which is triggered by the electronic atrial pacing signal sensed in the ventricle. If the P wave sensing fails for any reason, fixed-rate atrial pacing sets the AV sequential rate at 70 beats per minute. If for any reason the triggering signal from the atrium is not detected in the ventricle, the ventricular unit reverts to a backup system of fixed-rate ventricular pacing at its basic rate of 60 beats per minute (Fig. 11–7).[7]

We use triggered systems throughout in atrial programmed systems for two reasons. First, in atrial pacing, even after careful preoperative screening, some 20% or more of patients will later develop AV block. This can be readily detected during routine postoperative follow-up by the use of external or indirect overdrive (Fig. 11–8).[15] As the pacer rate is increased by overdrive, the onset of the Wenckebach phenomenon can be readily detected and the rate at which it occurs noted. If the phenomenon occurs at progressively lower rates, it is clear that the patient will need conversion either to ventricular or AV sequential pacing. The increasing use of rate programmability should make it possible to check AAI pulse generator function similarly, if less precisely.

The second advantage of the triggered mode is in the AV sequential system. Autoinhibition cannot occur as is possible in an inhibitory mode (DVI) if the atrial lead becomes misplaced.[16]

The AV sequential, ventricular-inhibited pacing device is controlled by the QRS signal. This represents a major advantage of the DVI system, since the R wave is a larger and more reliable cardial signal for sensing than the P wave. The DVI system requires a bipolar configuration for both the atrial and ventricular leads, and sensing occurs only through the ventricular lead.

The pacer is inhibited and reset when the patient's spontaneous ventricular beat is detected prior to the completion of the atrial escape interval of the pulse generator. An atrial output pulse is emitted to depolarize the atrium when the spontaneous R to R interval is exceeded. The ventricular output pulse is inhibited by a conducted R wave if the patient's PR interval is shorter than the AV sequential interval (atrial pacing mode). A ventricular stimulus is discharged if the atrial paced beat conducts with an excessive PR interval or not at all (AV sequential pacing mode).

The AV delay of the DVI device may be fixed* or programmed† (Fig. 11–9). The

---

*The American Pacemaker Corp., Woburn, Massachusetts.
† Byrel, Medtronic, Inc., Minneapolis, Minnesota.

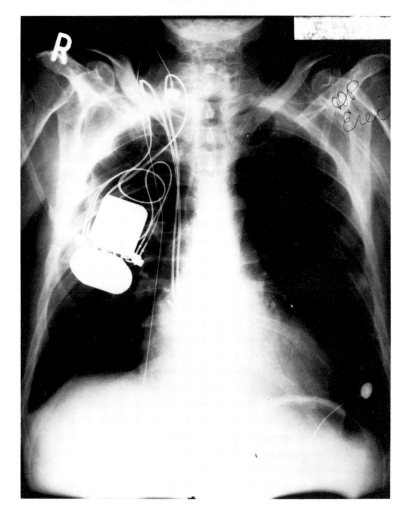

Fig. 11–10. Chest radiograph showing position of bipolar tined J lead in right atrial appendage and bipolar ventricular lead in right ventricle.

pacing lead system is designed to be bipolar. This minimizes unwanted pacer inhibition incident to sensing of the atrial signal by the ventricular lead. The implanted bipolar system is shown in Figure 11–10.

J-SHAPED LEAD VERSUS TINED J-SHAPED LEAD

In the postoperative period in the first series of patients there was a 20% incidence of lead dislodgment, loss of atrial sensing or capture, or both. Fifteen patients survived, 13 with atrial pacing (AAT or AOO), 1 with atrioventricular synchronized (VAT), and 1 with atrioventricular sequential pacing (DDT). All have been observed for 5 to 11 years and have complete stability of their pacing systems.

Despite the satisfactory record, it was nevertheless clear that better fixation of the lead was needed. The 20% incidence of lead dislodgment was believed to be too high to permit general use of this lead.

It seemed that a way had to be found to

anchor the lead in the right atrial appendage so that fixation would occur, ideally without scarring around the electrode. The J-shaped lead was therefore modified by the addition of three rows of silicone rubber tines (Fig. 11–11). It was felt that fixation might occur mechanically, at first by the tines tangling in the trabeculae and later by scarring around the tines, rather than around the electrode (Fig. 11–12).

Studies in dogs showed that at three months postinsertion the lead was firmly encapsulated in the right atrial appendage, with the preservation of P wave sensing and acceptable stimulating thresholds. Scarring occurred around the silicone rubber tines, with minimal scarring around the electrode.[17]

The tined J-shaped lead for human implantation is made with a preformed curve in the silicone outer covering and a preformed curve in the MP35N wire coil. The electrode is canted toward the inside of the J curve to enhance contact with the upper inner surface of the appendage. It is made of platinum-iridium and has a surface area of 12 mm^2.[*] The tines are trimmed prior to insertion of the lead, so that those nearer the electrode are shorter to enhance advancement of the tip of the lead into the appendage.

Clinical trials with the new tined J-shaped lead were begun in October 1974. Since then the lead has been used in 22 patients. Atrial pacing has been established in 16 patients (14, AAT; 1, AAI; and 1, AOO). AV synchronized (VAT) pacing has been established in 5 patients (Fig. 11–13), and AV sequential pacing (DDT) in 1 patient. In all the groups, intracavitary electrograms and stimulating thresholds were obtained when possible (Fig. 11–14). Recently we have used programmable versions of the special sensitive triggered pulse generators (Cordis Omni-Ectocor, Omni-Ventricor, and Omni-Atricor) (Table 11–1).

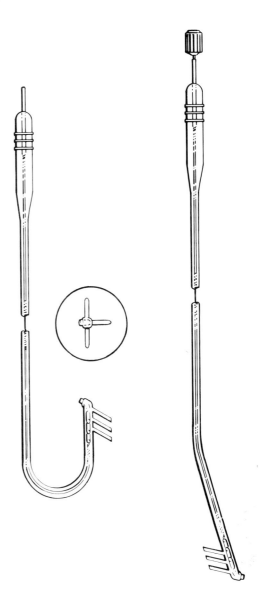

Fig. 11–11. Construction of new J lead with three rows of three Silastic tines and a canted electrode (see text).

In one patient with atrioventricular synchronized pacing, repeated supraventricular tachycardia occurred, apparently triggered by retrograde conduction. Anginal pain occurred with each of these episodes. For this reason the atrial lead was

---

*Medtronic Incorporated, Minneapolis, Minnesota.

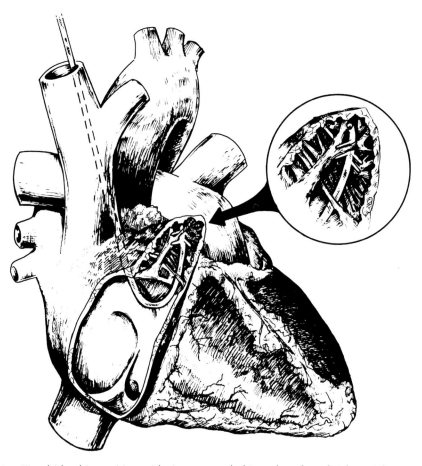

Fig. 11–12. Tined J lead in position with tines entangled in trabeculae of right atrial appendage.

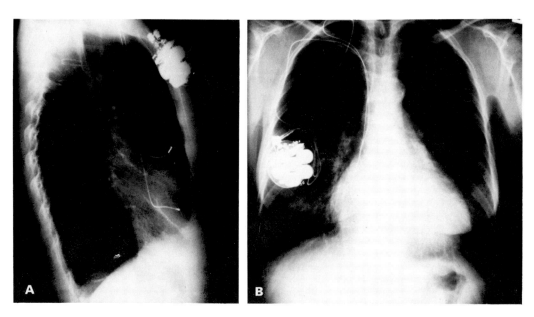

Fig. 11–13. A, Posteroanterior and B, lateral chest radiographs showing characteristic appearance of VAT (AV synchronized) pacing system.

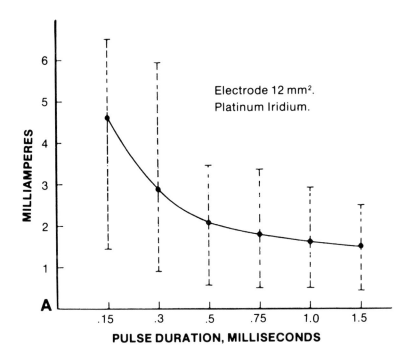

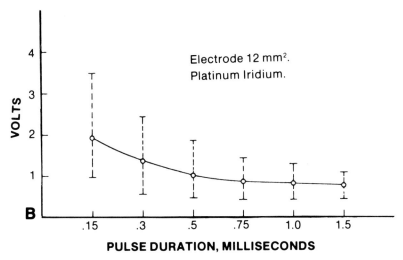

Fig. 11–14. A, Average "acute" strength duration curve for pacing current thresholds in 16 patients. Spread between maximum and minimum values is also indicated. B, Values in voltage, the same patients.

TABLE 11-1

Clinical Trials with Tined J Lead

PATIENT	AGE (yr.)	SEX	DIAGNOSIS	PEAK TO PEAK P-WAVE AMPLITUDE (mv)	I	R	LEAD	PULSE GENERATOR	PACING MODE
C.J.	74	M	Sick sinus node syndrome	±2.2	*		Tined atrial J-shaped lead	Cordis Ectocor (1 mv)	AAT
R.L.	62	F	Sick sinus node syndrome	±2.5	*		Tined atrial J-shaped lead	Cordis Ectocor (1 mv)	AAT
S.I.	53	M	Sick sinus node syndrome	±2.0	*		Tined atrial J-shaped lead	Cordis Omni-Ectocor (1 mv)	AAT
R.S.	64	F	Sick sinus node syndrome	±3.8	*		Tined atrial J-shaped lead	Cordis Ectocor (1 mv)	AAT
R.H.	67	M	Sick sinus node syndrome	±3.0	*		Tined atrial J-shaped lead	Cordis Ectocor (1 mv)	AAT
N.Z.	84	F	Second degree AV block	±2.8	*		Tined atrial J-shaped lead (Medtronic 6907-58 lead)	Cordis Atricor (1 mv)	VAT
H.B.	52	F	Complete heart block	±2.2	*		Tined atrial J-shaped lead (Cordis 2 mm lead)	Cordis Atricor (1 mv)	VAT
M.L.	61	F	Complete heart block	±3.0	*		Tined atrial J-shaped lead (Cordis 2 mm lead)	Cordis Omni-Atricor (1 mv)	VAT
M.S.	55	M	Sick sinus node syndrome	±5.9		*	Tined atrial J-shaped lead	Cordis Ectocor (1 mv)	AAT
E.B.	83	M	Sick sinus node syndrome	±1.5		*	Tined atrial J-shaped lead	Cordis Ectocor (1 mv)	AAT
E.P.	61	F	Sick sinus node syndrome	±8.0	*		Tined atrial J-shaped lead	Medtronic 5863 (1 mv)	AAI
M.G.	73	F	PAT alternating with sinus bradycardia	±4.2	*		Tined atrial J-shaped lead	Cordis Omni-Ventricor	AOO

M.G.	56	M	LAD, RBBB, cardiomyopathy, coronary ectasia	±7.5	*	Tined atrial J-shaped lead (Cordis 2 mm lead)	Cordis Omni-Ectocor (1 mv)	DDT
C.S.	70	F	IHSS and bradycardia	±4.5	*	Tined atrial J-shaped lead	Cordis Atricor (0.5 mv) Cordis Omni-Ectocor (1 mv)	AAT
M.T.	66	F	Sick sinus node syndrome	±4.0	*	Tined atrial J-shaped lead	Cordis Omni-Ectocor (1 mv)	AAT
D.D.	65	F	Sick sinus node syndrome	±2.0	*	Tined atrial J-shaped lead	Cordis Omni-Ectocor (1 mv)	AAT
C.W.	66	M	Sick sinus node syndrome	†	*	Tined atrial J-shaped lead	Cordis Omni-Ectocor (1 mv)	AAT
W.F.	69	M	Sick sinus node syndrome	±2.5	*	Tined atrial J-shaped lead	Cordis Omni-Ectocor (1 mv)	AAT
A.M.	74	M	Sinus bradycardia	±3.8	*	Tined atrial J-shaped lead	Cordis Omni-Ectocor (1 mv)	AAT
T.B.	76	M	Complete heart block	±5.5	*	Tined atrial J-shaped lead (Cordis 2 mm lead)	Cordis Omni-Atricor (0.5 mv)	VAT
D.M.	54	F	Sinus bradycardia	±2.75	*	Tined atrial J-shaped lead	Cordis Omni-Ectocor (1 mv)	AAT
C.E.	78	M	Complete heart block	±2.5	*	Tined atrial J-shaped lead (Cordis 2 mm lead)	Cordis Omni-Atricor (1 mv)	VAT

I = Initial implant; R = replacement of malfunctioning coronary sinus lead; † = P wave measurement impossible due to atrial fibrillation. Patients are listed in order of treatment.

capped at another hospital, and conventional ventricular pacing was established. P-wave amplitude was measured at this time and was 2.2 mv—the same as at the time of insertion of the lead four months earlier (Patient H.B., Table 11–1)—suggesting the absence of significant fibrosis around the electrode.

Of the patients now living with intact atrial programmed systems, there are 12 in the atrial paced group (AAT—AOO—AAI) and 5 in the AV synchronized (VAT) group. The longest follow-up is two years and nine months (C.J., Table 11–1). There has been no case of dislodgment of the lead from the appendage in the entire series.

The atrial tined J-shaped lead may provide the characteristics of satisfactory sensing and pacing with firm fixation, long sought in an atrial lead. Even with small numbers and a short follow-up period the stability of the tined J-shaped lead is clearly superior to that of the simple J-shaped lead used in the earlier series of cases. Satisfactory early results have also been obtained by another investigator who has inserted 86 tined J-shaped leads with a 7% incidence of dislodgment.[18]

ATRIAL OVERDRIVE PACING

Atrial overdrive pacing or rapid atrial stimulation (RAS) has been used for the electronic management of selected cases of recurrent, drug refractory supraventricular tachycardia (SVT). These pacing systems consist of an external, patient-activated transmitter and an implanted receiver without a battery which is connected by bipolar leads to the atrial myocardium.[19,20] The leads are usually implanted at thoracotomy. Various types have been used, usually of the epicardial type that is sutured to the atrium or atrial appendage. Simplified clip-on leads are also under study (Fig. 11–15). The bipolar tined atrial J-shaped lead will also be considered for use in this system.

Energy transmission between the transmitter and the implanted receiver is af-

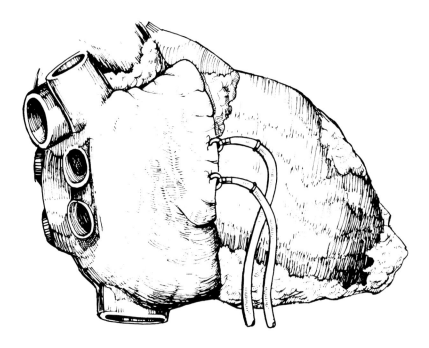

Fig. 11–15. Atrial clip-on leads in position on right atrial appendage.

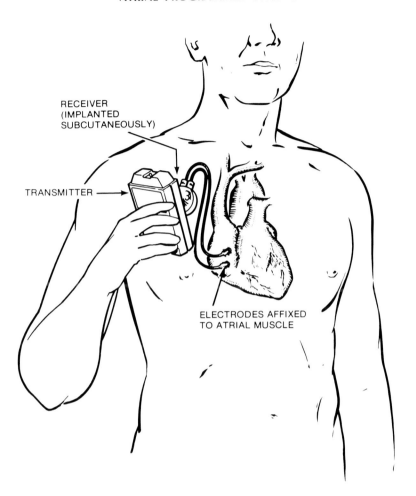

RECEIVER
(IMPLANTED
SUBCUTANEOUSLY)

TRANSMITTER

ELECTRODES AFFIXED
TO ATRIAL MUSCLE

Fig. 11–16. RAS atrial pacing system in operation.

fected by radiofrequency (R-F) coupling. During an episode of SVT, the patient places the transmitter directly over the receiver site and depresses the ON-OFF button to activate the system (Fig. 11–16). Pulsed R-F energy at a rate preset by the physician (between 50 and 400 pulses per minute) is detected and filtered by the receiver and conducted through the leads to the atrial myocardium. The mechanism by which rapid atrial stimulation terminates an arrhythmia may involve overdrive suppression of an ectopic focus, conversion of the arrhythmia to atrial flutter or fibrillation which spontaneously reverts to sinus rhythm, or the interruption of a reentry pathway.

FUTURE TRENDS

The problems of symptomatic bradycardia have essentially been met and mastered, whether pacing is done through the atrium or the ventricle. The real challenge in the future, however, lies with the electronic recognition and the electronic control of the tachyarrhythmias, particularly the supraventricular tachyarrhythmias.

The ideal pacemaker to cope with these

arrhythmias does not yet exist. In theory, this device should be completely implanted. It should be capable of recognizing the tachyarrhythmia and instituting the appropriate corrective paced rhythm. Furthermore, if this should fail, it should be capable of recognizing the failure and either repeating the therapeutic rhythm or changing to an alternate pacing mode until satisfactory correction of the arrhythmia is achieved. All of this should be done automatically and without risk to the patient.

A few years ago such a concept was unthinkable. However, with better understanding of the mechanism of conduction between the atrium and the ventricles and of the anatomy and physiology of aberrant conduction pathways, increased sophistication of pulse generator circuitry, and the development of improved atrial leads, the achievement of this goal is much closer.

REFERENCES

1. Kelley, D.T.: Comparison of right atrial and right ventricular single and paired pacing in the canine heart. Am. Heart J., 77:206, 1969.
2. Mitchell, J., and Shapiro, W.: Atrial function and the hemodynamic consequences of atrial fibrillation in man. Am. J. Cardiol., 23:556, 1969.
3. Samet, P., et al.: Hemodynamic results of right atrial pacing in cardiac subjects. Dis. Chest, 53:133, 1968.
4. Benchimol, A., and Goldstein, M.R.: A review of atrial pacing: Clinical and laboratory application. Ann. N.Y. Acad. Sci., 167:604, 1969.
5. Nathan, D.A., et al.: An implantable synchronous pacemaker for the long-term correction of complete heart block. Am. J. Cardiol., 11:362, 1963.
6. Castillo, C.A., et al.: Bifocal demand pacing. Chest, 59:360, 1971.
7. Smyth, N.P.D., et al.: Permanent transvenous sequential A-V pacing. Clin. Res., 23:305, 1974.
8. Carlens, E., et al.: New method for atrial-triggered pacemaker treatment without thoracotomy. J. Thorac. Cardiovasc. Surg., 50:229, 1965.
9. Kleinert, M.: Personal communication, March, 1976.
10. Moss, A.J., et al.: Transvenous left atrial pacing for the control of recurrent ventricular fibrillation. N. Engl. J. Med., 278:928, 1968.
11. Smyth, N.P.D., et al.: A permanent transvenous atrial electrode catheter. J. Thorac. Cardiovasc. Surg., 58:773, 1969.
12. Moss, A.J.: Therapeutic uses of permanent pervenous atrial pacemakers: A review. J. Electrocardiol., 8:373, 1975.
13. Smyth, N.P.D., et al.: Permanent transvenous atrial pacing: An experimental and clinical study. Ann. Thorac. Surg., 11:360, 1971.
14. Legato, M.J.: The correlation of ultrastructure and function in the mammalian myocardial cell. Progr. Cardiovasc. Dis., 11:391, 1969.
15. Smyth, N.P.D., Bacos, J.M., and Keller, J.W.: Experimental and clinical use of a variable parameter cardiac pacer. Dis. Chest, 53:93, 1968.
16. Furman, S., Reicher-Reiss, H., and Escher, D.J.W.: Atrioventricular sequential pacing and pacemakers. Chest, 63(5):783, 1973.
17. Smyth, N.P.D., et al.: Permanent pervenous atrial sensing and pacing with a new J-shaped lead. J. Thorac. Cardiovasc. Surg., 72:565, 1976.
18. Kleinert, M.: Personal communication, April, 1977.
19. Iwa, T., and Wada, J.: Electrical and surgical treatment of tachycardias. In Cardiac Pacing: Proceedings of the 4th International Symposium on Cardiac Pacing. Groningen. Edited by H. J. Th. Thalen. Assen, the Netherlands, Van Gorcum, 1973, pp. 376–383.
20. Kahn, A., Morris, J., and Citron, P.: Patient-initiated rapid atrial pacing to manage supraventricular tachycardia. Am. J. Cardiol., 38:200, 1976.

12

Pacemaker Therapy in Cardiac Surgery

CHARLES L. BYRD

Cardiac surgery encompasses a wide range of surgical procedures to treat both congenital and acquired heart disease. This chapter will be confined to cardiac surgical procedures requiring cardiopulmonary bypass. These procedures provide a dramatic and vivid demonstration of the need for and utility of pacemaker therapy, which has evolved into a technical and a highly specialized form of therapy that is applied to all patients undergoing cardiopulmonary bypass.

CARDIOPULMONARY BYPASS SURGERY

Cardiac surgical procedures may be conveniently divided into three phases: pre-bypass, bypass and post-bypass. Pre-bypass and noncardiac patients have identical physiologic stresses for the induction of anesthesia and surgery. It is unlikely that a serious conduction problem will arise spontaneously during this phase of surgery and create an emergency situation.

A small group of patients undergoing cardiopulmonary bypass surgery may have pacemakers for preexistent conduction problems. These patients are at some risk of pacemaker malfunction during the pre-bypass phase of surgery. The potential dangers are inadvertent transection of the lead, cautery effects, and defibrillation currents.

Cautery current can inhibit a demand pacemaker. If the underlying rhythm is unsafe, the pacer can be changed from a demand to a fixed-rate mode. Applying a magnet converts all pacemakers to a fixed-rate mode (20 to 30% rate increase with some pacers), and in a few sophisticated units the mode change can be programmed. Direct contact of a cautery to an exposed pacemaker and to cut or uncapped leads may cause fatal myocardial damage. Cardioversion at high power setting can damage the pacer, necessitating replacement of the unit.

Cardiopulmonary bypass is that unique period during surgery when the blood returning to the heart is diverted from the heart and lungs to a mechanical oxygenator and pump.[1] It is a state of controlled perfusion adequate for tissue survival but nevertheless abnormal and frequently approaching a shock state. During this period a specific surgical procedure is performed on the heart. Upon completion of the surgical procedure the patient is weaned off bypass. Any metabolic deficit incurred must be corrected, and physiologic cardiac perfusion must be reinstated and sustained.

The myocardium and/or the conduction system may be altered during bypass. Reversible ischemic changes, metabolic abnormalities, medications, and myocardial preservation techniques cause transient changes in both the myocardium and the conduction system. Permanent damage to the myocardium and/or conduction system may result from technical misadventures, irreversible ischemic changes, or inherent demands of the specific surgical procedure. The insult may be minimal and go unnoticed, or it may be major enough to threaten the patient's survival.

The post-bypass phase may last for several days. Upon completion of the operation, the patient must receive maximal support for the time necessary to correct the reversible metabolic and pathologic changes incurred in the lungs, peripheral circulation, and organ systems. In the post-bypass phase, the heart frequently functions at decreased efficiency, with maximal fluctuations in peripheral resistances and left ventricular filling pressure. The heart has two means of compensating to maintain an adequate cardiac output: heart rate and stroke volume. Pacing is beneficial in controlling heart rate. It may also enhance the stroke volume if the atrium can be paced appropriately.

Therapy in the postoperative period is directed toward total system recovery by attempting to keep all parameters (blood pressure, blood volume, blood gases, peripheral resistance, heart rate) within physiologic limits. Survival may be jeopardized if therapy is concentrated only on one or two parameters. It is obvious that correction of all these abnormalities is predicated on an effective cardiac output and

time to reverse the effects of injuries and metabolic insults.

LEAD SYSTEMS AND IMPLANTATION TECHNIQUES

All patients requiring cardiopulmonary bypass, regardless of the procedure performed, should have a temporary pacing electrode suitable for ventricular pacing. Many would benefit from the placement of an atrial electrode. A few patients will be candidates for the implantation of permanent electrodes during surgery. The need for pacemaker therapy is rare during the induction of anesthesia and for that portion of the operation prior to cardiopulmonary bypass. When this situation does arise, it constitutes an emergency for which special techniques must be employed.

Ventricular Implants

Three regions of the heart—two on the right ventricle, one on the left—are suitable for the placement of a ventricular electrode (Fig. 12–1). These sites are usually free from fatty tissue and devoid of significant coronary arteries. The site used depends upon the surgical approach, the type of electrode implanted, and the surgeon's personal experience. The most common incision for cardiac procedures is a median sternotomy. With this incision, sites on the right ventricle can be approached with the least manipulation of the heart. The left ventricular area is more accessible through a left thoracotomy.

Anatomically, the three usable regions of the heart are the anterior surface of the right ventricle, the diaphragmatic surface of the right ventricle extending towards the apex, and the anterior lateral aspect of the left ventricle between the left anterior descending and circumflex coronary artery systems. The anterior surface of the right ventricle (Fig. 12–1A) is the most accessible area from a median sternotomy incision, but is usually composed of a thin myocardial wall. This tissue is acceptable for short-term use with temporary electrodes but is not adequate for long-term implantation with a permanent electrode.

The bare area on the diaphragmatic surface of the right ventricle (Fig. 12–1B) is the next most accessible site. This is a triangular-shaped area with the base distal to the right atrium, extending towards the apex of the right ventricle. The basilar area of this triangle is of variable thickness and changes into a thick substantial region at the apex. The muscular portion of the septum and the diaphragmatic portion of the right ventricular wall join at the apex to form this thick tissue, which is suitable for any type of electrode implant.

The area on the anterior lateral aspect of the left ventricle (Fig. 12–1C) is composed of thick muscle and is suitable for all types of electrode implants. The manipulation required to expose this site with a median sternotomy incision frequently results in hemodynamic and/or arrhythmic sequelae.

The temporary epicardial ventricular electrode that is placed on the heart following cardiopulmonary bypass is frequently a prophylactic pacing electrode. To justify its implantation, the electrode must be simple to implant during surgery and easy to remove in a noninvasive fashion 36 to 72 hours after surgery. The most practical lead for this purpose is a braided wire electrode (Davis & Geck #2597–63) sutured to the epimyocardial layer of the heart. Securing the electrode with a U or tear drop suture configuration causes minimal trauma to the myocardium. The atraumatic needle is removed, and the cutting needle is then passed out to the skin. Within 36 hours a thin fibrous sheath has formed about the Teflon lead, and the electrode can be dislodged from the heart with gentle traction.

For bipolar pacing, a second electrode is placed in the same area of the ventricle 1.5 to 2.5 cm from the first. If the electrodes are placed too far apart, they will tend to sense extraneous signals in much the same fashion as does a radio antenna. The greater the distance between the electrodes, the greater the likelihood that this "antenna effect" will occur. In a radio, this phenomenon produces annoying but harmless static. In a pacemaker, the extraneous signals may be put through the sensing circuit and identified as a myocardial potential, causing inhibition of pacemaker function. The antenna effect becomes especially significant in atrioventricular systems.

Permanent epimyocardial leads were the first lead systems used in pacing. Two basic types of electrodes are available today: one made of Elgiloy and the other of platinum-iridium. The Elgiloy electrode is suitable only as a cathode for unipolar pacing systems. Long-term use as an anode, or with any biphasic wave form having an anode phase of greater than 0.75 volts, will result in corrosion of the electrode and exit block.[2] Platinum-iridium electrodes are more versatile and function well as cathode or anode.

Electrodes are available in both the suture-in and sutureless configurations. The implantation technique for the suture-in electrode is to incise the epicardium and implant the electrode directly into the myocardium. The electrode is secured by suturing the Silastic sheath directly to the myocardium. The corkscrew design or sutureless electrode can be implanted in a less traumatic manner by screwing the electrode directly into the myocardium.

The diaphragmatic apical portion of the right ventricle and the anterior lateral area of the left ventricle are the best sites for permanent implants. The anterior surface of the right and left ventricles must be avoided. The right ventricle is too thin for a secure atraumatic implant, and the left ventricular surface is usually covered with fat, which obscures the left anterior descending coronary artery system. Also, in patients

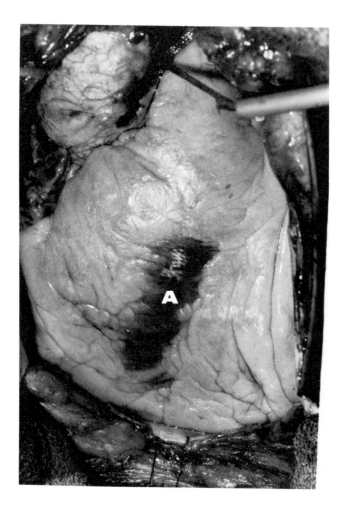

Fig. 12–1. Multiple views of heart as shown at operation with standard median sternotomy incision. Typical fat distribution is shown with the accessible pacing areas labeled as A, B, and C. A is bare area on anterior surface of heart. This area is suitable for implantation of only temporary short-term pacing wires. B is diaphragmatic surface of heart (shown in relation to area A). Muscle toward apex is thick and suitable for all types of pacing. C is left anterolateral portion of heart between two branches of left anterior descending coronary arteries (shown in relation to anterior surface). Heart is supported on pad and rotated out of mediastinum to demonstrate maneuver required to attach lead to this portion of heart. This region is most easily approached from a left thoracotomy. It is suitable for any type of pacemaker electrode implant.

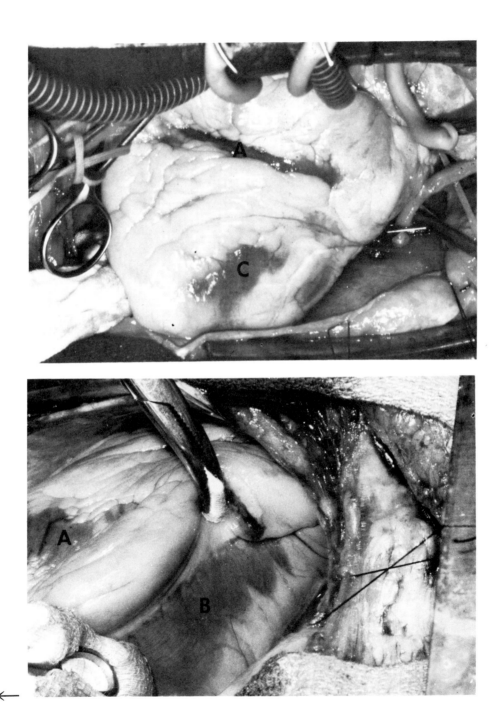

with a median sternotomy incision or with loss of the pericardium, anterior electrodes become entrapped in the cicatrization process. This results in the electrode becoming fixed to the rigid chest wall while attached to a pliable beating heart. The entrapment of the electrode in scar tissue is normal and of no consequence as long as the lead can move freely with the heart. The right diaphragmatic pacing site places the lead in opposition to the diaphragm; the left ventricular pacing site places the lead in opposition to the pleura.

The permanent electrode should be applied as atraumatically as possible. The suture-in electrode has a certain amount of trauma inherent in the incision of myocardium and in suture technique. This can be kept to a minimum.

The sutureless electrode has three variables which must be controlled for optimum implantation. First, the electrode should never be screwed tightly into the myocardium. The screwing action will compress and eventually tear the myocardium. To eliminate this possibility, the electrode initially should be detorqued about one quarter of a turn. Second, the electrode should be inserted perpendicular to the surface. Angular insertions may not eliminate the tension on the lead, causing it to erode out of the myocardium. Third, the electrode depth must be controlled to avoid penetration of the myocardium into the ventricular chamber. If the electrode is placed in the ventricular cavity, the electrical measurements will be unsatisfactory.

The lead is passed from the mediastinum to a subcutaneous pocket. An expeditious method of accomplishing this is to reflect the pleura and tunnel through the muscular portion of the intercostal space to the subcutaneous tissue on the chest wall. A small Penrose drain passed through the tunnel provides an excellent sheath for transporting the lead through the tunnel without injuring the lead. Care must be taken to avoid the internal mammary artery and vein and to stay out of the pleura. Following cardiopulmonary bypass, coagulation is frequently abnormal. Meticulous hemostasis must be obtained to avoid hematoma formation. The passage of the lead through the intercostal muscle tunnel may be helpful in preventing the blood in the mediastinum from tracting along the lead into the subcutaneous pocket.

Atrial Implants

The atrial lead should be placed only in conjunction with a ventricular lead. Placement of a temporary prophylactic atrial electrode is not absolutely essential, but is considered sound practice in patients with an atrial contraction.[3] At present the indication for a permanent atrial epicardial lead is rare.

Epicardial atrial implants are technically difficult and demand considerable judgment and experience to achieve successful implantation consistently. The right atrium is thin and the tissue is easily damaged during an implant. The potential pacing sites around the right atrial appendage are usually damaged by the venous return cannulae during cardiopulmonary bypass (Fig. 12–2). The remaining lateral wall of the right atrium is too thin for a reliable implant. The site that has given consistently reliable pacing is the median aspect of the right atrium just anterior to the left atrium (Fig. 12–2, site A). Temporary electrodes can also be placed just anterior to the superior cava in this region. The electrode is supported and protected by the ascending aorta resting against this portion of the right atrium. The trauma that the relatively tenuous right atrial tissue receives is probably the critical factor in the long-term survival of the electrode.

The same type of temporary wire electrode used for the ventricle is adequate for temporary atrial pacing. The lead is large and must be placed in substantial atrial tissue. The same type of lead in a finer wire has been used in an attempt to lessen the trauma of implantation.

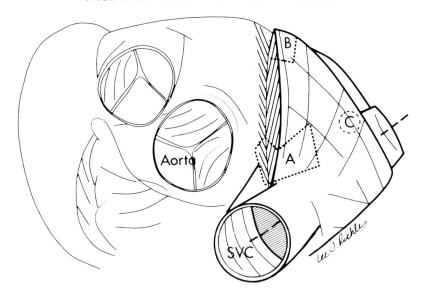

Fig. 12–2. Atrial epicardial pacing sites. Site A gives optimum results for long-term pacing with noninvasive surface electrodes. It is also suitable for temporary electrodes. Site B is atrial appendage which is usually obliterated by a cannulae pursestring suture but may function as an electrical ground. Site C is right atrial lateral and inferior wall. This area is usually too thin for reliable long-term atrial pacing. SVC is the superior vena cava.

The permanent epicardial atrial leads range from simple noninvasive loops that lie on the atrial surface to the conventional ventricular epicardial designs. Invasive models (including pinch-on leads) have not given consistent results. Noninvasive epicardial surface electrodes provide the theoretical benefit of minimal trauma and have given excellent results. However, the number of such implants is too small for conclusive results to be drawn. Intracavitary electrodes that screw into the septal wall and are brought out through pursestring sutures in the atrium have also had good short-term results.

At present, bipolar pacing is the only safe method of pacing in the acute postoperative period. Current external atrioventricular pacemakers (external or permanent DVI*) function appropriately only with a bipolar atrial lead arrangement. Use of a bipolar ventricular lead arrangement is also advisable. Other benefits of bipolar atrial pacing are a redundant lead and the ease of obtaining an atrial electrogram. Unipolar DDI* pacing systems, atrial synchronous pacers, and straight atrial pacers will function satisfactorily with a unipolar lead arrangement.

Temporary-Permanent Lead Extension

Once the permanent leads are attached to the heart and brought out to a subcutaneous tissue pocket, three alternatives are available. The permanent leads may be connected to a permanent pacemaker or a temporary extension device (Fig. 12–3),[4] or they may be capped and sealed. If the decision is made to insert the permanent pacemaker during this operation, it is wise to attach a temporary epicardial ventricular electrode to provide access to other pacing modalities.

---

*DVI: Double chamber pacing–ventricular sensed–inhibited mode.
DDI: Double chamber pacing–double chamber sensing–inhibited mode.

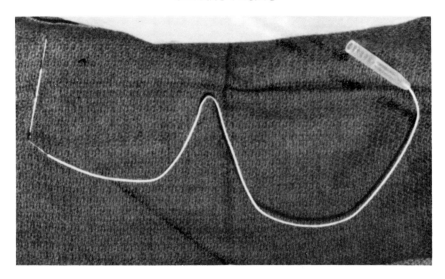

Fig. 12–3. Temporary permanent electrode extension (Medtronic lead shown) connects to permanent lead in subcutaneous pocket. Temporary extension is removed by traction, leaving permanent lead capped and sealed. Permanent lead is ready for future use if necessary.

The second alternative, a temporary extension lead, connects to the permanent lead and passes out to the skin where it functions as a temporary lead throughout the immediate postoperative period. The temporary extension lead is pulled out, and the permanent lead is left capped and sealed for future use. This method avoids losing the use of an excellent lead during the postoperative period.

Emergency Pacing Techniques

The sudden onset of profound refractory bradycardia, creating a need for emergency pacing, is definitely an exceptional event for a surgeon. In today's operating room environment, most surgeons have not been exposed to this clinical situation. A more common problem is the sudden loss of pacing in a pacemaker-dependent patient, requiring decisive action to reinstitute pacing. Depending on the gravity of the problem, two types of approaches are available. First, if time permits, a temporary transvenous lead can be passed into the right ventricle. Second, in extreme situations the heart can be punctured with a percutaneous needle and/or an open epicardial implant.

The simplest technique for the rapid passage of a temporary right ventricular pacing lead is to use a subclavian central venous pressure line as a conduit, to pass a fine electrode, or to insert a transvenous lead introducer system (8 French or larger) that will pass a larger transvenous electrode. The electrodes can be inserted rapidly into the right ventricle with blind manipulation. When time permits, accurate positioning with fluoroscopy is desirable to obtain maximal stability of the electrode. This technique is also applicable to the common femoral vein and the external or internal jugular vein.

The direct approach to the heart with a percutaneous needle is definitely more radical and has a greater potential for complications. This technique should be used without hesitation in emergency situations as a means of pacing until a less traumatic route for pacing can be obtained.

The safest technique is to insert a long needle just to the right of the xiphoid, pointing it towards the back of the left shoulder. With this approach, the needle has a greater chance of penetrating the heart along the diaphragmatic surface in the apical region of the right ventricle. The only major complication from this approach is a myocardial tear and subsequent bleeding. This need not be a fatal complication, and the risk is justified by the gravity of the clinical situation.

An open epicardial electrode implant is reserved for life-or-death situations. Profound bradycardia in the immediate postoperative period can degenerate rapidly into an emergency and, frequently, cardiac arrest. The most expeditious and ultimately the safest method of handling this problem within the limited time available is to open the median sternotomy incision and implant an electrode directly on the heart. Fortunately, this sequence of events cannot occur if the prophylactic electrodes are correctly placed on the heart.

ELECTRICAL MEASUREMENTS

Measuring the minimum energy required to stimulate the heart and the electrical potential generated by a spontaneous heart beat is essential for determining the pacing and sensing capabilities of the implanted electrode. The concept of the energy delivered to the heart eliminates many problems in understanding the idiosyncrasies of the complex pacing systems available today. Once the basic electrophysiology is mastered, any pacing system can be reduced to a few simple parameters that are easy to measure and understand.

The application of Ohm's law (voltage=current × resistance) to a simple electric circuit serves as a satisfactory model for demonstrating the principles involved (Fig. 12–4). All modern testing equipment functions either as an ammeter or voltmeter, that is, the voltage is known and the current is measured, or vice versa. With one variable known and another measured,

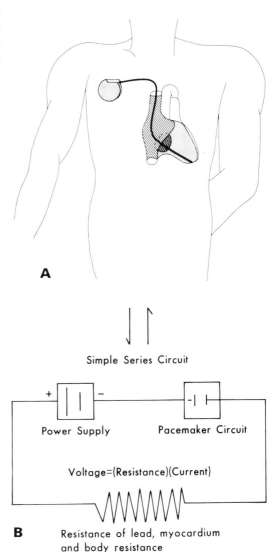

A

Simple Series Circuit

Power Supply   Pacemaker Circuit

Voltage=(Resistance)(Current)

B   Resistance of lead, myocardium and body resistance

Fig. 12–4. Pacemaker system, whether unipolar or bipolar, can be presented as a simple electrical circuit. This circuit has power supply and pacemaker circuit which can be considered as single unit. Pacemaker discharges through lead into heart. Following stimulation of the heart, current flows back to anode (+ pole) via body tissue. This can be a small volume of tissue or blood for a bipolar lead and a large volume of tissue in a unipolar lead. The resistance of the lead, myocardium, and body tissue represent the total resistance of the circuit in this simple model. The circuit obeys Ohm's law (voltage = resistance × current).

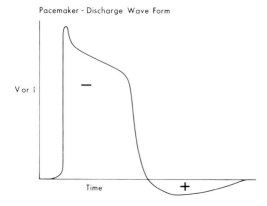

Pacemaker - Discharge Wave Form

V or i

Time

Fig. 12–5. Schematic representation of electrical discharge of pacemaker. Amplitude can be measured either as voltage (V) or current (I). The other coordinate is time. The area under the (−) curve is the total voltage or current delivered to the heart. The time required to deliver this voltage or charge is called pulse width. Energy delivered to the heart is pulse width × current × voltage.

the third can be calculated using Ohm's law. For example, if the minimum voltage required to pace the heart is 0.5 volts and the current measured is 1.0 mA, the circuit has a resistance of 500 ohms. Although the measured current accurately reflects the threshold current, it may not represent the energy delivered to the heart.

The energy delivered to the heart is a function of voltage, current, and time (energy = voltage × current × time). The waveform of the pacemaker's electrical discharge pulse (Fig. 12–5) has two parameters—current or voltage and pulse width. The pulse width represents the time necessary to deliver a pulse of electrical energy to the heart. The longer the pulse width, the greater the energy delivered to the heart at the same current or voltage amplitude.

At surgery, the voltage, current, and pulse width must be known to determine the *stimulation threshold*—the minimum energy needed for cardiac stimulation. Two techniques exist for measuring the stimulation threshold. One involves varying the

voltage or current and keeping the pulse width constant. The result is the *standard threshold*—the minimum voltage and current required to stimulate the heart at a predetermined pulse width (usually the pulse width of the pacemaker). The second technique involves holding the voltage and current constant (usually at the same values as the pacemaker) and varying the pulse width to determine the minimum pulse width for cardiac stimulation. This alternative threshold is established easily in a noninvasive fashion by progammable pacers in which pulse width is a variable.

The threshold values change during the maturation of the implanted electrode.[5] If the acute or chronic threshold exceeds the maximal energy output of the pacemaker generator, the heart cannot be stimulated. This phenomenon is called exit block. In general, a pacemaker output of three to four times the acute threshold is an adequate safety margin. Therefore, a threshold of 1 volt or below for a constant voltage system and 2 mA or below for a constant current system is within this range for permanent 4 to 5 volt constant voltage and 9 to 10 mA constant current pacemakers (Fig. 12–6). External temporary pacemakers are constant current and have more power (9 volt batteries and current outputs of 25 to 30 mA).

A 5 volt pacemaker will generally have a pulse width threshold of less than 0.1 msec. Therefore, a pulse width of 0.5 msec. should provide an acceptable safety margin for ventricular pacing.[6] This increases to 1.0 msec for atrial pacing.

The electrical potential generated by the heart during depolarization (R wave) must have sufficient amplitude and slope to be detected by the sensing circuit of the pacemaker.[8] A generated potential with an inadequate amplitude and/or slope will not be sensed. A safety margin of two to three times greater amplitude than the minimum sensing capability of the pacemaker will provide reliable sensing. In general, sensing circuits designed for ventricular pacemak-

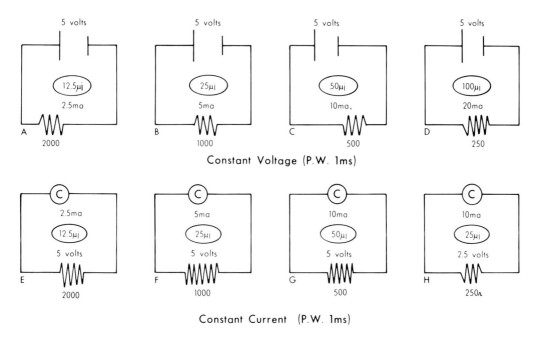

Fig. 12–6. Theoretical behavior of constant current and constant voltage pacemakers at various resistances. Constant current and voltage systems behave the same at high resistances since voltage is the limiting factor. Energy delivered to the heart is 12.5 microjoules. At low resistances the constant current system is current-limited and thus delivers less energy at 250 ohms than the constant voltage system (100 vs 25 microjoules). Therefore constant current systems are at risk in low resistance implants.

ers are not sensitive enough for atrial sensing.

CLINICAL APPLICATIONS

Pacemaker therapy offers three potential modalities of therapy: rate control, management of arrhythmias, and augmentation of cardiac output. The objective of pacing in this environment is to help achieve and maintain the most effective cardiac function possible by providing an optimal heart rate and by pacing the heart at a site that gives the maximal physiologic response.

Rate Control

A slow heart rate should not be classified as bradycardia unless the heart rate fails to respond to the normal regulatory mechanisms. Heart rate is one of the four factors controlling cardiac output. The others are contractility of the heart, preload, and afterload. The maintenance of a satisfactory heart rate is essential to the management of the patient following cardiopulmonary bypass. Failure to maintain an appropriate heart rate will frequently result in heart failure despite an optimal filling pressure and afterload. This is especially true of patients with an enlarged left ventricle and a poor ejection fraction.

At operation, bradycardia of neurogenic origin is most common. It usually responds at once to atropine or similar compounds. Respiratory insufficiency secondary to inadequate ventilation produces a refractory bradycardia which usually reverts back to normal with restoration of ventilation.[9]

Patients with a clinically significant

bradycardia secondary to a sick sinus syndrome, a complete AV block, and atrial fibrillation should have a temporary or permanent pacemaker implanted prior to surgery. Patients with intermittent complete AV block or the potential of AV block from some of the more exotic His bundle lesions may not be detected prior to surgery. These patients are at risk of developing profound bradycardia following cardiopulmonary bypass and in the immediate postoperative state.

Brady-tachyarrhythmia syndromes are common. Irritable ventricular foci result from an insult incurred at surgery and serve as the origin for premature contractions and tachyarrhythmias. The heart rate may be sufficient for adequate tissue perfusion but not rapid enough to suppress these irritable foci. Bradycardia following an acute myocardial infarction at surgery is usually a manifestation of massive muscle injury and is frequently fatal.

Pacing is the preferred treatment for bradycardia. Ventricular pacing is applicable to all types of bradyarrhythmias and is the most common application of pacing. Ventricular pacing forms the foundation for all types of pacing. It is effective, reliable, and technically feasible in all patients. Bradycardias are reversed by pacing the heart at an appropriate rate and the tachy-bradyarrhythmias are usually suppressed by the application of overdrive pacing.

The atrial component, if present, is lost with ventricular pacing. Because the heart usually compensates for the loss of atrial function, it may be of no clinical significance. However, the compensating mechanism in some patients is not sufficient. The acute loss of the atrial component in patients with severe left ventricular dysfunction from either left ventricular failure or a significant decrease in ventricular compliance will result in a marked reduction in cardiac output. This is especially true following bypass and in the early postoperative period due to the inability to respond to the physiologic extremes of filling pressure and systemic resistance.

Tachyarrhythmia Control

Control of tachyarrhythmia encompasses the diagnosis and treatment of ventricular and atrial arrhythmias. The ventricular arrhythmias are the sequelae of premature ventricular contractions. These are most effectively diagnosed by a conventional electrocardiogram. The atrial tachyarrhythmias include atrial flutter, fibrillation, and the supraventricular tachycardias. They are best analyzed by an atrial electrogram or a complete conduction study. In contrast to bradyarrhythmias, drug therapy is the primary modality of treatment. Pacing is used in conjunction with medication and is frequently reserved for the refractory arrhythmias.

Ventricular tachyarrhythmias range from ventricular premature beats to ventricular tachycardia and are managed primarily with myocardial suppressive medication. Overdrive suppression pacing is an excellent adjunct to this therapy.[10] The combined approach is highly effective in managing postoperative patients with transient myocardial irritability of a magnitude that cannot be managed by medication alone.

The atrial tachyarrhythmias consist of atrial flutter and supraventricular tachycardia. They have diverse etiologies and are more difficult to diagnose and treat.[11] Diagnosis has been made easier by the routine use of atrial electrograms, even in the presence of atrioventricular block. The precise analysis of supraventricular tachycardias into either automatic or AV nodal reentrant mechanism frequently requires a right heart catheterization with a complete electrophysiologic study. Four methods of treatment are effective: medication, rapid atrial stimulation, atrial pacing, and cardioversion. Drug therapy is frequently successful in the management and stabilization of acute and chronic atrial arrhythmias and is often successful in the conversion and stabilization of the atrial rate. Aggressive pacing techniques are justified for serious arrhythmias that often lead to critical clinical deterioration.

Atrial flutter and supraventricular reentrant tachyarrhythmias frequently respond to rapid atrial stimulation and overdrive atrial suppression. The atrial electrode is used to obtain an electrogram as well as to pace. The ectopic supraventricular tachyarrhythmias are more difficult to manage, but overdrive suppression may be a useful adjunct to treatment.

Cardioversion is frequently the only method to manage the refractory arrhythmias. In life-threatening situations there should be no hesitation in using this mode of therapy.

Cardiac Output

Enhanced cardiac output is another potential benefit from pacing. The atrial component or "atrial kick" has been shown to be effective in increasing the stroke volume. The mechanism of this action is probably related to the increased filling pressure in the ventricle following an atrial contraction.[12-14]

The relationship between the atrial component and the cardiac output becomes apparent if two variables are included—the *effective left ventricular filling pressure* (passive component + atrial component) and *systemic resistance* (Fig. 12–7). A low effective filling pressure on the first portion of Starling's curve (cardiac output/filling pressure) and a loss of the atrial component produces a maximal change in the cardiac output. A miminal systemic resistance shifts the ventricular function curve to its peak cardiac output with respect to filling pressure.

The cardiovascular system compensates for an acute or a chronic loss in the atrial

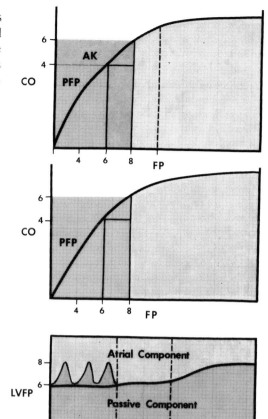

Fig. 12–7. Starling's curve is used to demonstrate relationship between cardiac output (CO) and left ventricular filling pressure (LVFP) at constant pressure and systemic resistance. A, The acute loss of the atrial component is depicted with resultant loss in cardiac output. The cardiac output change will be greater on the first portion of the curve (maximal slope) and less on the flat portion. B, Model compensation following loss of the atrial component to the filling pressure by increasing the passive filling component. The net result is a restoration of cardiac output and loss of cardiac reserve. C, Effective left ventricular filling pressure (passive component + atrial component) is plotted against time.

component by increasing the systemic resistance and/or the passive left ventricular filling pressure. The increase in the systemic resistance maintains a physiologic blood pressure but lowers the cardiac output. An increase in the passive filling pressure increases the cardiac output and decreases the cardiac reserve. Therefore, an acute or chronic loss in the atrial component is manifest as a loss of the cardiac output and/or loss of cardiac reserve.

When possible, it seems logical to preserve the superior hemodynamic state afforded by AV synchrony. At present, a demand atrioventricular sequential pacer (DVI) is a proven, effective, safe, and reliable method of restoring AV synchrony. It functions as an atrial pacer when needed and as a standby ventricular pacer if the atrial contraction is ineffectual. It encompasses all of the advantages of atrial pacing with the assurance of the proven ventricular pacer.

Only two forms of atrioventricular pacers, DVI and DDI, meet the aforementioned criteria. They pace both the atrium and the ventricle. The DVI senses only ventricular activity; the DDI senses in the atrium as well as in the ventricle.

The magnitude of the surgical procedure and the associated operative morbidity must be considered and justified prior to implanting a DVI pacemaker. The current multichambered pacers are bipolar and require a more extensive surgical procedure to implant. This is especially true for implanting bipolar atrial epimyocardial leads. Transvenous bipolar atrial and ventricular leads are also large and need larger veins for implantations. However, from the experience to date, a simple reduction in size and the rapid evolution of the unipolar pacers should solve these problems.

Clinically, the primary criterion for selection of patients for this modality of pacing is the need for the superior hemodynamic benefits of AV synchrony. Physiologic testing to demonstrate the sequelae of decreased cardiac output with loss of the atrial component has been nonproductive. All patients placed in the appropriate hemodynamic state can exhibit almost any cardiac output and/or blood pressure

TABLE 12–1

Atrial and Ventricular Pacing in the Immediate Postoperative Period

PACING	ATRIAL PACING	VENTRICULAR PACING
Cardiac output	3.5 l/min.	2.5 l/min.
Mean systemic blood pressure	100 mmHg	65 mmHg
Central venous pressure	10 mmHg	15 mmHg
Pulmonary artery diastolic pressure	14 mmHg	20 mmHg

Summary:
  Acute change from atrial to ventricular pacing results in a marked drop in the cardiac output (averages about 1 l/min.).
  Systemic pressure falls.
  Acute compensatory rise in the left atrial filling pressure.

change desired. Most patients in whom the atrial component is essential have left ventricular failure and are in danger of developing congestive heart failure with ventricular pacing. Patients immediately following cardiopulmonary bypass are subject to transient left ventricular failure and/or decreased compliance coupled with changes in blood volume, circulating catecholamines, and pulmonary resistance. These hemodynamic changes are reflected in an altered left ventricular function curve, left ventricular filling pressure, and peripheral resistance. Patients in this unique group benefit dramatically from restoration of AV synchrony (Table 12–1).[15]

Future Trends

The future trend for pacing as an adjunct to cardiopulmonary bypass surgery is towards atrial and, especially, atrioventricular pacing rather than ventricular pacing alone. Atrioventricular pacing combines effectively the potential for all three prospective benefits of pacing: rate control, tachyarrhythmia control, and increase in cardiac output.

Omni external pacing devices will soon be available. These devices combine into one system the multitude of devices in use today. The omni devices will offer the potential for sophisticated analysis of atrial and ventricular arrhythmia and treatment and will provide an ideal perioperative pacing system that will be easy to attach to the patient, safe to operate, and reliable for accurate analysis of data.

REFERENCES

1. Clower, G.H.A.: Bypass of the heart and lungs with an extracorporeal circulation. Gibbon's Surgery of the Chest, 3rd ed. Edited by D.C. Sabiston and F.C. Spencer. Philadelphia, W.B. Saunders Company, 1976.
2. Kraska, R.E.: Anodic behavior of Cordis Elgiloy electrodes in Medtronic and Cordis pacemakers. (Internal communications, Medtronic, Inc.)
3. Waldo, A.V., et al.: Use of temporary placed epicardial atrial wire electrodes for diagnosis and treatment of cardiac arrhythmias following open-heart surgery. J. Thorac. Cardiovasc. Surg., 71:500, 1978.
4. Nathan, M.J., Yahr, W.Z., and Greenberg, J.J.: Temporary-permanent pacemaker lead for cardiac surgery. J. Thorac. Cardiovasc. Surg., 64:957, 1972.
5. Szabo, Z., and Solti, F.: The significance of the tissue reaction around the electrode on the late myocardial threshold; Doenecke, P., Flothner, G., and Bette, L.: Studies of short-and long-term threshold changes. In Advances in Pacemaker Technology, Vol. I. Edited by M. Schaldach and S. Furman. New York, Springer-Verlag, 1975, pp. 273–296.
6. Tobias, J.: Pacing at a very short pulse width. Ann. Thorac. Surg., 26:27, 1978.
7. Calvin, J.W.: Intraoperative pacemaker electrical testing. Ann. Thorac. Surg., 26:165, 1978.
8. Furman, S., Hurzler, P., and DeCaprio, V.: The ventricular endocardial electrogram and pacemaker sensing. J. Thorac. Cardiovasc. Surg., 73:258, 1977.
9. Katz, R.L., and Bigger, J.T.: Cardiac arrhythmias during anesthesia and operation. Anesthesiology, 33:193, 1970.
10. Freidberg, C.K., Lyon, L.J., and Donoso, E.: Suppression of refractory recurrent ventricular tachycardia by transvenous rapid cardiac pacing and antiarrhythmic drugs. Am. Heart J., 79:44, 1970.
11. Cogren, T.B., Mac Lean, W.A.H., and Waldo, A.L.: Overdrive pacing for supraventricular tachycardia. A review of theoretical implications and therapeutic techniques. Pace, 1:196, 1978.
12. Gesell, R.A.: The effect of auricular tone and amplitude of auricular systole on ventricular systole and ventricular output. Am. J. Physiol., 38:404, 1916.
13. Samet, P., et al.: Atrial contribution to cardiac output in complete heart block. Am. J. Cardiol., 16:1, 1965.
14. Ogawa, S., et al.: Hemodynamic consequences of atrioventricular and ventriculoatrial pacing. Pace, 1:8, 1978.
15. Hartz, G.O., et al.: Hemodynamic benefits of atrioventricular sequential pacing after cardiac surgery. Am. J. Cardiol., 40:232, 1977.

13

Cardiac Pacing in Infants and Children

DENNISON YOUNG
SEYMOUR FURMAN

Although much less frequently required than in adults, permanent artificial cardiac pacing in children and adolescents for selected life-threatening aspects of heart block and sinus nodal dysfunction is of firmly established value. The complexities of the growing, active child and the paucity of electronic equipment suited to his needs, however, make the problems of pacemaker therapy greater than those for the adult. Nevertheless, implanted pacemakers not only have been lifesaving but also have sustained a quality of physical and emotional well-being that has been gratifying to both patient and parent. The ultimate fate of the child or adolescent with a pacemaker is unknown. Experience to date, however, while occasionally disturbing and often arduous, allows for continued optimism.

INDICATIONS FOR PACEMAKER IMPLANTATION

Indications for permanent pacemaker implantation in children and adolescents can be therapeutic or prophylactic in a number of conditions associated with complete heart block or sinus nodal dysfunction.

Therapeutic

SYNCOPAL ATTACK OR RECURRENT DIZZINESS. The occurrence of syncope in a child with complete heart block, whether congenital, idiopathic, inflammatory, or late postoperative, should be considered an emergency. Additional studies to eliminate other causes of syncope, such as cerebral disease, hypoglycemia, aortic or pulmonary stenosis, or pulmonary hypertension are rarely required.

The electrocardiographic diagnosis of complete heart block is usually, although not always, immediately obvious. Some children and adolescents who have intermittent complete heart block may on initial observation demonstrate only first or second degree block. Such patients may require Holter monitoring and elec-

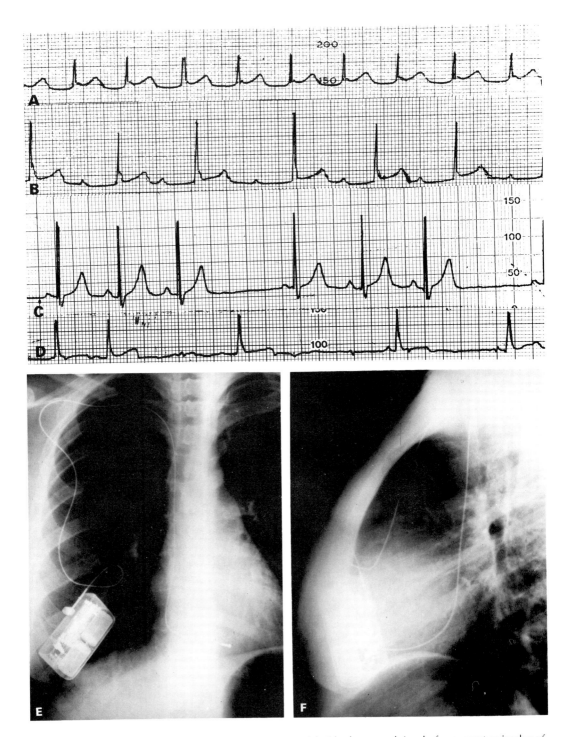

Fig. 13–1. Sinus nodal dysfunction in a sixteen-year-old girl who complained of recurrent episodes of dizziness and syncope over four-month period. There was no associated heart disease. Resting electrocardiograms showed only a sinus bradycardia at rate of 60/min. and PR interval of 0.16 sec. Holter monitoring: A, nodal rhythm at a rate of 100/min.; B, prolongation of PR interval up to 0.42 sec.; C, Wenckebach periodicity with sinoatrial block; D, periods of sinus arrest. His bundle study confirmed the presence of sinoatrial and atrioventricular nodal disease. E and F, Anteroposterior and lateral radiographs after retromammary implant of transvenous ventricular inhibited pacemaker. Patient has been entirely asymptomatic since.

trophysiologic study to establish the presence of complete heart block or significant parameters of disturbed atrioventricular conduction.

The decision for pacemaker implantation in children with sinus nodal dysfunction of presumed congenital or idiopathic origin is often difficult despite a history of syncope or dizziness. The initial electrocardiogram which commonly shows only mild sinus bradycardia and sinus arrhythmia with or without PR interval prolongation only sug-

gests the apparent cause of symptoms. Often exercise stress testing, repeated Holter monitoring, electrophysiologic study, and clinical or laboratory elimination of other diseases is required for convincing evidence of a causal relationship (Fig. 13–1).

CONGESTIVE HEART FAILURE CAUSED BY A SLOW VENTRICULAR RATE. Congenital complete heart block in infancy, with or without associated cardiac defects, is often incompatible with survival due to congestive

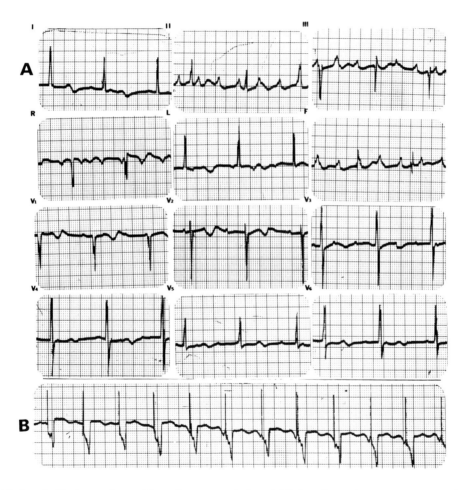

Fig. 13–2. A, Electrocardiographic pattern present since birth in a boy who was asymptomatic until two years of age when he had recurrent syncopal attacks. Cardiac catheterization showed L-transposition and insufficiency of both atrioventricular valves. The electrocardiogram shows complete heart block with an atrial rate of 150/min. and a ventricular rate of 60/min. The presence of Q waves in leads 3 and V_1 and their absence in leads 1, AVL, and the left precordial leads are consistent with L-transposition. B, No further attacks have occurred subsequent to the institution of transvenous pacing at a rate of 90/min.

heart failure. Most who survive remain asymptomatic until late in childhood when syncope or, less likely, congestive heart failure may occur in a relatively small number (Fig. 13–2). Congestive heart failure due to complete heart block in other than infancy, therefore, is primarily a complication of complex intracardiac surgical procedures. Heart failure due to sinus nodal dysfunction is exclusively a postoperative complication and not a sequela of this otherwise idiopathically occurring arrythmia.

Congestive heart failure resulting from the slow heart rate of either complete heart block or sinus nodal dysfunction requires urgent pacemaker implantation. The younger the child, the greater the potential for the development of heart failure and frequently the greater the severity and the more rapid is its occurrence (Fig. 13–3).

INADEQUATE CARDIAC OUTPUT DURING MODERATELY STRENUOUS EXERCISE. Most children and adolescents with complete heart block show a junctional rhythm of 50 to 60/min. and can increase the rate approx-

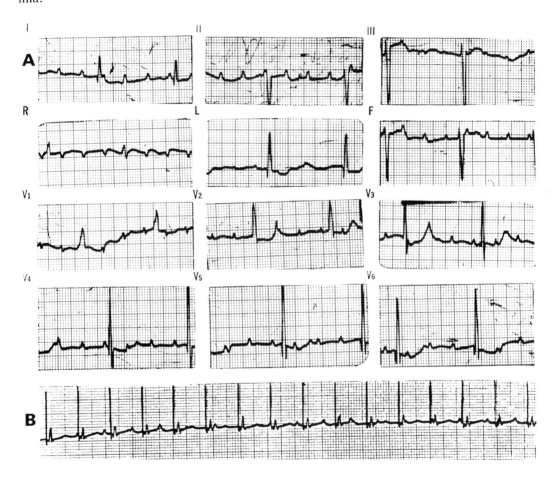

Fig. 13–3. A, Electrocardiographic pattern present since birth in four-week-old infant admitted in severe congestive heart failure and no associated heart disease. There is complete heart block with an atrial rate of 188/min., a ventricular rate of 52/min., a frontal plane QRS axis of −70° and QRS in V₁ of 0.08 sec. which is the upper limit of normal for her age. The electrocardiogram suggests the presence of trifascicular block. B, Radiofrequency pacemaker was immediately implanted via thoracotomy at a rate of 125/min. with rapid disappearance of the congestive failure.

imately 10% on exercise. Occasional patients, however, may even double the heart rate. Usually the small increase in rate, in view of the large stroke volume, is adequate to maintain output under stress. Some, however, become symptomatic and benefit from pacemaker implant. We prefer to confirm this with stress testing and physiologic examination in the cardiac catheterization laboratory prior to implantation.

DRUG-RESISTANT SINUS NODAL DYSFUNCTION. The brady-tachycardia syndrome occurs more commonly with sinus nodal dysfunction than with complete heart block in children. Drug therapy, although notoriously poor as treatment for either cerebral insufficiency or the brady-tachycardia syndrome in sinus nodal dysfunction, should be tried first. Suppression of the supraventricular tachycardia with digitalis or propranolol may also depress sinus node activity or atrioventricular conduction, however, and thus enhance the escape mechanism. Atropine accelerates the rate of sinus node discharge and velocity of atrioventricular conduction but may also intensify the escape mechanism represented by the supraventricular tachycardia in such patients. Drug therapy becomes much more effective, or may not be required, once permanent pacing is initiated.

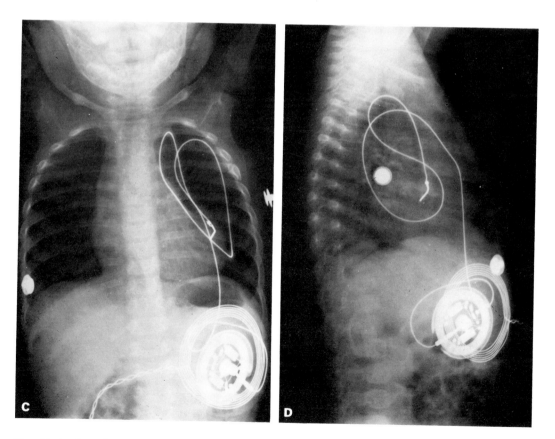

Fig. 13–3 (Cont'd).   C, Posteroanterior and D, lateral roentgenographic views of the chest showing abdominally implanted radiofrequency module with radiopaque components, external transmitting antenna, the braided wire, with its connection to external generator. A large amount of slack in the myocardial electrode has been left to allow for growth.

Prophylactic

QRS COMPLEX GREATER THAN 0.10 SEC AND A HEART RATE OF 35 to 40/MIN. A greater potential for sudden death exists for children with complete heart block with a ventricular focus than for those who maintain ventricular activity at a higher atrioventricular nodal center. The electrocardiogram is readily recognizable (Fig. 13–4), and further diagnostic study is not required. Although the arrhythmia may remain stable for many years, pacemaker implantation is indicated regardless of lack of symptoms or the normality of other physiologic parameters.

RAPID ATRIAL RATE AND A SLOW VENTRICULAR RATE. The predictability of the development of congestive heart failure in infants with complete heart block and an atrial rate of approximately 150/min. and a ventricular rate of 50/min. is quite certain. In the infant particularly, adequate cardiac output under stress is maintained by in-

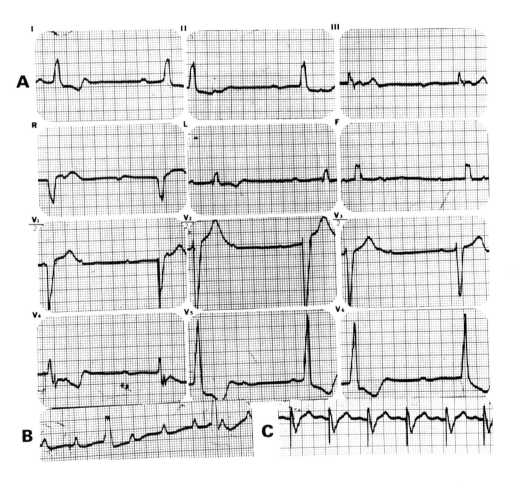

Fig. 13–4. Electrocardiographic pattern known to have been present since early infancy in a seventeen-year-old boy who had developed exertional dyspnea. There was no associated heart disease; a low cardiac output on exercise was demonstrated on cardiac catheterization. A, Complete heart block with an atrial rate of 60/min. and a ventricular rate of 32/min.; the QRS measures 0.14 sec. B, On exercise, atrial rate increases to 107/min. but ventricular rate is unchanged. C, Implantation of atrial synchronous pacemaker allowed return to normal physical activity.

creasing the heart rate, and congestive failure ensues if this is not possible, so that prompt institution of pacemaker implantation is required.

POSTOPERATIVE COMPLETE HEART BLOCK. Myocardial electrodes usually are implanted prior to closure of the chest in children undergoing complex cardiac operative procedures and those who demonstrate immediate postoperative heart block or significant arrhythmias (sinus or nodal bradycardia, supraventricular or ventricular tachycardia). An external cardiac pacemaker is attached for use immediately or on a standby basis. Use of the pacemaker will then depend on optimal rate and rhythm necessary for maintenance of adequate cardiac output. If there is no further concern about rhythm or adequacy of cardiac function without pacing, the myocardial electrodes are preferrably removed after three to four days.

If, however, by two weeks postoperatively, there is significant second degree block (Wenckebach block, especially with a slow rate, or 2:1 block or greater) or complete heart block, even though the child is asymptomatic, pacemaker implantation is indicated. If there seems to be a reasonable expectation that the arrhythmia will end, pulse generator implantation is not necessary at this time. Implantation of a radiofrequency receiving module to be used with an external generator is a relatively simple approach. The receiving unit is readily removable at a later date.

POSTOPERATIVE ARRHYTHMIAS OR SIGNIFICANT SINUS BRADYCARDIA. Because of better comprehension of the anatomy of the conduction system, availability of electrical methods for determination of the sites of its vulnerability and interruption, and improved surgical techniques, the incidence of postoperative complete heart block and symptomatic sinus nodal dysfunction has decreased drastically since the initial days of repair of congenital cardiac lesions. Permanent postoperative heart block now occurs only after the most complex operative

repairs, but delayed onset of heart block (up to 14 years postoperatively) still remains a potential problem.

Other predictability factors, in addition to the electrocardiographic pattern of right bundle branch block, left anterior hemiblock, and prolonged atrioventricular conduction, are early postoperative transient complete heart block and later appearance of arrhythmias (Fig. 13–5). Unfortunately complete heart block may also occur late in patients who have a normal postoperative electrocardiogram. Although electrophysiologic studies have shown two subgroups of surgically-induced right bundle branch block patterns, the demonstration of prolonged right ventricular activation time or H-V interval does not currently constitute an indication for prophylactic pacemaker implantation.

MANAGEMENT OF PACEMAKER IMPLANTATION

Many difficulties may be encountered in the management of children and adolescents who require pacemaker implantation. No solution is totally satisfactory. There are four major problems: (1) the size of the pacemaker relative to the child's size; (2) growth which stresses the lead system; (3) the fragility of the lead system resulting from the child's vigorous activity; (4) the short life of pacemakers hitherto available.

Division of childhood into three relatively distinct but overlapping periods is helpful in the understanding and attempted resolution of each problem.

Infancy to Age 2 Years. Because of the pacemaker's size and the rapidity of the child's growth, virtually no pacemaker designed for adults will be easily useful.

Age 2 to 10 Years. With progression of age, the problem of size diminishes and a variety of pulse generators can be used.

Age 10 to 18 Years. Most pulse generators, especially the smaller adult units, can be used. The problem of the

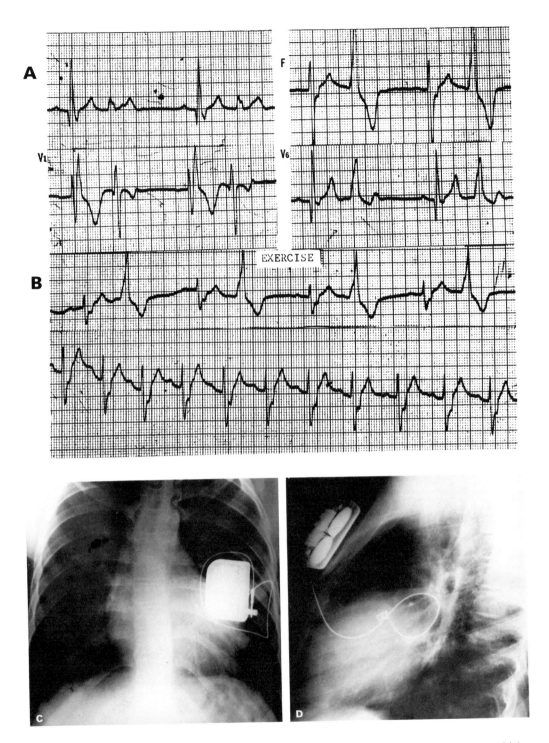

Fig. 13–5. Left anterior hemiblock and right bundle branch block occurred in nine-year-old boy subsequent to operation for tetralogy of Fallot. A, PR interval was prolonged and at 18 months postoperatively sinus rate decreased to 30/min. with ventricular escape. B, On mild exercise sinus rate increased to 88/min. with elimination of parasystolic focus. Although he was asymptomatic, "prophylactic" implantation of a ventricular inhibited pacemaker at a rate of 84/min. was performed. C and D, Thoracic implantation of pacemaker with myocardial electrode attachment via thoracotomy.

child's growth is twofold. During the first half of this period lower torso growth is rapid and that of the thorax less so, with the thorax reaching 90% of adult size by the time the child is twelve years of age. The problem of growth can be ameliorated by placement of the pulse generator in the subcutaneous tissue of the chest to take advantage of the smaller increase in its linear dimension during growth.

The thoracic volume increase, which is at the fourth power of linear increase, is relatively less important because the electrode, stressed by growth, is more sensitive to linear (height) than to volume growth. Despite the value of pacemaker implantation in the subcutaneous tissue of the abdomen earlier in childhood, where both the skin and the muscles of the abdominal wall yield to accommodate the pacemaker, during the later years when growth is rapid such implantation can present a serious problem.

Transvenous Versus Transthoracic Implantation

Implantation with thoracotomy has been considered superior to transvenous implantation largely because fixation of the myocardial electrode prevents its displacement and consequent cessation of pacing and because the venous system in the child is alleged to be too small for transvenous implantation. Although suture fixation to the myocardium is more secure than the fibrous fixation of the transvenous electrode, the transvenous route is both useful and successful, and we use it in almost all patients. Retromammary implantation of the unit in adolescent girls has been accomplished with an unusually good cosmetic result that is far superior to abdominal implantation.

In the child or adolescent with a relatively normal-sized right ventricle and normal right ventricular pressures, transvenous implantation offers no difficulties. The cephalic, external, or internal jugular vein

is usually of adequate size. If one is uncertain, a contrast medium can be injected to visualize the veins prior to the procedure.

A moderate amount of electrode slack, usually inappropriate, can remain in the right ventricle to allow for growth. Serial x-ray films at six-month intervals will indicate consumption of the extra length and tension on the point of intraventricular fixation. Before demonstrated electrode movement or tension, perhaps after one and a half to two years of growth, reexploration allows the introduction of additional electrode length and concomitant replacement of the pulse generator.

Implantation by thoracotomy offers similar growth problems. Growth places tension on the lead system fixed at the myocardium and the point of attachment of the lead to the pulse generator. Without movement of the generator, the electrode that lies in the mesothelial-lined subcutaneous tunnel cannot accommodate growth and it, too, requires revision by adding electrode length. If necessary, the pulse generator can be replaced at this time.

A technique, unused by us, is that of implantation by thoracotomy with fixation of the electrodes at the myocardium and placement of redundant electrode wire in the subcutaneous tissue within a Teflon bag. The redundant electrode is thus not fixed by an ingrowth of tissue and plays out as growth occurs.

Pacemaker Size

Fortunately the large-sized adult pacemakers of 150 to 200 gm weight and 80 to 100 ml volume no longer exist. Much smaller units are now manufactured and thus lessen the surgical problems of implantation. With rapid technologic development in decreasing pacemaker size the surgeon must therefore acquaint himself with the hardware available at the time of use. We have implanted in infants and small children a radiofrequency module, which weighs 18 gm and has a volume of 13 ml. Manufacture has been discontinued, but a few such modules are available at our institution for limited use, as these still remain the smallest pacemakers obtainable.

Problems with size have resulted in pulse generators being placed in the subcutaneous tissue, the retroperitoneal space, the pelvis, the properitoneal abdominal space, and within the thorax. Because of the relatively short life span of all but a nuclear generator and the need for electrode remanipulation, it is not advisable to implant the generator so deeply as to make a secondary procedure difficult.

Selection of Pulse Generator and Pacing Mode

Most children with complete heart block have fixed block with no evidence of atrioventricular conduction, few premature contractions, and a junctional focus with a rate of 50 to 60/min. Syncopal attacks are usually episodic and unpredictable. Many are not constantly pacemaker-dependent so that sudden cessation of pacemaker function does not necessarily result in immediate syncope or sudden death. The potential for syncope is even less in those symptomatic due to sinus nodal dysfunction. In children paced to maintain cardiac output because of slow heart rates caused by either complete heart block or sinus nodal dysfunction, failure of pacemaker function has even less imminent danger.

Asynchronous (VOO)*

Almost all children with complete heart block can be managed with an asynchronous pacemaker. Children with sinus nodal

---

* The three-letter code for pacemaker terminology is used as suggested in the report on Cardiac Pacemakers of Inter-Society Commission on Heart Disease Resources.

dysfunction who require a more rapid rate for maintenance of cardiac output and for whom sensing of cardiac rate is not important can also be handled with this modality. Two types have been available: radiofrequency and wholly implanted pacemakers.

RADIOFREQUENCY PACING. One of the earliest pacemakers available, the passive radiofrequency implantable capsule, receives energy by transmission across the skin from a pulse generator and antenna carried externally. The implantable module can be attached to an endocardial or myocardial electrode. The external generator contains rate and output adjustment controls, is large, and is carried in a garment. Batteries in the external module are consumed rapidly but are readily replaced when exhausted. The rate can be varied as necessary, and pacing can be discontinued, yet held in readiness should it be required. At maximum the output of this unit is greater than that of any of the small wholly implantable units.

There are two major disadvantages, however. Only an asynchronous pacing mode is available; no noncompetitive (VVI) circuitry has been developed and none seems likely. Also, only children who are not pacemaker-dependent can be managed with radiofrequency pacing because the antenna must be removed during bathing and it frequently falls from the skin. The implantable capsule, despite its simplicity of construction, has not been more reliable than conventional units and the associated antenna and external pulse generator have been subject to mechanical and electronic failures.

WHOLLY IMPLANTED UNIT. The smallest of the implantable pulse generators previously available has been a mercury-zinc unit weighing 78 gm and of 45 ml volume. Presently 57 gm lithium cell generators for pediatric use exist. A noninvasively programmable lithium unit weighing 80 gm, with rates of 30 to 120 beats per minute, is newly available.

Noncompetitive Pacemakers (VVI)

Ventricular inhibited (VVI) units of small size have also recently become available. Pacemakers at pediatric rates (80 to 110/ min.) with ventricular inhibited circuitry, weighing 50 to 75 gm, now exist. Since units with modern ventricular inhibited circuitry are no larger than asynchronous units, ventricular inhibited generators are preferred.

Atrial Synchronous (VAT)

Atrial control of ventricular rate, retaining both the atrial contribution and physiologic rate variability, seems desirable, especially in children who are free of significant myocardial disease and have stable, physiologically responsive atrial activity. Unfortunately, no atrial synchronous pacemaker of truly pediatric size has been manufactured and those available present a significant surgical problem for smaller children because of size. The smallest programmable atrial synchronous unit weighs 92 gm (Omni Atricor 192, Cordis Corporation, Miami, Florida).

Of equal importance is the difficulty with which an atrial synchronous pacemaker synchronizes to produce a ventricular rate of 150 or more per minute. The atrioventricular delay and refractory period in older units allows a maximum rate of 140/min. and yields poor synchronization and an erratic ventricular rate at an atrial rate of 170 to 190/min., especially if intermittent ventricular conduction exists. An atrial synchronous, ventricular noncompetitive pacemaker is now available and may display superior characteristics.

Although we have not performed cardiac output studies on children during atrial synchronous and single rate pacing, clinical benefits from atrial synchrony have not been observed. The one child in our series who was changed from atrial synchronous (VAT) to ventricular inhibited (VVI) pacing has had no alteration in clinical state or in normal exercise tolerance. Adult patients who have been changed from atrial synchronous (VAT) pacemakers to single rate pacing, either noncompetitive (VVI) or asynchronous (VOO) units only infrequently have shown symptomatic or physiologic deterioration. The conversion from single rate to atrial synchronous pacing seems beneficial only in special circumstances.

Pacemaker Longevity

Interest in prolonged pulse generator longevity, although well founded in adults, is of far less importance in children, inasmuch as the major problems are pacemaker size and the child's growth. Because of the problems induced by growth and the need for introducing greater electrode length, prolonged generator longevity is not necessarily an asset, for generator replacement can readily be accomplished at the time of modification of electrode position or length.

For these reasons we have seen no great necessity to implant nuclear-powered generators. One has been implanted in a 17-year-old boy who had probably reached maximum growth and was not physically active, on the presumption that this would obviate subsequent recurrent operative procedures. We have been reluctant to install nuclear materials in a growing child and especially in a retromammary position in adolescent girls, despite the manufacturers' assurances.

Pulse Generator Rate

Only single rate generators in pediatric size have been obtainable. Programmable units weighing 70 to 80 gm are now becoming available. For children aged less than two years, rates of 100 to 125/min. have been used; from 2 to 10 years, rates of 90 to

100/min. at the earlier ages and of 80 to 85/min. at later ages; and for children aged 10 or more years, rates of 75 to 80/min. During later adolescence, the conventional adult rate of 70/min. has been selected. These rates, though not totally physiologic, seem to allow adequate cardiac output under stress and physical activity. The ventricular inhibited mode allows for the increase in sinus rate on activity in children paced because of symptomatic sinus nodal dysfunction and in the occasional child or adolescent with complete heart block who may have a significant increase in junctional rate in response to physical activity.

MANAGEMENT POSTIMPLANTATION

Immediate postimplantation care is relatively simple. Little other than observation for pacemaker function and follow-up chest

TABLE 13–1

Indications for Operation in 21 Patients with Cardiac Pacemakers

INDICATION	INSTANCES (no.)
Generator insertion or change	
Initial implantation	21
Routine replacement	21
Manufacturer's recall	2
Reimplantation	3
Electronic modification	7
Change in pacing mode	
(2 cases)	
Electronic failure	
(5 cases)	
Electrode fracture	6
Pacing discontinued (removal)	2
Wound revision	1
Infection	8
7 procedures (1 patient—	
same infection)	
1 procedure (1 patient)	
TOTAL	71

roentgenograms for determination of retention of the position of the transvenously implanted electrode in the apex of the venous ventricle is required. Prior to discharge, five days for patients with transvenous implants and seven to ten days for those with myocardial implants by thoracotomy, a final pacemaker check is made.

Usually patients are then recalled one month following hospital discharge for operative wound and pacemaker evaluation. Thereafter monitoring is by telephone, particularly for those living at a distance, and by repeated clinic visits at intervals of three to four months until battery depletion is imminent. During the period of rapid growth, x-ray evaluation of the length of and tension on the intraventricular or myocardial electrode is made at six-month intervals. Except for contact sports which are discouraged in an effort to minimize electronic failure due to direct trauma, participation in normal physical activity is allowed.

PROBLEMS AND COMPLICATIONS

Because of frequent monitoring and therefore early detection of electronic failure, and despite precautions to avoid trauma, rehospitalization has been frequent. Thus in 21 patients over an 11-year period, with an average duration of pacing of 60 months, 71 operative procedures have been required (Table 13–1). The relatively recent availability of improved hardware has, however, reduced the incidence of such intervention.

Operative procedures have always necessitated rehospitalization. Although routine replacement of the pacer generator has been the most frequent cause (ranging from 18 to 40 months), electronic failures and electrode fracture have been relatively common and proportionately more frequent than in adults. Infection, with one exception, due to too large a pacemaker which no longer would be used, has not been a significant problem.

Three children have had too large a pacemaker. One was initially referred for wound revision of an impending skin breakdown over an adult-sized pacemaker; another, who also underwent implantation elsewhere with an adult-sized unit, showed skin tightening and required generator replacement to relieve the tenuous integrity of the skin. The third, a two-year-old child with an atrial synchronous pacemaker placed in the subcutaneous tissue of the abdomen, sustained a size-related wound breakdown that led to infection and ultimately death from sepsis.

LONG-TERM RESULTS

It must be emphasized that the ultimate fate of the child with a pacemaker implant is unknown. Maximal duration of implantation has been 11 years and mean duration 6 years. Eighteen of the 21 patients are well and pursue normal physical activity except for contact sports.

Only one patient, now three years since implant, requires digoxin. Her electrocardiogram, acquired after cardiac catheterization, indicates diffuse infarction of the anterior myocardial wall, and the echocardiogram shows evidence of significant left ventricular dysfunction.

Three patients in our series have died, only one as a result of pacemaker implantation with subsequent infection. In the other two patients, death could not be attributed to implantation or pacemaker failure. One four-year-old girl paced postoperatively died two months later of advanced heart disease inadequately corrected surgically. The other, who was not pacemaker-dependent, died at age 21 years of unknown cause after four years of pacing. The original indication for pacemaker implantation had been an idioventricular rhythm at a rate of 30/min. and a low cardiac output on moderate exercise. Gross postmortem ex-

amination did not reveal the cause, but the pacemaker was operating normally.

In two asymptomatic children, permanent pacing was instituted postoperatively because of anticipated persistence of complete heart block. Spontaneous reversion to sinus rhythm in both allowed removal of the radiofrequency pacemaker three and two months after implantation. The children have since remained in sinus rhythm for seven years and two years. In the latter, His bundle study one year postoperatively showed prolongation of both A-H and H-V intervals at atrial pacing rates slower than those that yield a normal response in children. This may have some ominous portent for the future.

In an 18-month-old child, who had postoperative sinus nodal dysfunction with intermittent Wenckebach phenomenon and consequent congestive heart failure because of the slow ventricular rate, the radiofrequency pacemaker was continued at a rate of 90 to 100/min. for one year. When the pacemaker was inactivated, the patient's heart rate ranged from 70 to 150 beats/min. with intermittent Wenckebach periods. The faster rates did not necessarily occur at times of stress, but no evidence of congestive heart failure developed. Because electrophysiologic study revealed prolongation of the A-H interval, persistent Wenckebach conduction at slow atrial pacing rates, and a markedly variable spontaneous atrial rate, the radiofrequency receiver and transvenous leads were left in place, but pacing was held in abeyance.

Despite the requirements of frequent telephone monitoring, direct examination, repeated periods of hospitalization, a distorted physical appearance from the implanted pacemaker, and operative scars and knowledge of the dependence of cardiac function on an electronic apparatus, these children and adolescents have shown a gratifying degree of emotional health. Fear of pacemaker failure has not been verbally expressed nor manifested by regressive or dependent behavior.

Early indoctrination of the patient, and especially the parents, is required. The parental attitude of overprotectiveness toward the child is readily recognizable and understandable. It is important, therefore, to spend considerable time to assure the parents of the protective aspects of the pacemaker implant but still to emphasize the necessity for frequent surveillance. Once the parent is freed of excessive concern, the child readily returns to normal physical activity and peer group participation.

SELECTED READINGS

Benrey, J., et al.: Permanent pacemaker implantation in infants, children and adolescents. Long-term follow-up. Circulation, 53:245, 1976.

Campbell, M., and Emanuel, R.: Six cases of congenital complete heart block followed for 34–40 years. Br. Heart J., 29:577, 1967.

Dodinot, D., Dupuis, C., and Pernot, C.: Indications et techniques de l'entrainement electrosystolique chez l'enfant. Ann. Cardiol. Angeiol. (Paris), 21:371, 1972.

Furman, S., and Young, D.: Cardiac pacing in children and adolescents. Am. J. Cardiol., 39:550, 1977.

Galdston, R., and Gamble, W.J.: On borrowed time. Observations on children with implanted pacemakers and their families. Am. J. Psychiatry, 126:104, 1969.

Glenn, W.W.L., et al.: Heart block in children: treatment with radio-frequency pacemaker. J. Thorac. Cardiovasc. Surg., 58:361, 1969.

Lindesmith, G.G., et al.: Experience with an implantable synchronous pacemaker in children. Ann. Thorac. Surg., 6:358, 1968.

Liu, L., Griffiths, S.P., and Gerst, P.H.: Implanted cardiac pacemakers in children. Am. J. Cardiol., 20:639, 1967.

Michaëlsson, J., and Engle, M.A.: Congenital complete heart block: an international study of the natural history. Cardiovasc. Clin., 4:85, 1972.

Molthan, M.E., et al.: Congenital heart block with fatal Adams-Stokes attacks in childhood. Pediatrics, 30:32, 1962.

Parsonnet, V., Furman, S., and Smyth, N.P.D.: Implantable cardiac pacemakers. Status report and resource guideline. Circulation, 50:A21, 1974.

Radford, D.J., and Izukawa, T.: Sick sinus syndrome. Symptomatic cases in children. Arch. Dis. Child., 50:879, 1975.

Reiffer, J.A., et al.: Ability of Holter electrocardiographic recording and atrial stimulation to detect sinus nodal dysfunction in symptomatic and asymptomatic patients with sinus bradycardia. Am. J. Cardiol., 40:189, 1977.

Scott, O., Macartney, F.J., and Deverall, P.B.: Sick sinus syndrome in children. Arch. Dis. Child., 51:100, 1976.

Siddons, H.: Transvenous pacing in the child. Ann. Cardiol. Angeiol. (Paris), 20:445, 1971.

Stanton, R.E., Lindesmith, G.G., and Meyer, B.W.: Pacemaker therapy in children with complete heart block. Am. J. Dis. Child., 129:484, 1975.

Steeg, C.N., et al.: Postoperative left anterior hemiblock and right bundle branch block following repair of tetralogy of Fallot. Clinical and etiological considerations. Circulation, 51:1026, 1975.

Sung, R.J., et al.: Analysis of surgically-induced right bundle branch block pattern using intracardiac recording techniques. Circulation, 54:442, 1976.

Vanetti, A., et al.: Techniques et indications de l'entrainement electrosystolique chez l'enfant. Arch. Mal. Coeur, 65:805, 1972.

Young, D., et al.: Wenckebach AV block (Mobitz type I) in children and adolescents. Am. J. Cardiol., 40:393, 1977.

14

Cardiac Pacing for Refractory Arrhythmias

PETER R. FOSTER
DOUGLAS P. ZIPES

Cardiac pacing, alone or in combination with various drugs, has been used to terminate acutely recurrent tachyarrhythmias resistant to antiarrhythmic agents, as well as to prevent them on a chronic basis. This chapter (1) reviews briefly the present understanding of the genesis of cardiac arrhythmias to provide a rationale for pacing, (2) discusses the different modes of pacing that can be used, (3) evaluates the response of various tachyarrhythmias to cardiac pacing, and (4) offers some indications when pacing might be used to treat tachycardias.

GENESIS OF TACHYARRHYTHMIAS

A knowledge of the mechanisms involved in the genesis of arrhythmias is necessary to understand and utilize fully the concepts of pacing to treat arrhythmias. In general, arrhythmias may be characterized as arising from disorders of impulse formation (automaticity), impulse conduction, or a combination of the two. Automaticity is the unique property of pacemaker cells which maintains a rhythmic spontaneous depolarization and is due to diastolic (phase 4) depolarization. Since this usually occurs most rapidly in the sinus node, sinus rhythm normally is present. Diastolic depolarization may be either abnormally decreased or enhanced by a variety of factors. Bradycardia or asystole may result from decreased automaticity of the sinus node and latent escape pacemakers and is easily treated with a pacemaker.

Enhanced automaticity may take many different abnormal forms and affect any pacemaker tissue. Since tachyarrhythmias due to enhanced automaticity depend on the increase in rate of diastolic depolarization, which is self-perpetuating from cycle to cycle, therapy ideally consists of removing any physiologic or pharmacologic precipitating factors or of using antiarrhythmic drugs to decrease phase 4 depolarization. Enhanced automaticity at times may be controlled by pacing which may suppress the automatic focus by several mechanisms. Thus, overdrive pacing occasionally suppresses rhythms felt to be automatic, although definite proof that a particular tachycardia in man is due to an automatic mechanism is extremely difficult to obtain.

Disorders of impulse conduction may present as first, second, or third degree heart block, most commonly recognized at the level of the atrioventricular (AV) node or distal His-Purkinje system. When symptomatic bradycardia due to AV block is diagnosed, artificial pacing is the accepted therapy. However, impaired conduction may also lead to reentry and tachyarrhythmias. The concept of a "circus movement" dates back at least to the early 1900s, when Mayer observed that a single stimulus could initiate constant cyclic reexcitation in the rings of jelly fish. Since that time, many investigators have contributed greatly to the understanding of the mechanisms involved in reentry, but the basic characteristics, outlined initially by Mayer, Mines, Erlanger, and Schmitt, have not been altered significantly.

The electrophysiologic prerequisites to establish a reentrant circuit include the presence of at least two functionally separate pathways with unidirectional block in one and slow conduction in the other. De-

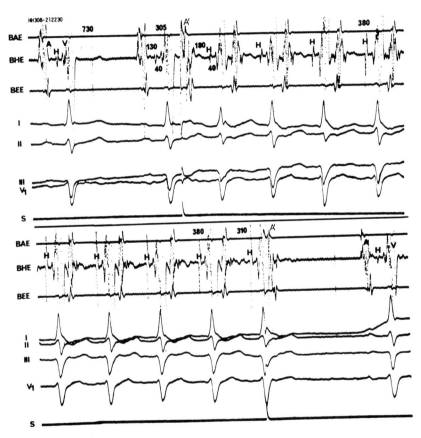

Fig. 14–1. Initiation and termination of paroxysmal supraventricular tachycardia (PSVT) by premature atrial stimulation. Top panel, premature atrial stimulation (A') 305 msec after the last spontaneous sinus beat initiated PSVT. During PSVT, premature atrial stimulation 310 msec after the last spontaneous atrial depolarization restored sinus rhythm (bottom panel).
    BAE, bipolar atrial electrogram; BHE, bipolar His electrogram; BEE, bipolar esophageal electrogram; I, II, III, V₁, surface ECG leads I, II, III, V₁; S, stimulus channel; A, atrial depolarization; H, His bundle deflection; V, ventricular depolarization. Paper speed, 100 mm/sec. All numbers in msec.

layed excitation distal to the site of block may lead to reexcitation proximal to the site of block if the conduction time for a complete circuit exceeds the refractory period of the tissue proximal to the block. When these prerequisites are met, reentry may occur within the atrium, the AV junction, the ventricle, or over two anatomically discrete pathways such as in the Wolff-Parkinson-White (WPW) syndrome. In some patients without evidence of accessory bypass tracts, the presence of "dual AV nodal pathways" that exhibit different functional properties has been suggested as a possible basis for supraventricular tachycardia.

Onset of a reentrant tachyarrhythmia by a critical degree of conduction delay in one pathway and block in an alternate pathway is most frequently initiated by one or more premature systoles (Fig. 14–1). With critical timing, a single reentrant beat may be followed by a tachycardia which continues in a self-perpetuating manner. One or more critically timed pacemaker stimuli will effectively interrupt a reentrant circuit, similar to the effects of direct current cardioversion, by depolarizing and thus blocking one of the reentrant pathways, so that the returning impulse encounters a refractory pathway and cannot continue to propagate (Fig. 14–1).

The response of a tachyarrhythmia to single premature or multiple stimuli has been used to differentiate between the mechanisms of reentry and automaticity. If an arrhythmia can be initiated or terminated by premature stimulation, it is assumed to be due to reentrant excitation. Although clinically this criterion is still useful, experimental evidence indicates that the coronary sinus, AV valves exposed to catecholamines, and Purkinje fibers exposed to acetylstrophanthidin exhibit the property of "triggered automaticity." In these tissues, single or multiple stimuli applied to a quiescent fiber may initiate a series of spontaneous depolarizations caused by an unusual form of automaticity. Premature stimulation may also terminate the "tachycardia." At this time, however, this type of arrhythmia has not yet been demonstrated in man.

When a supraventricular tachycardia

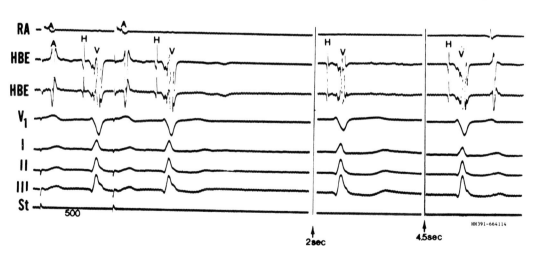

Fig. 14–2. Prolonged sinus node recovery time. Right atrial pacing at a cycle length of 500 msec for 2 minutes was suddenly discontinued (last two paced beats are shown). Over 2 minutes elapsed before an escape beat, originating in or near the His bundle, resulted. Approximately 7 seconds following cessation of right atrial pacing, the first sinus impulse occurred (last impulse in right panel). Ventriculoatrial block of the escape beats was present. Sections of the tracing have been cut out (arrows). Conventions as in Figure 14–1.

suddenly terminates, the cardiac pacemaker with the fastest intrinsic rate (usually the sinus node) regains control and establishes the cardiac rhythm. However, overdrive suppression of the sinus node may occur when sinus node disease is present and significant periods of asystole may result before the sinus node resumes discharging or a subsidiary pacemaker escape occurs (Fig. 14–2). This syndrome of alternating periods of slow and rapid heart rate has become known as the bradycardia-tachycardia syndrome and frequently requires combined treatment with a pacemaker (to prevent bradycardia) and drugs. Another form of the brady-tachycardia syndrome occurs in patients with advanced AV block and slow heart rates punctuated by bouts of ventricular tachyarrhythmias (Fig. 14–3). Ventricular pacing at more rapid rates usually eliminates the ventricular tachyarrhythmias. The most likely explanation for these ventricular tachyarrhythmias occurring in association with bradycardia seems to be that a greater disparity in duration of action potential and refractory periods exists at slow heart rates. This creates temporal dispersion of the recovery of excitability, which may be accentuated by premature extrasystoles, leading to inhomogeneous areas of conduction delay and block which favors re-entry. Pacing at faster rates during nonischemic conditions may improve the synchrony of recovery and alleviate the ventricular arrhythmias.

It is important to note that accelerating the heart rate in the presence of ischemia may increase the degree of conduction delay present in the ischemic area and therefore increase the temporal dispersion of refractoriness. These changes may result in ventricular tachycardia and fibrillation and therefore caution should be used when pacing patients who have a myocardial infarction to find an optimal heart rate that alleviates the arrhythmia but does not exacerbate the ischemia or provoke new arrhythmias.

MODES OF PACING

Temporary cardiac pacing is performed transvenously, whereas permanent pacing can be accomplished using electrodes placed endocardially via a transvenous route or epicardially via thoracotomy. The leads generally used have unipolar or bipolar electrodes. Leads with multiple electrodes are often employed during diagnostic electrophysiologic (His bundle) studies in order to use one lead to simultaneously record intracardiac electrocardiograms during pacing.

Pacing, either temporary, using an exter-

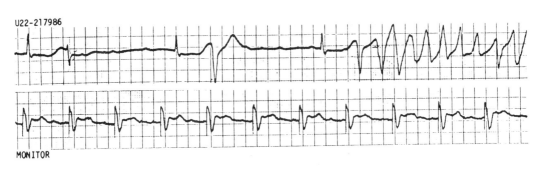

Fig. 14–3. Complete heart block and ventricular tachycardia. Complete heart block with an independent ventricular escape focus, coupled ventricular extrasystoles, and a run of ventricular tachycardia are seen in the top strip. Right ventricular pacing at a rate of 75/minute (bottom panel) prevented recurrence of ventricular extrasystoles and ventricular tachycardia.

nal unit, or permanent, using an implanted unit, may be performed in a number of different ways, depending on the needs of a specific situation. Demand pacing provides a noncompetitive mode of pacing during which spontaneous depolarizations inhibit the pacemaker or trigger the pacemaker to discharge harmlessly into the refractory period of the spontaneous beat. During fixed-rate pacing, the pacemaker discharges repetitively, unaffected by the spontaneous cardiac rhythm. A magnet held over some demand pacemakers will cause them to function in a fixed rate mode.

Many external units and some newer permanent pacemakers can provide coupled or paired pacing. Coupled pacing consists of delivering a stimulus to the heart at a preselected coupling interval following a spontaneous beat; paired pacing provides a series of two sequential stimuli, either coupled to the intrinsic rhythm or delivered in a regularly recurring competitive manner.

Most pacemaker units for temporary ventricular pacing have a maximum rate of approximately 150 to 180/minute. Some relatively new atrial pacemakers will discharge at rates exceeding 1000 times per minute. These should not be used for ventricular pacing because of the danger of inducing ventricular fibrillation.

A number of recent advances in pacemaker technology have been applied to control tachyarrhythmias on a permanent basis. A bifocal demand pacemaker with both atrial and ventricular pacing, but only ventricular sensing, or a newly developed pulse generator that senses atrial and ventricular activity, but only paces the ventricle, provides the capability for sequential atrioventricular contraction with an adjustable AV delay. In certain instances, these units have been found to prevent paroxysmal reentrant, supraventricular tachycardias, possibly by eliminating retrograde conduction to the atrium during ventricular pacing.

Other pacing approaches to terminate tachyarrhythmias include a rate scanning pacemaker which, when activated by a magnet held over the skin externally, increases its rate each successive beat over a two-minute period from 165 to 300/minute or until inactivated by removal of the magnet. A different type of scanning pacemaker provides single or double atrial or ventricular stimuli at an initial predetermined coupling interval which increases by 5 milliseconds after each beat up to 100 milliseconds or until cessation of the tachycardia. A dual demand pacemaker is essentially a demand pacemaker modified to discharge at a fixed rate of approximately 70 times per minute when a spontaneous heart rate falls below 70 or exceeds 150/minute. It may be used to terminate supraventricular tachycardia. Radiofrequency pacemakers, activated by the patient with an external transmitter at the onset of supraventricular-tachycardia, provide rapid atrial stimulation at adjustable rates for selected patients with recurrent paroxysmal supraventricular tachycardia (PSVT) (Fig. 14–4) and, at times, for patients with recurrent ventricular tachycardia. Many of the more recent

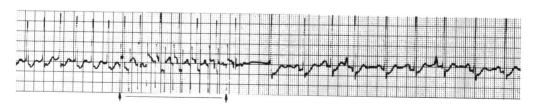

Fig. 14–4. Termination of PSVT by activation of radio frequency atrial pacing (250 minutes). In the left portion of the tracing, PSVT at a rate of 210/minute can be seen. Between the arrows, the patient activated a radio frequency pacemaker which promptly restored sinus rhythm.

pacemakers may be programmed externally so that some of the pacemaker features such as rate, stimulus intensity or duration, or various pacing intervals may be altered noninvasively.

A new orthorhythmic pacemaker has been introduced in the United States. At the present time this unit consists of an external temporary pacemaker that can function in either the fixed rate or demand mode and provide coupled stimulation with a coupling interval fixed either in milliseconds or as a specific percentage of the preceding R-R interval. This percentage may be chosen between minus 70% and plus 30% of the preceding R-R interval, whether spontaneous or paced. It can also be programmed to initiate from 1 to 10 consecutive stimuli separated by a preset interval to follow the coupled stimulation. This programmed cardiac stimulation may be triggered manually or initiated automatically when a predetermined number of spontaneous R-R intervals fall within a preset rate. In Europe, this orthorhythmic programmable cardiac stimulator has met with initial success in the termination of supraventricular as well as ventricular arrhythmias.

Various types of arrhythmias require different methods of pacing for successful suppression. To attempt overdrive suppression of an intermittent rhythm such as ventricular ectopy unresponsive to drugs, the rate of pacing is gradually increased to a level at which the ectopy decreases to an acceptable degree. Likewise, an optimum rate may be determined for correcting a bradycardia conducive to reentrant arrhythmias. The degree of success and optimum rate for arrhythmia suppression must be determined on a temporary basis before any thought is entertained of implanting a permanent pacemaker. Complicating the problem is the possibility that pacing parameters successfully suppressing tachycardia during an electrophysiologic study may be different in the ambulatory patient.

When interrupting a reentrant tachyarrhythmia, single or multiple stimuli may be delivered randomly or coupled to the spontaneous rhythm at precise intervals in an attempt to preexcite one limb of the circuit and render it refractory to the returning impulse. Stimulating close to the site of the reentrant pathway increases the chance of successfully initiating and terminating reentrant tachycardias and may require stimulating a specific chamber, a specific site within a chamber, or two chambers (atrium or ventricle) simultaneously.

Paired pacing may be more advantageous than single pacing when the refractory period at the site of stimulation is long or the stimulus is delivered far from the reentrant pathway and penetrating the reentrant pathway is difficult. In this situation, the first of two stimuli may preexcite and "peel back" the refractory period of the atrium or ventricle, thus providing the second stimulus an earlier, excitable gap to enter the reentrant circuit.

Rapid atrial pacing may terminate effectively many atrial arrhythmias, either by interrupting the reentrant circuit or by inducing atrial fibrillation. In some situations, atrial fibrillation purposely is induced because, as a less stable rhythm, it will usually revert to sinus rhythm, within a short time. In addition, because of the phenomenon of repetitive concealed conduction into the AV node, the ventricular rate usually slows when atrial fibrillation occurs and is generally easily controlled by administration of digitalis. Similarly, rapid atrial stimulation or paired atrial stimulation has also been employed to produce 2:1 or greater degrees of AV block and thereby slow the resultant ventricular rate.

ATRIAL FLUTTER

The ventricular rate during atrial flutter is often difficult to control with digitalis alone, and atrial pacing is used relatively early to treat this arrhythmia. Stimuli are delivered most frequently at rates faster than the atrial flutter rate in an attempt to interrupt this presumably reentrant rhythm. Following interruption of the atrial flutter, pacing is terminated, and approximately 50 to 75% of patients will develop normal sinus rhythm either immediately or later following the termination of an intervening unstable rhythm such as atrial fibrillation. Because a variable period of asystole may occur after terminating the tachycardia because of overdrive suppression of the sinus node, the investigator should be prepared to treat this when necessary with the atrial pacemaker already in place.

Some patients fail to convert to sinus rhythm or atrial fibrillation with pacing alone. However, before a patient is considered a failure, the position of the pacing electrode should be evaluated fluoroscopically to assure good endocardial contact has been accomplished. In other patients carotid sinus massage or other vagal maneuvers concomitant with atrial pacing may successfully terminate the atrial flutter when pacing alone fails. This treatment probably succeeds because the increase in vagal tone shortens the atrial refractory period and may allow the pacing stimuli to penetrate the reentrant pathway. Failure to terminate apparent atrial flutter with rapid atrial pacing may indicate the presence of dissimilar atrial rhythms such as atrial fibrillation in one atrium and atrial flutter in the other. In our experience with these patients atrial flutter cannot be terminated with pacing and direct current cardioversion is required. It may be conjectured as well that some failures in terminating presumed atrial flutter may be secondary to the presence of an automatic rather than a reentrant rhythm responsible for the tachycardia.

ATRIAL FIBRILLATION

Atrial pacing has not been reported to successfully terminate atrial fibrillation which generally requires either drug therapy or DC cardioversion. The reason for this is multiple, randomly advancing wave fronts that probably cause atrial fibrillation and create marked temporal dispersion of excitation and recovery so that even the capture of small areas of atrial muscle by pacing fails to terminate the overall rhythm. Simultaneous depolarization of a large portion of both atria is required for conversion to normal sinus rhythm.

PAROXYSMAL ATRIAL AND JUNCTIONAL TACHYCARDIA

Paroxysmal atrial tachycardia (PAT) and paroxysmal junctional tachycardia (PJT) are both assumed to be due to reentry in the atrium and/or the AV junction and generally may be easily terminated by atrial pacing and, in some patients, by ventricular pacing. The distinction between PAT and PJT may be difficult, and they are often unceremoniously lumped together and called PSVT. Pacing has been reported to terminate approximately 85% of spontaneously occurring episodes of PSVT (Figs. 14–1, 14–4). Most of these patients will develop normal sinus rhythm directly, and the remainder will develop normal sinus rhythm after a transient period of atrial fibrillation. A small number of patients will convert back to PAT or PJT. In the His bundle, laboratory pacing almost uniformly terminates paroxysmal atrial or junctional tachycardia which has been initiated during electrophysiologic studies.

In addition to the experience with temporary pacing to terminate PSVT, permanent atrial and ventricular pacing has been used chronically for long-term treatment. Competitive atrial or ventricular pacing, usually initiated by a magnet held over a demand unit, represented the initial approach, sometimes combined with drug therapy, and in selected patients was quite successful. More recently, atrial synchronous pacemakers with adjustable AV delay, paired atrial pacing with induced 2:1 AV block, rate scanning pacemakers, continuous rapid atrial pacing, dual demand pacemakers, patient-activated radiofrequency pacemakers (Fig. 14–4), and orthorhythmic pacing have been used and have met with a high incidence of success in terminating PSVT. In general these patients have been carefully selected on the basis of electrophysiologic studies performed prior to insertion of a permanent pacemaker.

The initial assessment of the patient being considered for therapy with a permanent pacemaker usually includes invasive electrophysiologic (His bundle) studies during which refractory periods of the atrium, AV node, and ventricle are determined, the echo zone and mechanism of the tachycardia are established, and the tachycardia is initiated and terminated on multiple occasions. The echo zone is the interval during which premature stimulation of the atrium or ventricle initiates the tachycardia. During these episodes, various sites in the atrium, coronary sinus, and ventricle are paced to establish a successful approach to terminate the PSVT. The pacing site may be critical, so that right ventricular pacing may successfully terminate the tachycardia, but left ventricular pacing may not or, similarly, left atrial pacing may be successful, but right atrial pacing may not. These factors must be determined on a temporary basis prior to insertion of the permanent pacemaker.

Many ectopic atrial tachycardias, nonparoxysmal junctional tachycardia, and multifocal atrial tachycardia are rhythms thought possibly to be associated with increased automaticity, and pacing may be of limited value in their control. Theoretically, atrial pacing to convert multifocal atrial tachycardia (chaotic atrial rhythm) to atrial fibrillation may be of occasional value in more easily controlling the ventricular rate with digitalis. Paired ventricular pacing has been used following open heart surgery to control the rapid ventricular rate during a presumed automatic AV junctional tachycardia. Paired ventricular pacing in-

volves delivering a stimulus to the ventricle at a premature interval too short to produce mechanical contraction, thus effectively halving the heart rate. Such premature ventricular stimulation may precipitate ventricular fibrillation in the setting of ischemia, electrolyte imbalance, hypoxia, or digitalis intoxication. To minimize this possibility, the premature stimulus should be of short duration (less than 1 to 2 milliseconds) and of minimum intensity (less than twice the diastolic threshold). Continuous electrocardiographic and intra-arterial pressure monitoring is recommended during this procedure.

SINUS TACHYCARDIA

Sinus tachycardia may be an undesirable tachyarrhythmia when it markedly impairs ventricular function and cardiac output during certain disease states or jeopardizes the preservation of ischemic myocardium in the presence of acute myocardial infarction. Paired or coupled atrial pacing may effectively slow the ventricular rate by introducing the premature atrial stimulus when the AV node is still refractory. This results in 2:1 AV block and effectively reduces the ventricular rate. To accomplish this reduction the refractory period of the AV node must exceed the refractory period of the right atrium.

WOLFF-PARKINSON-WHITE SYNDROME

Therapy of reentrant supraventricular tachycardias in patients who have the Wolff-Parkinson-White (WPW) syndrome creates special problems because of the presence of one or more accessory bypass tracts, which circumvent the safety features of slow AV nodal conduction. Because of the increased conduction velocity in the accessory pathway, very rapid ventricular rates are possible during atrial fibrillation, atrial flutter, or rapid atrial pacing. Caution

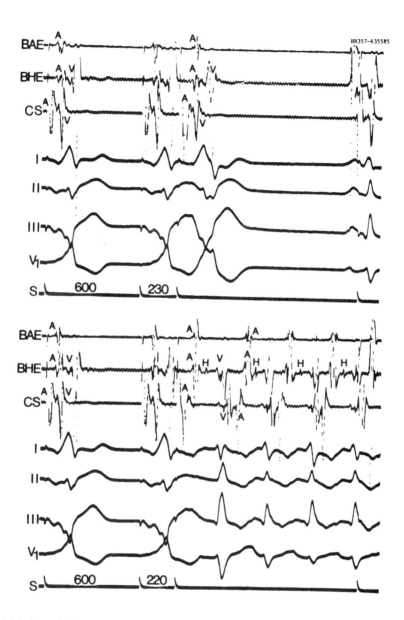

Fig. 14–5. Initiation of PSVT in patient with Wolff-Parkinson-White syndrome. Last two beats of a regular train at 600 msec and premature stimulus are shown. Top recording, premature left atrial stimulation at cycle length of 230 msec was followed by conduction over accessory pathway to ventricle. Bottom panel, shortening premature interval to 220 msec was followed by conduction to ventricle over normal pathway (antegrade block occurred in accessory pathway) and initiation of supraventricular tachycardia. Note that during supraventricular tachycardia, sequence of atrial activation was earliest in left atrium (CS, coronary sinus recording), followed by low right atrial (BHE) and high right atrial (RA) activation. This finding is consistent with retrograde atrial activation over a left-sided bypass tract. Conventions as in Figure 14–1.

should always be exercised during atrial pacing at short cycle lengths in patients with the WPW syndrome, not only because each stimulus may be conducted to the ventricles, but because of the potentially serious consequences of inducing atrial fibrillation or atrial flutter with rapid ventricular rates. On occasion, ventricular fibrillation may result owing to rapid ventricular rates during atrial fibrillation or atrial flutter.

Most commonly, during paroxysmal supraventricular tachycardia in patients with the WPW syndrome, the impulse travels over a circuit in which antegrade conduction (from the atrium to the ventricle) is over the AV node and retrograde conduction (from ventricle to atrium) is over the accessory pathway (Fig. 14–5). Interruption of this reentrant rhythm may be accomplished by prematurely stimulating either the atrium or the ventricle with stimuli appropriately timed to render one limb of the pathway refractory to the returning impulse. In some patients, "concealed WPW" may exist, during which the accessory pathway conducts only in a retrograde direction. The lack of antegrade conduction obviates evidence of WPW in the scalar 12 lead electrocardiogram, and the diagnosis is usually made only by invasive electrophysiologic studies. Naturally, these patients will not develop excessively rapid ventricular rates during atrial fibrillation or atrial flutter.

It is obvious that careful analysis of the number and location of accessory pathways and their role in initiation and maintenance of the reentrant supraventricular tachycardia, as well as the optimum site and rate of stimulation needed to terminate the tachyarrhythmia, must be obtained in the electrophysiologic laboratory and assessed on a temporary basis prior to permanent pacing. The potential risks of initiating atrial flutter and atrial fibrillation should be assessed, as well as the patient's ability to tolerate the resultant ventricular rates.

BRADYCARDIA-TACHYCARDIA SYNDROME

The syndrome of alternating bradycardia and tachycardia, called the "brady-tachy syndrome," has become familiar to most physicians. Tachycardias most frequently take the form of atrial fibrillation, atrial flutter, or PSVT; however, ventricular tachyarrhythmias may also occur. The patient's symptoms may at times be due to the bradycardia, the tachycardia, or to both. Therapy presents a special problem in that drugs most likely to suppress or slow the supraventricular tachycardias, such as digitalis, quinidine, or propranolol, may actually accentuate the asystole or bradycardia following termination of the tachycardia. Similarly, drugs such as atropine, isoproterenol, or ephedrine, which are used to treat the sinus bradycardia or asystole, may exacerbate the tachyarrhythmias. Pacing will prevent the bradycardia, but in most instances must be combined with drug therapy to treat the tachycardia. It has been shown that there is a high frequency of AV node disease coexisting with the sinus node disease in these patients, and, therefore, ventricular rather than atrial pacing is usually indicated. In some patients, synchronized atrioventricular pacing may be useful.

If AV nodal conduction is not severely depressed, stable atrial fibrillation often will relieve the episodes of bradycardia associated with sinus node disease, and digitalis may be used when necessary to slow the ventricular rate. Therefore, stable atrial fibrillation should not be converted to sinus rhythm electrically or pharmacologically when it occurs in the setting of the brady-tachycardia syndrome.

VENTRICULAR TACHYCARDIA

Ventricular pacing to suppress ventricular arrhythmias was first described in patients with complete heart block who experience Stokes-Adams syncope due to recurrent episodes of ventricular tachycardia or ventricular fibrillation. It was found that increasing the ventricular rate prevented the ventricular arrhythmias and subsequent Stokes-Adams attacks. Following that early experience, pacing was used to suppress recurrent ventricular tachycardia in patients without bradycardia, and numerous reports have described the use of atrial and/or ventricular pacing to treat ventricular arrhythmias chronically.

The pacing rate providing optimal suppression of ventricular ectopy varies with the patient and, of necessity, must be determined on a temporary basis a number of days prior to permanent pacing. This rate most commonly is in the range of 80 to 140 beats/minute. Exceptionally, very rapid pacing at rates of 300/minute for short periods may be used to terminate a ventricular tachycardia (Fig. 14–6). This method naturally runs the risk of initiating

ventricular fibrillation. As with the studies performed in patients with recurrent PSVT, invasive electrophysiologic evaluation must be accomplished during which the ventricular tachycardia may be precipitated by premature or rapid ventricular and at times atrial pacing (Fig. 14–7). In this way electrophysiologic determinants of the ventricular tachycardia can be established, the response to drug therapy evaluated, and the most effective pacing approach to terminate the ventricular tachycardia determined. Most frequently, the right ventricle is paced, although right atrial pacing has become more popular since the advent of more stable permanent endocardial atrial pacing electrodes and, at times, is successful when ventriculat pacing fails.

Atrial pacing provides certain advantages not found with ventricular pacing. Augmentation of ventricular filling with sequential atrioventricular contraction will often improve the cardiac output, and this benefits patients with hemodynamic problems. This

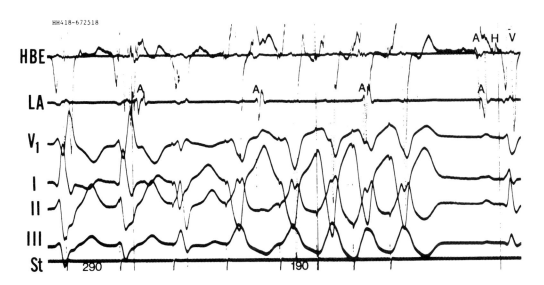

Fig. 14–6. Termination of ventricular tachycardia by rapid ventricular pacing. First two QRS complexes represent spontaneously occurring ventricular tachycardia. Right ventricular pacing at cycle length of 290 msec created fusion beat (3rd QRS complex) and then captured the ventricle for two consecutive QRS complexes. Pacing cycle length was abruptly shortened to 190 msec for three consecutive beats, and pacing was then terminated, with restoration of sinus rhythm. Conventions as in Figure 14–1.

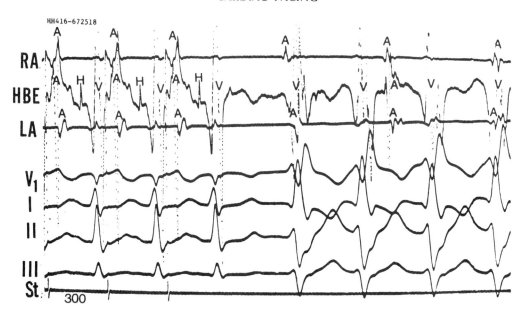

Fig. 14–7. Same patient as in Figure 14–6. Initiation of ventricular tachycardia during rapid right atrial pacing. Right atrial pacing at a cycle length 300 msec was abruptly discontinued and was followed by ventricular tachycardia (midportion of figure). Note presence of A-V dissociation and absence of His deflection preceding ventricular depolarization during ventricular tachycardia (right). Conventions as in Figure 14–1. (Reproduced with permission from Zipes, D.P., et al.: Atrial induction of ventricular tachycardia: re-entry versus triggered automaticity. Am. J. Cardiol. In press.)

avoids inadvertent stimulation during the vulnerable period of ventricle and the ventricular ectopy which occur from mechanical stimulation of the myocardium by a loose pacing lead. Atrial pacing may create more uniform repolarization following the normal sequence of depolarization and may be important in preventing some arrhythmias. In determining whether to use atrial, ventricular, or atrioventricular sequential pacing, the integrity of AV conduction and the response of arrhythmias to pacing at various sites must be determined. At times a combination of cardiac pacing and antiarrhythmic drugs is successful when neither alone will suppress the arrhythmia. As mentioned before, caution should always be used when pacing patients who have myocardial ischemia or infarction because rapid heart rates may increase localized delay in myocardial conduction and

initiate ventricular tachycardia or ventricular fibrillation.

INDICATIONS

The efficacy of ventricular and atrial pacing to treat many cardiac tachyarrhythmias is now well established. Pacing may control or terminate arrhythmias of supraventricular as well as ventricular origin and may be used alone or in combination with various antiarrhythmic medications. In emergent situations when a tachycardia produces rapid hemodynamic decompensation, DC cardioversion is the preferred therapy. However, when the situation permits more therapeutic flexibility, cardiac pacing offers certain advantages to DC shock in managing patients with drug-resistant arrhythmias.

The tachyarrhythmias most commonly treated with pacing include atrial flutter, paroxysmal atrial or junctional tachycardia, PSVT in the presence of the Wolff-Parkinson-White syndrome, the bradycardia-tachycardia syndrome and ventricular arrhythmias refractory to antiarrhythmic medication. At times atrial pacing may be used in the presence of rapid ectopic automatic tachycardias or sinus tachycardia in a manner that produces AV block and slows the ventricular rate. By far the most common use of pacing is to terminate reentrant tachyarrhythmias.

Pacing may be used to treat tachyarrhythmias in situations of suspected digitalis intoxication, when DC shock may cause serious ventricular arrhythmias and should be avoided if at all possible. When the arrhythmia to be suppressed recurs frequently, in spite of optimal drug therapy and metabolic balance, repeated external shock is not only impractical and painful at times, but may cause myocardial damage; pacing may be a better choice of therapy. Pacing may also be preferable to DC shock in children and pregnant women with tachyarrhythmias. In acute self-limited stiuations, such as those occurring during cardiac catheterization or electrophysiologic studies, pacing, when feasible, is preferred because DC cardioversion and drug therapy will alter the hemodynamic and/or electrophysiologic parameters under study. When successful in suppressing an arrhythmia, pacing also offers the advantage of providing on a chronic basis the means of rapidly controlling each episode by patient activation of a permanently implanted pacemaker.

Although a better knowledge of the mechanisms and pathogenesis of arrhythmia and the development of new pacing techniques may establish pacing as the treatment of choice in more situations than at the present time, the continued introduction of more effective antiarrhythmic agents may decrease the need for pacing or surgical intervention to control otherwise resistant tachyarrhythmias.

SUGGESTED READINGS

Batchelder, J.E., and Zipes, D.P.: Treatment of tachyarrhythmias by pacing. Arch. Intern. Med., *135*:1115, 1975.

Cohen, H.E., et al.: Treatment of refractory supraventricular arrhythmias with induced permanent atrial fibrillation. Am. J. Cardiol., *28*:472, 1971.

Davidson, R., et al.: Electrically induced atrial tachycardia with block: A therapeutic application of permanent radiofrequency atrial pacing. Circulation, *44*:1014, 1971.

Dreifus, L., et al.: Use of atrial and bifocal cardiac pacemakers for treating resistant dysrhythmias. Eur. J. Cardiol., *3*:257, 1975.

Fischer, J., Furman, S., and Mehra, M.: Ectopic ventricular tachycardia treated with bursts of pacing at 300 per minute from an implanted ventricular pacemaker. Circulation, *51–52*:182, 1976.

Goyal, S.L., et al.: Refractory re-entrant atrial tachycardia. Successful treatment with a permanent radio frequency triggered atrial pacemaker. Am. J. Med., *58*:586, 1975.

Haft, J.I., et al.: Termination of atrial flutter by rapid electrical pacing of the atrium. Am. J. Cardiol., *20*:239, 1967.

Haft, J.I.: Treatment of arrhythmias by intracardiac electrical stimulation. Prog. Cardiovasc. Dis., *16*:539, 1974.

Hunt, N.C., et al.: Conversion of supraventricular tachycardias with atrial stimulation. Circulation, *38*:1060, 1968.

Kahn, A., Morris, J.J., and Citron, P.: Patient initiated rapid atrial pacing to manage supraventricular tachycardia. Am. J. Cardiol., *38*:200, 1976.

Kitchen, J.G., and Goldreyer, B.N.: Demand pacemaker for refractory paroxysmal supraventricular tachycardia. N. Engl. J. Med. *287*:596, 1972.

Krikler, D., Curry, P., and Buffet, J.: Dual-demand pacing for reciprocating atrioventricular tachycardia. Br. Med. J., *60*:1114, 1976.

Lister, J.W., et al.: Treatment of supraventricular tachycardias by rapid atrial stimulation. Circulation, *38*:1044, 1968.

Mandel, W.J., et al.: Recurrent reciprocating tachycardias in the Wolff-Parkinson-White syndrome: control by the use of a scanning pacemaker. Chest, *69*:769, 1976.

Massumi, R.A., Kistin, A.D., and Tawakkol, A.A.: Termination of reciprocating tachycardia by atrial stimulation. Circulation, *36*:637, 1967.

Preston, T.A., and Kirsh, M.M.: Permanent pacing of the left atrium for treatment of WPW tachycardia. Circulation, *42*:1073, 1970.

Ryan, G.F., et al.: Paradoxical use of a demand pacemaker in treatment of supraventricular tachycardia due to the Wolff-Parkinson-White syndrome. Circulation, *38*:1037, 1968.

Sowton, E., et al.: Long-term control of intractable supraventricular tachycardia by ventricular pacing. Br. Heart J., *31*:700, 1969.

Spurrell, R., and Sowton, E.: Pacing techniques in the management of supraventricular tachycardias. J. Electrocardiol., *9*:89, 1976.

Spurrell, R.A., and Sowton, E.: Proceedings: management of paroxysmal supraventricular tachycardia using a scanning pacing system. Br. Heart J. *38*:536, 1976.

Vergara, G.S., et al.: Conversion of supraventricular tachycardias with rapid atrial stimulation. Circulation, *46*:788, 1972.

Waldo, A.L., et al.: Continuous rapid atrial pacing to control recurrent or sustained supraventricular tachycardias following open heart surgery. Circulation, *54*:245, 1976.

Waldo, A.L., et al.: Ventricular paired pacing to control rapid ventricular heart rate following open heart surgery. Observations on ectopic automaticity. Report of a case in a four-month-old patient. Circulation, *53*:176, 1976.

Weiner, L., and Dwyer, E.M.: Electrical induction of atrial fibrillation: an approach to intractable atrial tachycardia. Am. J. Cardiol., *21*:731, 1968.

Wellens, H.: Electrical Stimulation of the Heart in the Study and Treatment of Tachycardia. Baltimore, University Park Press, 1971.

Zeft, H.J., et al.: Right atrial stimulation in the treatment of atrial flutter. Ann. Intern. Med., *70*:447, 1969.

Zeft, H.J., and McGowan, R.L.: Termination of paroxysmal junctional tachycardia by right ventricular stimulation. Circulation, *40*:919, 1969.

Zipes, D.P., et al.: Artificial atrial and ventricular pacing in the treatment of arrhythmias. Ann. Intern. Med., *70*:885, 1969.

Zipes, D.P.: The contribution of artificial pacemaking to understanding the pathogenesis of arrhythmias. Am. J. Cardiol., *28*:211, 1971.

Zipes, D.P., et al.: Treatment of ventricular arrhythmias by permanent atrial pacemaker and cardiac sympathectomy. Ann. Intern. Med., *68*:591, 1968.

15

Pacemaker Complications

WILLIAM C. BOAKE
GEORGE M. KRONCKE

Cardiac pacemakers were first implanted at the University of Wisconsin Hospitals in 1961. This chapter is drawn from our 17 years of experience with the diagnosis and treatment of problems associated with cardiac pacing. Most pacemaker complications can be diagnosed by a conventional electrocardiogram (ECG) and chest roentgenograms. In difficult situations, a 24-hour Holter monitor, fluoroscopy with spot films of the pacemaker-lead system, and appropriate intraoperative electrical testing using a pacing system analyzer (PSA) are necessary.

EARLY FAILURE TO PACE

The causes of early pacing failure following transvenous lead installation include lead displacement, ventricular perforation by the electrode, and increased endocardial stimulation threshold. In reviewing the histories of 600 patients with transvenous pacemaker systems from 1967 to 1975 at the University Hospitals in Madison, endocar-dial lead displacement was the most common cause of early pacing failure. This occurred in approximately 5% of patients reviewed from 1974 to 1976. In other reported series, the average incidence of lead displacement was 8% and ranged from 2% to 18%. Pacemaker spikes without capture were usually seen within three days of implantation and all before six weeks (Fig. 15–1). One lead displacement was noted at six months incident to "twiddler's syndrome".

The diagnosis of lead displacement is usually established by a chest roentgenogram that shows electrode migration to an area other than its initial apical right ventricular site. The lead can displace into the pulmonary artery (Fig. 15–2) or the right atrium, but any slight electrode movement of 1 to 2 cm may change the effective electrode contact with endocardium and result in failure to pace.

The following points are emphasized during lead installation in order to avoid electrode displacement. The lead is advanced into the pulmonary artery and then with-

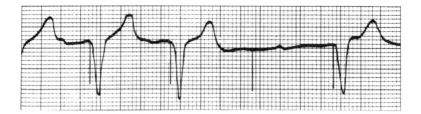

E.C.G. showing intermittent capture

Fig. 15–1. ECG showing failure to capture with all pacer impulses.

drawn into the right ventricle. This maneuver eliminates inadvertent placement into the coronary sinus or cardiac vein. On fluoroscopy, the lead tip can be seen to bend slightly with each cardiac systole and should be stable on deep inspiration and coughing.

Perforation of the right ventricle occurred in 10 of 250 consecutive new implants (4%) from 1974 to 1976. Forceful placement of the endocardial lead within the apex of the right ventricle may account for this complication (Fig. 15–3).

An increase in the endocardial pacing

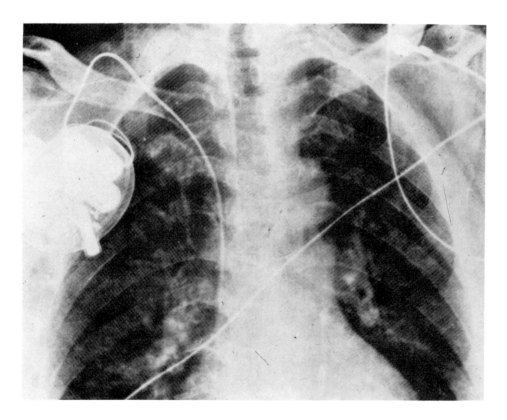

Fig. 15–2. Endocardial lead displaced into pulmonary artery.

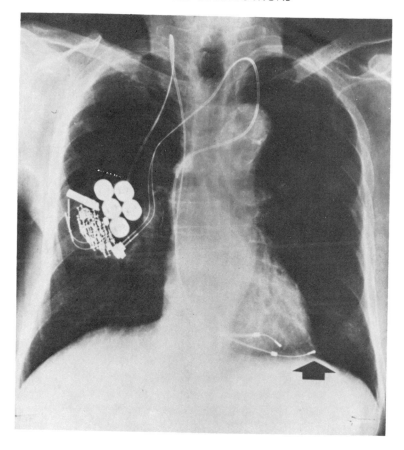

Fig. 15–3. Endocardial lead (arrow) penetrating right ventricle and lying in pericardial cavity. Compare with second lead in proper position.

threshold may have many causes. We have seen a significant increase in stimulation threshold from electrolyte imbalance due principally to lower serum potassium concentration. High doses of quinidine, lidocaine, or procainamide used for arrhythmias may also produce abnormally high pacing thresholds. Other causes include endocardial edema and hematoma secondary to the trauma of lead installation.

The normal increase of 1.5 to 2 V (2 to 4 mA) in stimulation threshold during the first six weeks after an implant should not result in failure to pace, since most pulse generators have an output of 5 to 6 V (9 to 11 mA). We have encountered, however, excessive threshold elevation of 6 to 8 V (11 to 16 mA) in the first six weeks after lead implantation. The diagnosis may be resolved by obtaining serum levels of electrolytes, quinidine, or lidocaine. The final diagnosis is established by intraoperative electrical measurements using a PSA.

Management of early pacing failure involves the following measures: (1) lead reposition, (2) restoration of physiologic parameters, (3) conversion to unipolar pacing, (4) steroids, and (5) a high output pulse generator. In the patient who is not pacemaker-dependent, one can attempt noninvasive methods of management. These include restoration of electrolyte balance and a dosage reduction of antiarrhythmic drugs. A short course of steroids might be helpful, but this therapy was effective in only one of 250 new implants. In most patients the lead must be repositioned under fluoroscopic control. Time-consuming trials of the electrode guided into several endocardial sites is sometimes necessary.

For initial implants, a stimulation threshold of 0.7 V (1.0 mA) or less is recommended. Higher pacing thresholds usually indicate poor electrode position or endocardial contact. A stimulation threshold above 1.2 V (1.5 mA) should not be accepted. In these patients an epicardial pacing system is recommended. A small left anterior thoracotomy is preferred and the electrodes are installed on the high left ventricle, since this area usually has a satisfactory threshold. In elderly or debilitated patients, a thoracotomy may be dangerous.

The proximal electrode of a bipolar lead may offer a satisfactory pacing threshold and can be used as a unipolar stimulating electrode. In a few seriously ill patients a high output pulse generator may be indicated; on occasion the current output is increased to 18 to 24 mA or approximately twice the stimulation threshold.

LATE FAILURE TO PACE

The causes of late failure to pace include depletion of the pulse generator battery, pulse generator component failure, lead fracture, lead insulation break, and increased endocardial stimulation threshold or exit block. The diagnosis may be initially suspected from the following ECG findings: (1) abnormally prolonged pacemaker pulse interval consistent with battery depletion; (2) absent pacemaker spikes, consistent with component failure; (3) intermittent absence of pacemaker spikes and/or intermittent decrease of pulse artifact amplitude, consistent with lead fracture; (4) pacemaker spikes without capture, consistent with high stimulation threshold; and (5) varying spike amplitude and altered vector of pacer stimuli, consistent with lead insulation break.

The most common indication for pulse generator replacement is battery depletion. All pacemakers have a programmed rate decrease concomitant with depletion of the power source. In some units there is a gradual decline throughout pacer life, and in others the rate remains constant for most of the battery life and then decreases 5 to 10% shortly before complete battery depletion. All pulse generators will eventually fail from battery depletion, but failure is dependent upon chronic threshold variations and the duration of pacing.

Random component failure should be less than 1% per year. Battery depletion may be accelerated or pacemaker output function may cease abruptly when capacitors or transistors fail or an internal short circuit occurs. Unusual manifestations of component failure can be precisely determined by the pacemaker manufacturer.

The patient with a lead fracture may have syncope. ECG monitoring may demonstrate intermittent loss of pacer spikes (Fig. 15–4). Separation of the coiled wire fragments incident to heart, body, or pacer movements can reproduce the ECG and clinical findings. Wire fragment separation

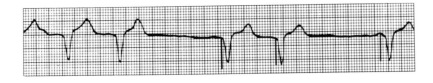

Fig. 15–4. Intermittent interruption of pacer impulses.

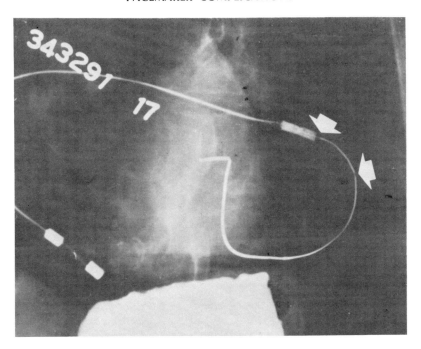

Fig. 15–5.   Spot films of old myocardial lead showing multiple areas of wire fracture (arrows) near old splice.

can also be induced to duplicate the ECG findings by percutaneous manipulation of the pulse generator. The weight of the pulse generator can have the same effect when the patient assumes the upright position. In the early days of pacing, lead fractures were relatively common and leads were repaired repeatedly (Fig. 15–5). Present leads are more resistant to disruption, but fractures still do occur on occasion at stress points.

Normal leads have a resistance that ranges between 250 and 1200 ohms.* Intraoperatively, broken leads exhibit an increased wire resistance. A lead resistance over 1200 ohms is considered unacceptable and consistent with an impending or existing lead fracture. Using a constant-voltage PSA, a simple test can determine lead integrity. The output voltage of the PSA is

increased until the current digital readout is 10 mA, and the resultant voltage is then multiplied by 100 to provide an estimate of lead resistance. Lead impedance can also be calculated using Ohm's law when voltage and current threshold are measured simultaneously using a PSA and expressed in the formula

$$R = \frac{E}{I}$$

where E = volts (V), I = current (mA) and R = resistance (ohms). A lead resistance below 250 ohms is consistent with a lead insulation break.

A high stimulation threshold is seen in 10% of chronic leads at the time of pulse generator replacement. A threshold greater than 4.0 V is unacceptable and a new lead system is indicated. Rarely, as in an elderly patient, a high output pulse generator may

---

*Except with a ball-tip electrode which may normally have a resistance up to 1500 ohms.

be used. Battery depletion or component failure are indications for pulse generator replacement. On occasion, the proximal electrode of a bipolar lead provides an acceptable stimulation threshold and may therefore be successfully converted to a unipolar pacing system.

FAILURE TO SENSE

The causes of failure to sense may be related to problems associated with the lead, the pulse generator, the myocardium, skeletal muscle, or electromagnetic interference. Failure to sense may be divided into two major categories: undersensing and oversensing.

Undersensing

Asynchronous or fixed-rate pacing characterized all early pacemakers. Competitive or fixed-rate pacing may produce ventricular tachycardia when a pacemaker stimulus falls within the vulnerable period of the heart (ascending limb or peak of the T wave). Although rarely seen, peer pressure and medical-legal considerations have influenced widespread preference for the demand or ventricular inhibited pulse generator. The sensing circuit of a ventricular demand pulse generator detects the intrinsic QRS activity and inhibits the pacemaker, and competition between the spontaneous and the pacer rhythm is eliminated.

Undersensing is readily diagnosed from the ECG when the pacemaker output pulse is not inhibited by the intrinsic QRS wave. The incidence of undersensing has been less than 1% in our patients. Undersensing may be more common in an epicardial bipolar lead system because of inadequate separation between the implanted electrodes. Conversion to a unipolar pacing system with the positive pole represented by the indifferent electrode plate of the pulse generator may offer an improved cardiac signal and satisfactory QRS sensing.

Intraoperative R-wave measurements from the implanted leads are obtained with a PSA. QRS signals of 5 mV or more indicate a good lead position. The lead must be repositioned if this sensing measurement is not obtained. A high sensitivity pulse generator may be used for marginal cardiac signals that are measured at pulse generator replacement. Occasionally, component malfunction of the pulse generator may also result in sensing failure.

The sensing function of a demand pulse generator can be tested by proper connection to a PSA using, for example, the Medtronic Model 5300. A train of 4.0 mV simulated R-waves at a rate of 150 PPM are emitted when this unit functions in the Pulse Amplitude mode and the R-wave test switch is depressed. This maneuver should inhibit the pulse output of a normally operating pulse generator. Replacement of the pulse generator is indicated if sensing malfunction is apparent. An increased distance between the myocardium and the electrode due to edema or fibrosis can also cause undersensing, which, if persistent, requires replacement of the lead system.

Oversensing

Oversensing is related to extraneous signals that cause pacer inhibition after detection by the sensing circuit. Sophisticated circuit filters of modern pacemakers usually reject most signals other than the normal QRS activity. Pacemaker inhibition may rarely occur with P or T wave sensing. Strong external electromagnetic interference is another cause of pacemaker oversensing. Patients should be instructed in the hazards to pacemaker function by such devices as microwave ovens, radar, and powerful electrical generators. Less powerful motors with defective brushes in appliances such as saber saws, hair driers, and electric razors can produce sufficient pulsed energy to inhibit pacemakers. Muscle potentials arising from contraction of the pectoralis major or the diaphragm have also been reported to inhibit pulse generators. Pacer inhibition from myopotentials is rare and usually seen only in the unipolar configuration.

Oversensing may be confirmed by Holter monitor or telemetry and absence of pacer spikes during exposure to electromagnetic interference (EMI). Placement of a magnet over the pulse generator will induce a fixed-rate pacing mode and disable sensing function when oversensing is present.

Management is dependent upon the specific factor causing oversensing. Obvious sources of EMI should be avoided. Conversion to a bipolar pacing system, transfer of the pulse generator site, or enclosure of the pulse generator with a Parsonnet pouch will eliminate oversensing due to pectoral muscle voltage potentials.

INFECTION

The cause of pacemaker infection is not always apparent. Contributing factors include poor tissue viability, tissue interaction with a foreign material, or an infraction of sterile technique. The diagnosis is suspected when fever develops and becomes obvious when redness and swelling appear over the pacemaker pocket. Bacterial etiology may be confirmed from the fluid aspirated from the pacemaker pocket. A febrile reaction may also occur when a sterile hematoma collects in the pacemaker pocket. Erosion of the skin due to the pressure of the underlying lead or pulse generator may also occur with localized infection (Fig. 15–6).

Meticulous surgical preparation of the selected pacemaker site and routine use of antibiotics have considerably reduced the incidence of pacemaker infection. Severe wound infection requires removal of the pacing system, drainage of the area, and administration of appropriate antibiotics. A new pacing system is implanted in another area during antibiotic administration when extensive infection or bacteremia is present. The lead and pulse generator are also

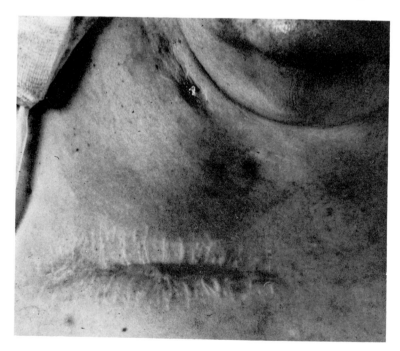

Fig. 15–6.   Lead eroding through skin of neck with secondary infection of pacemaker pocket.

replaced when skin erosion is the result of infection. Irrigation with a bactericidal antibiotic solution for 3 to 5 days followed by secondary closure will usually suffice when the infection is confined to the pacemaker pocket with a well-formed fibrotic lining.

MUSCLE STIMULATION

The causes of skeletal muscle stimulation may arise from the pulse generator, electrode malposition incident to myocardial perforation, or lead insulation break. Subtle or marked contractions of the pectoral or intercostal muscle coincident with the pacemaker pulse stimulus may appear. Diaphragmatic muscle stimulation has been more common in our experience and has been seen in 10 of 250 new pacer implants (4%). In most patients, this complication was secondary to myocardial perforation by the electrode. Diaphragmatic stimulation in all lead installations is evaluated by stimulating with a PSA pulse amplitude of 10 volts while palpating the abdomen. The lead is repositioned to a new site when this maneuver provokes diaphragmatic stimulation.

Chest roentgenograms are obtained when diaphragmatic pacing occurs 12 to 24 hours after a new pacer implant. The patient may be observed if the lead tip position is unchanged and myocardial perforation is not manifest. Diaphragmatic stimulation may then subside in 3 to 5 days. A decreased energy output can be established noninvasively to maintain myocardial capture without diaphragmatic stimulation when the pulse generator output is programmable. With a bipolar lead system, the ring electrode may be used if this pole offers a satisfactory threshold. Cardiac tamponade, not seen in our patients, may occur with right ventricular perforation. Immediate surgical drainage is indicated when a fall in blood pressure is associated with a narrow pulse pressure and echocardiographic evidence of cardiac tamponade.

Pectoral and intercostal muscle stimulation is most common with a unipolar pulse generator. Active contraction may develop when the positive electrode plate or case of the pulse generator is in close apposition to these muscles. Pacemaker enclosure with a Dacron pouch or Silastic sleeve or medial placement of the pulse generator can eliminate chest wall muscle stimulation. A lead insulation break with current leakage in proximity to the intercostal muscles may also stimulate muscles. The lead must be replaced or repaired. Failure to insert nylon screws or Silastic plugs over the Allen screws that secure the lead to the pulse generator may also produce stimulation of the pectoral or abdominal muscles.

PACEMAKER MIGRATION

The causes of pacemaker migration include hematoma, poor tissue turgor, and pulse generator weight. Hematoma of the pacemaker pocket is the most common cause of early pacemaker motion or migration. A low grade fever and swelling are usually present, and the surrounding tissues may be ecchymotic. The pulse generator can rotate in a large pocket with liquefied hematomas. Pectoral muscle stimulation may then occur with a unipolar generator. Withdrawal and displacement of the lead (twiddler's syndrome) may also occur as the pulse generator turns within its pocket (Fig. 15–7).

Adequate hemostasis at operation will usually prevent this problem. Muscle bleeders often require suture ligatures. Development of a pocket that follows the avascular plane between the deep layer of superficial fascia of the skin and the pectoral fascia reduces hematoma formation. An elastic bandage (Elastoplast or Ace) pressure dressing for 24 hours postoperatively is recommended. If a large hematoma develops, reopening the incision and evacuation of blood clot under strict aseptic conditions will decrease morbidity and speed recovery.

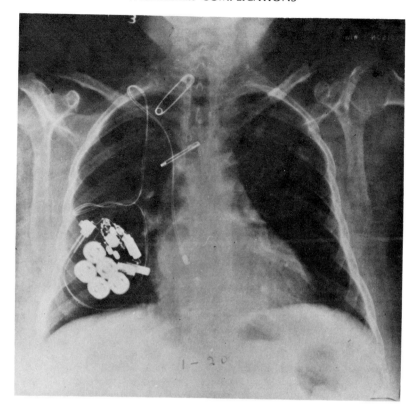

Fig. 15–7. Twiddler's syndrome (note multiple twists of lead in pocket and tip of lead pulled back into right atrium).

Using the suture hole or placing the suture around the boot may prevent pacemaker twisting in the pocket. A Dacron mesh pocket (Parsonnet pouch) can be sewn to the tissues, particularly in the elderly patient who has poor connective tissue turgor. This may prevent migration of the pulse generator by tissue dissection into the axilla or other regions of the chest wall.

COMPLICATIONS OF TRANSTHORACIC IMPLANTATION

All pacemaker implantations were initially transthoracic. This approach was used infrequently after the introduction of the transvenous method for cardiac pacing in 1965. Other operative approaches have gained popularity recently with the advent of the sutureless electrode. These include epigastric or parasternal extrapleural methods of electrode placement on either the right or left ventricle. Complications of these approaches include pericarditis, pleuritis, and effusion.

Laceration of the ventricular wall as a result of electrode insertion is the most serious complication. When this occurs, the exposure must be enlarged and the laceration closed with interrupted sutures; Dacron or Teflon pledgets may be necessary. Cardiopulmonary bypass has been employed to control hemorrhage and permit repair of severe laceration of the inferior wall of the right ventricle.

Adequate operative exposure and sound surgical techniques that avoid injury to muscles or the coronary artery during electrode installation will reduce the morbidity and mortality associated with the transthoracic approach. A satisfactory pacing site offers a low stimulation threshold and a high sensing measurement.

The pericardial tissues are reapproximated loosely over the implanted leads. This procedure protects the leads and provides adequate drainage from the pericardial to the pleural space. A large chest tube through a lower interspace is used for adequate dependent drainage.

PACING COMPLICATIONS IN CHILDREN

The most common causes of pacemaker dysfunction in children are lead fracture and displacement. Extremely forceful myocardial contractions in children disrupt the lead wire and electrode more commonly than in adults. The growth of the patient stresses the lead traversing the chest wall. This stress shortens redundant coils and engenders kinking of the lead and subsequent fracture. Chest roentgenograms should be taken every six months to identify lead kinking, and the pacing system should be revised when this is detected.

We prefer the transthoracic approach for permanent lead implantation on the high left ventricle in children under 16 years of age or before full growth has been reached. Redundant lead coils are placed within the chest cavity. In infants the pulse generator is implanted in the abdominal wall. In older children the pacemaker is placed deep beneath the pectoralis major muscle. Some pacemakers are implanted in a Teflon mesh pocket inside the left pleural space. The newer lithium pacemaker has an improved weight-sized ratio and can be adequately covered even in small children. The problems of pulse generator migration and skin erosion are therefore considerably reduced.

UNUSUAL PACEMAKER COMPLICATIONS

Less frequent causes of pacemaker failure, intermittent or complete, include capacitor failure, defective sensing bandpass filter, faulty hermetic sealing, lead pin corrosion, and faulty magnetic reed switch. The pacemaker output pulse ceases abruptly when component failure occurs.

Modern pulse generators have not been associated with the runaway pacemaker rate. The literature contains reports of other rare complications such as fractured leads that perforate the atrial and bronchial walls and subsequent infection associated with bronchocutaneous fistulae. Thrombi occur commonly in the cephalic or axillary veins but rarely produce a swollen upper extremity or pulmonary emboli. The tricuspid valve may be damaged during lead placement and predispose to bacterial valvulitis. Additionally, the endocardial lead can induce ventricular arrhythmias by mechanical stimulation of the myocardium.

SELECTED READINGS

Furman, S., and Escher, D. (Editors): Modern Cardiac Pacing. Bowie, Maryland, The Charles Press, 1975.

Kennelly, B.M., and Piller, L.W.: Management of infected transvenous permanent pacemakers. Br. Heart J., 36(11):1133, 1974.

Kostianess, S.: Complications of transvenous and transthoracic electrodes. Acta Med. Scand. Suppl., (596): 40, 1976.

Mansour, K.A.: Complications of cardiac pacemakers. Ann. Surg., 43(2):1316, 1977.

Schaldach, M., and Furman, S. (Editors): Advances in Pacemaker Technology. New York, Springer-Verlag, 1975.

Spence, M.I., and Lemberg, L.: Cardiac pacemakers. IV. Complications of pacing. Heart Lung, 4(2):286, 1975.

16

Transvenous versus Transthoracic Cardiac Pacing

JAMES J. MORRIS, JR.

The insertion of a permanently implanted cardiac pacemaker is a well-established and oftentimes dramatic therapeutic intervention. Conversely, the failure of a pacing system is a dangerous and frustrating medical experience for the patient and the physician.

The complete pacing system consists of a pulse generator, a lead system, and the patient in whom the lead system must be implanted with minimal effort and safety and with maximal certainty of long range efficiency. After two decades of clinical experience and engineering and design modifications, the most reliable method of lead implantation is still debated. The information supplied is from personal and institutional experience at Duke University and is not intended to be an exhaustive review of the literature.

SURGICAL METHODS

The original pacing systems required direct attachment of pacing leads to the epicardial surface of the heart by thoracotomy,[1-3] referred to as the transthoracic method. These systems were fraught with failures principally because of early fracture of the lead material which in large part was due to material problems and mechanical fatigue. With changes in material and design, leads became more reliable, and the major problems centered around pulse generator malfunctions.

As time passed and pacing systems were modified, it became apparent that formal thoracotomy was associated with inherent risks and operative complications. Limited surgical approaches were devised. An extrapleural technique, referred to as the transmediastinal approach, was used to avoid the pleural space.[4-7] To further minimize surgical exposure, the subxiphoid approach, a technique of exposing the epicardial surface of the heart by an epigastric transdiaphragmatic approach was then introduced.[8-9] Leads were modified from those requiring direct suturing to the epimyocardium for permanent implantation to the sutureless screw-in lead designed to be self-affixing to the heart.[8-12]

While these surgical approaches were being pursued, it also became apparent that the stimulating electrode could be passed into the venous system to effectively stimulate the heart from the endocardial surface. The transvenous approach, achieved by the passage of a pacing electrode into the venous system, avoids the necessity for entering the pleural or mediastinal space. The outstanding advantages of the endocardial method of pacing were a limited surgical intervention and use of local rather than general anesthesia.

Thus two general approaches for establishing a permanent lead system are available: (1) the direct epicardial approaches: transthoracic (TT), transmediastinal (TM) and subxiphoid (SX) and (2) the transvenous (endocardial) approach. This chapter will focus upon the comparative merits and disadvantages of these methods for pacing lead implantation.

As a general statement, transvenous leads may be characterized as a simple system in application, low in acute complications, and usually relatively high in problems principally from early or late migration or movement of the endocardial lead. Failures of the endocardial electrode have been reported to vary from 5% to 38%.[13-26] Although electrode failures of greater than 5% have been viewed as excessive,[27] many institutions installing pacemakers report a greater incidence. The surgical methods have uniformly been reported to be associated with fewer electrode failures, but a higher incidence of morbidity and mortality.

SHORT-TERM LEAD PERFORMANCE

The experience gleaned at Duke Medical Center with electrode implantation has been reported on two occasions, in 1967 and in 1974, and is updated in this chapter by the addition of unpublished results from 1973 to 1976.[18,28] Each of these reports has focused upon the risks and short-term effectiveness of different lead systems.

Transvenous Electrodes

Transvenous leads were implanted in 51 patients between 1961 and 1966 and in 129 patients between 1967 and 1970 (Table 16-1). The ages, associated illnesses, and other pertinent data concerning these patients, which were included in the original reports, can be considered rather typical of most patient populations who have been subjected to permanent transvenous pacemaker installation.

The incidence of major complications in the two series was rather low; most were transient and hospital mortality was low. Major complications during hospitalization included pericardial tamponade, cerebral vascular accidents, infections, serious cardiac arrhythmias, acute myocardial infarction, pulmonary complications, serious

TABLE 16-1

Transvenous Electrodes

	1961–1966	1967–1970
Time period		
Number of Patients	51	129
Major in-hospital complications	8%	19%
Permanent electrode failure	16%	22%
Temporary electrode failure	14%	16%
Mortality: Hospital	2%	2%
Late	6%	23%
Period of follow-up	1–6 years	2 years

TABLE 16–2

Epicardial Electrodes

METHOD	TRANSTHORACIC		TRANSMEDIASTINAL*		SUBXIPHOID*
Time period	1961–1966	1967–1970	1961–1966	1973–1976	1973–1976
Number of patients	35	50	68	43	72
Major in-hospital complications	35%	44%	35%	33%	18%
Permanent electrode failure	3%	2%	7%	0%	1%
Temporary electrode failure	0%	5%	9%	5%	2%
Mortality: Hospital	0%	0%	1%	0%	4%
Late	6%	4%	22%	7%	4%
Period of follow-up	1–6 years	2 years	2 years	1 year	1 year

* Sutureless epicardial leads.

bleeding, and thromboembolic phenomena (pulmonary and systemic).

Permanent electrode failure, in which the electrode system failed to achieve pacing, required replacement in 16% of the patients in the first series and in 22% in the second series. Although in some instances failure to pace was caused by lead fracture or myocardial infarction, in most instances it was caused by dislodgment of the electrode and/or elevation of the stimulation threshold.

Temporary electrode failure, or loss of satisfactory capture, was corrected by reoperation and remanipulation of the pacing leads in 14% of the patients in the first series and 16% in the second. The total permanent and temporary electrode failures, 30% in the 1961 to 1966 series and 38% in the 1967 to 1970 series, suggest that the transvenous method of electrode insertion, though easy to perform with relatively low hospital complications, carries a surprisingly high permanent and temporary failure rate in the early years after implant.

Epicardial Electrodes

In the first series reported thoracotomy was used for implantations; in the second series transthoracic and transmediastinal insertions were compared (Table 16–2). In a third series of epicardial implantations from 1973 to 1976 transmediastinal and subxiphoid approaches were used. In this later series the sutureless myocardial lead (Medtronic model 6917) was employed. The incidence of hospital complications was higher with transthoracic and transmediastinal approaches than with the subxiphoid approach.

The frequency of permanent and temporary electrode failures was low in the brief follow-up periods reported, and hospital mortality was low. Thus the epicardial approaches do carry a high in-hospital complication rate, but are extremely reliable with a low incidence of electrode problems. The subxiphoid approach using the sutureless electrode seems to have reached the desired goal, namely, relatively low rates of hospital complications and of permanent and temporary lead failure.

Tined Leads

The ideal lead would be one inserted by the tranvenous route, have a low rate of in-hospital complications, and be nondislodgable. To accomplish this purpose several "adherent" or "attachable" transvenous leads have been designed. The tined lead has Silastic tines which protrude from the catheter and are designed to become anchored within the trabeculae of the right ventricle.

TABLE 16–3

Transvenous Electrodes

TYPE	CONVENTIONAL	TINED
Time period	9/76 to 8/77	9/76 to 8/77
Number of patients	27	26
Major in-hospital complications	15%	8%
Permanent electrode failure	4%	0%
Temporary electrode failure	15%	4%
Mortality: Hospital	4%	0%
Late	0%	8%
Period of follow-up	4–14 months	4–14 months

A random trial involving patients allocated to conventional transvenous leads and tined leads (Medtronic models 6901 and 6950, respectively) was carried out between 9/76 and 8/77 (Table 16–3). The implanting physicians were the same, and no obvious differences were apparent in the two groups of patients. Permanent and temporary lead failures were still noted to be high with the conventional lead, and not dissimilar from our previous experience (Table 16–2). The tined leads, however, showed a low incidence of permanent and temporary lead failures. Although these results are preliminary and the follow-up period short, they are encouraging.

Conclusions

The patients studied at the Duke University were not randomized; in fact, the selection tended to favor older and more debilitated patients for the transvenous method of electrode implantation. However, the following conclusions are clear from our experience: (1) transvenous electrodes are easier to implant, but show a high tendency to fail in follow-up; (2) epicardial leads are much less likely to fail in follow-up, but carry a higher hospital complication rate. The subxiphoid approach with use of the sutureless electrodes seems to have reduced the in-hospital complications and also has maintained the advantage of a low rate of electrode failure. Long-term studies will be required to settle the question of electrode performance. However, at the present time, there is no evidence that either epicardial or endocardial lead implants will differ in late performance.

Most authors agree that lead dislodgment is a significant problem in maintaining satisfactory pacing with transvenous pacing electrodes. Our experience with transvenous leads supports this position (Tables 16–2 and 16–3). Our experience also supports the view that epicardial placement assures firmer lead fixation and fewer electrode failures, but yields higher in-hospital complications.

Significant advances have occurred in both epicardial and transvenous electrode implantations. The subxiphoid epicardial approach using the sutureless electrode has reduced in-hospital complications and also maintained lead performance. The use of the tined transvenous lead has been associated with a minimum of major in-hospital complications and appears to significantly reduce the incidence of lead dislodgment. These advances are in their preliminary stages of development and therefore require confirmation of their advantages by long-term follow-up. Given continued success, it would seem that these two methods—transvenous using the tined lead and subxiphoid using the sutureless lead—offer equally good approaches to a safe and effective lead system.

LONG-TERM LEAD PERFORMANCE

We have undertaken a long-range prospective study of lead performance. The following is a preliminary report of that study. All patients who had pacing electrodes implanted between 9/69 and 12/71 have been followed at six-month intervals.

One hundred and fifty of the original 151 patients have been followed continuously for six years. Endocardial leads (Medtronic

TABLE 16–4

Six-Year Electrode Experience

	NO. PATIENTS	%
Implanted	151	
Lost to follow-up	1	
Expired by 6 years	53/145	37
Lead failure by 6 years	31/145	24
Alive by 6 years who experienced lead failure	31/92	33
Endocardial leads	57	
Epicardial leads	94	

TABLE 16–5

Lead Failures

CAUSE OF FAILURE	NO. OF PATIENTS	TIME (MONTHS) FAILURE OCCURRED
Threshold elevation	10	1, 6, 7, 11, 14, 17, 28, 29, 38, 71
Sensing failure	2	10, 28
Infection	2	17, 21
Fracture	7	15, 15, 18, 53, 65, 67, 72
Perforation	2	1, 40
Dislodgment	7	1, 1.5, 7, 10, 32, 74, 78
Unknown	1	9
Total	31	

models 5818 and 6901) were implanted in 57 patients and epicardial leads (Medtronic models 5814 and 6914) in 94 patients. Table 16–4 lists the status of these patients: 5 patients had their pacing systems removed and not replaced; 53 patients had expired; and 31 patients experienced lead failure corrected with implantation of a new lead system. Lead failure rate at six years was 24%; however, if one considers only those patients who survive six years, 33% will require a new lead system by that time.

These are revealing statistics when one considers the need for "long-life" pulse generators. Since 37% of the studied patients expired and 24% required reoperation for a new lead insertion, fewer than 50% of the patients would have been able to maintain their long-life generators if these generators were available in 1969–1971.

The reasons for the 31 lead failures are shown in Table 16–5, but a clear separation of lead failure due to stimulation threshold elevation or dislodgment is difficult in certain patients. Of special interest is the not uncommon occurrence of lead fractures (22.5%) as a cause of lead failure. Most lead failures seem to emanate from poorly defined and ill understood biologic problems, rather than from strict design or material causes. It should be clearly understood that the leads in this study are currently outmoded, but this study does offer a baseline for the comparison of present leads and those of the future which will presumably be better.

THE FUTURE

As engineering and designs of pacemaker systems advance and clinical demands increase, the need and application for atrial pacing, atrial synchronous pacing, dual-chamber pacing, dual-chamber sensing and pacing will multiply. Continual improvement in the methods of application—epicardial, endocardial, or coronary sinus—will require further refinements. The methods of fixation to the heart that avoid undue biologic reactions such as the sutureless or tined leads will also need further refinements. The ideal lead will undoubtedly be an endocardial lead that will provide certainty of fixation, minimal inherent resistance, smallness of size, and easy application and be virtually free of biologic reactivity and be indestructible. If past performance reflects future behavior, improvements in pacemaker systems can be expected in the near future.

REFERENCES

1. Chardack, W.M., Gage, A.A., and Greatbatch, W.: Transistorized, self-contained, implantable

pacemaker for the long-term correction of complete heart block. Surgery, 48:643, 1960.

2. Zoll, P. M., et al.: Long-term electric stimulation of the heart for Stokes-Adams disease. Ann. Surg., 154:330, 1961.

3. Kantrowitz, A., et al.: Treatment of complete heart block with an implanted controllable pacemaker. Surg. Gynec. Obstet., 115:415, 1962.

4. Frank, H.A., Zoll, P.M., and Linenthal, A.J.: Surgical aspects of long-term electrical stimulation of the heart. J. Thorac. Cardiovasc. Surg., 57:17, 1969.

5. Jude, J.R., Mobin-Uddin, K., and Callard, G.M.: Long-term follow-up of a new method of pacer lead implantation. J. Thorac. Cardiovasc. Surg., 58:783, 1969.

6. Reed, G.E., et al.: A new technique for pacemaker implantation: Extrapleural, intramyocardial. J. Thorac. Cardiovasc. Surg., 57:507, 1969.

7. Dixon, S.H., et al.: Transmediastinal permanent ventricular pacing. Ann. Thorac. Surg., 14:206, 1972.

8. Stewart, S.: Placement of the sutureless epicardial pacemaker lead by the sub-xiphoid approach. Ann. Thorac. Surg., 18:308, 1974.

9. Naclerio, E.A., and Varriale, P.: "Screw-in" electrode. New method for permanent ventricular pacing. N.Y. State J. Med., 74:2391, 1974.

10. Buffle, P. J.: Ventricular pacing with epigastric transdiaphragmatic electrodes. J. Thorac. Cardiovasc. Surg., 72:126, 1976.

11. Mansour, K.A., Fleming, W.H., and Hatcher, C.R.: Initial experience with a sutureless screw-in electrode for cardiac pacing. Ann. Thorac. Surg., 16:127, 1973.

12. Hunter, S.W., et al.: A new myocardial pacemaker lead (sutureless). Chest, 63:430, 1973.

13. Green, C.D., et al.: A four year review of cardiac pacing in Glasgow: 181 Medtronic generators implanted in 127 patients. Am. Heart J., 83:265, 1972.

14. Goldstein, S., et al.: Transthoracic and transvenous pacemakers: A comparative clinical experience with 131 implantable units. Br. Heart J., 32:35, 1970.

15. Conklin, E. F., Grannelli, S., and Nealon, T.F.: Four hundred consecutive patients with permanent transvenous pacemakers. J. Thorac. Cardiovasc. Surg., 69:1, 1975.

16. Bernstein, V., Rotem, C.E., and Peretz, D.I.: Permanent pacemakers: 8 year follow-up study. Ann. Intern. Med., 74:361, 1971.

17. McLaughlin, J.S.: et al.: Permanent transvenous catheter pacing; Six year experience. J. Thorac. Cardiovasc. Surg., 66:771, 1973.

18. Morris, J.J. Jr., et al.: Permanent ventricular pacemakers comparison of transthoracic and transvenous implantation. Circulation, 36:587, 1967.

19. Quetmit, A.S., Klatt, K.M., and Kroncke, G.M.: Permanent transvenous pacing. A report of 70 patients. J. Thorac. Cardiovasc. Surg., 62:307, 1971.

20. Fishman, J.H., et al.: Permanent transvenous pacing for senile heart block. Am. J. Surg., 120:187, 1970.

21. Sowton, E., Hendrix, G., and Roy, P.: Ten year surgery of treatment with implanted cardiac pacemakers. Br. Med. J., 3:155, 1974.

22. Seremetis, M.G., et al.: Cardiac pacemakers. Clinical experience with 289 patients. Am. Heart J., 85:739, 1973.

23. Torrensani, J., et al.: Clinical experience in transvenous and myocardial pacing. Ann. N.Y. Acad. Sci., 167:995, 1969.

24. Kahn, O.: Prosthetic cardiac pacers in community hospitals. Am. Heart J., 88:656, 1974.

25. Furman, S., Escher, D.J.W., and Solomon, N.: Experiences with myocardial and transvenous implanted cardiac pacemakers. Am. J. Cardiol., 23:66, 1969.

26. Parsonnet, V.: A decade of permanent pacing of the heart. Cardiovasc. Clin., 2(No. 2):182, 1970.

27. Parsonnet, V.: Permanent pacing of the heart: A comment on technique. Am. J. Cardiol., 36:268, 1975.

28. Brenner, A.S., et al.: Transvenous, transmediastinal and transthoracic ventricular pacing: A comparison after complete two year follow-up. Circulation, 49:407, 1974.

17

Electrical Testing in Cardiac Pacing

PHILIP VARRIALE
RAYMOND P. KWA
JOSEF NIZNIK
EMIL A. NACLERIO

Electrophysiologic studies during pacemaker implantation and reoperation will provide crucial information relative to the function of the complete pacing system. Initial intraoperative electrical testing establishes guidelines for the selection of an optimal electrode site and permits accurate assessment of lead and pulse generator performance. At reoperation, it ascertains chronic lead integrity and facilitates analysis of the causes of and solutions to a variety of problems incident to pacing malfunction.

The technique of electrical testing for cardiac pacing has been firmly established by the introduction of multipurpose testing devices termed pacing system analyzers (PSA) (Fig. 17–1). These sophisticated battery-operated devices are designed to measure a variety of important electrical parameters that relate to pacing function and to myocardial electrical responsiveness.

FUNDAMENTAL CONSIDERATIONS

A successful approach to pacing analysis is contingent upon a thorough comprehension of electrophysiologic concepts and their appropriate application to pacemaker therapy. The authors will therefore first consider these fundamental pacing concepts and then follow with a description of the essential steps in intraoperative testing.

Stimulation (Pacing) Threshold

The stimulation threshold for cardiac pacing is the minimal electrical energy that consistently produces propagated depolarization outside the refractory period of the heart. The stimulus is measured in milliamperes (mA) as *current threshold*, or in volts (V) as *voltage threshold*. The current threshold is considered to be a more physiologic measurement because it pro-

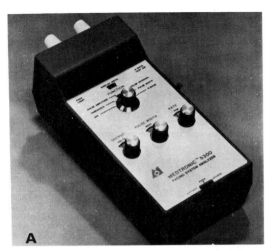

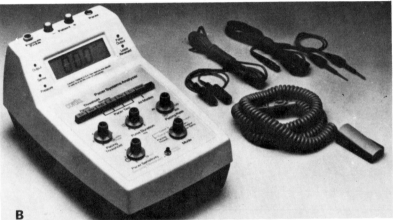

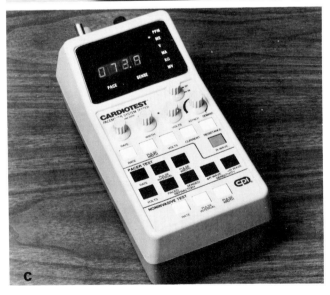

Fig. 17–1. Three currently available pacing system analyzers (PSA). A, Medtronic Model 5300; B, Cordis Model 209A; C, CPI Model 2200. All are external battery-operated multipurpose testing devices that generate a constant-voltage pulse and simultaneously digitally displayed current during stimulation. A constant-current stimulation pulse is also incorporated in the Cordis model. A sensing modality detects the cardiac signal available for sensing as an electronic digital readout. The PSA also permits measurement of electrical parameters of permanent pulse generator.

vides the necessary flow of ions across the cardiac cell membrane to induce depolarization and reflects the density of current responsible for stimulation. Practically, both current and voltage thresholds should be determined simultaneously to permit calculation of *lead impedance* (resistance) using Ohm's law (E = IR) where E = voltage, I = current and R = resistance. A *constant-voltage* or *constant-current* threshold or preferably both may be obtained with an external pulse generator as exemplified by the currently available pacing system analyzers.

It is recommended that the independent stimulation parameter for threshold determination be selected in accordance with properties of the output circuit of the implantable pulse generator. A constant-voltage external pacing device is most applicable, since most implantable units are designed as constant-voltage output circuitry; the leading edge of the voltage pulse remains constant within the limits of load (Fig. 17–2). Constant-voltage output may not remain constant when the resistance load falls below 200 ohms. A low load impedance of this magnitude is an unusual clinical occurrence.

With a constant-voltage stimulator, the voltage leading edge is adjusted independently. Current, as a function of resistance in the lead system, becomes displayed as a digital readout simultaneously and instantaneously.

Pulse generators, whose output circuitry is designated as "current-limited," are constant-current with low resistance and become, in effect, constant-voltage pulses as the resistance increases and the limit of voltage supply is reached. A constant-current external pacing device is used in these situations to provide current threshold as the independent parameter and voltage as a function of the resistance of the lead system.

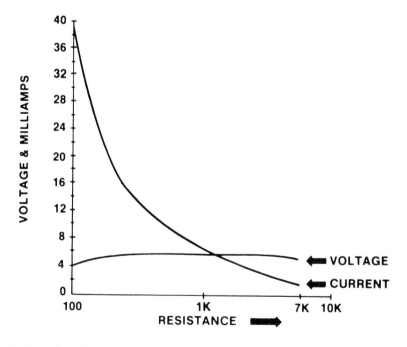

Fig. 17–2. Relationship of current output to lead impedance in a constant-voltage pulse generator. Leading edge of voltage pulse remains constant above resistance load of 200 ohms. Current pulse progressively decreases as lead impedance increases and becomes identical numerically to voltage pulse at 1000 ohms (1K). Lead impedance is shown in log scale.

Current or voltage threshold varies as a function of the duration of the stimulus pulse; this is readily defined and understood by the strength-duration curve. As a general principle the current or voltage threshold remains constant at a pulse duration of 1.0 to 1.5 milliseconds (rheobase) and rises as the stimulus pulse duration becomes less. The pacing threshold should always be measured with the stimulus whose pulse duration is equal to that of the implanted pulse generator.

The acute voltage threshold should be below 1.0 V or ideally 15% or less of the implantable pulse generator output, when tested with a constant-voltage PSA and measured at the same pulse width as the permanent pacemaker. A properly determined and satisfactory stimulation threshold reflects not only lead function and optimal electrode position but also the safety margin between the patient's threshold and the output capability of the permanent pulse generator.

The pacing system—unipolar or bipolar—may also affect testing measurements. Since current threshold is a function of the stimulating cathodal electrode in contact with the myocardium, its measurement is identical whether that electrode represents a part of the unipolar or the bipolar system. A bipolar pacing system presents a higher lead resistance because of the small size of the anodal electrode. As a result, the voltage stimulus required to deliver threshold current will be variably higher up to 30%.

Other Threshold Measurements

The current threshold of stimulation with a given pulse duration varies according to the surface area of the cathodal electrode. A more accurate and reproducible measurement is expressed as current density; that is, the current threshold divided by the effective surface area of the electrode. It also permits a valuable comparison of stimulation thresholds when electrodes of various sizes are used in different patients. With a fixed current pulse, the current density decreases chronically as the active tissue-electrode interface enlarges. The human heart requires a current density of approximately 3.0 mA/cm^2 for acute stimulation and 8 to 10 mA/cm^2 for chronic stimulation independent of electrode size.

Charge threshold, a measurement seldom used, is expressed in microcoulombs as the product of current threshold (mA) and pulse duration (msec). Unlike current or voltage threshold, the charge stimulation threshold decreases with shorter pulse durations. A comparison of the charges of the pulse generator output and its battery may be of some value in the calculation of generator longevity.

The total energy necessary for cardiac stimulation, *energy threshold* (Et), is determined from the product of voltage, current, and pulse duration and is expressed in microjoules. The energy threshold of stimulation at primary lead implantation or pulse generator replacement allows a safety margin measurement when compared to the energy output (Eo) of the implanted pulse generator.

Chronic Threshold

An expected progressive rise in stimulation threshold occurs during the first week or more after electrode placement. A decline from this peak then ensues so that a stabilized chronic threshold is established three weeks or more after implant. Given an intact and stable lead, this predictable rise in threshold is explained by the formation of nonstimulatable fibrotic tissue around the electrode. A decrease in current density in propinquity to viable cardiac tissue is apparent, since the effective electrode size that includes both the electrode and fibrotic tissue increases. In a majority of patients, long-term stability of the electrode threshold may be expected to reach a level two to three times above the acute stimulation measurement. In a recent study by Furman and co-workers, approximately 20% of thresholds increased progressively over the life of the lead to exceed pacemaker output in six to seven years.

Ideally, the chronic energy threshold of stimulation should not exceed one third of the energy output of the pulse generator to allow for the expected stimulation threshold rise with time and threshold variation with long-term stable electrodes. With a 5 V pulse generator, the highest acceptable chronic voltage threshold at 70% of the pulse generator output is 3.5 V and corresponds to a 2:1 energy ratio. A chronic voltage threshold at 60% of the pulse generator output, or 3.0 V, yields a more favorable safety margin with an energy ratio of 3:1.

Lead Impedance (Resistance)

Electrical testing must include the calculation of lead impedance or load on the pacing system when the electrode stimulates the heart. Impedance is derived from Ohm's law ($R = E/I$) when voltage and current threshold are measured simultaneously with a PSA during stimulation studies. As an independent measurement, lead impedance bears no relationship to the patient's stimulation threshold or to the selection of an optimal electrode site. Determination of lead impedance assists in the diagnosis of a defective lead, such as impending or existing lead fracture or insulation break.

Pacemaker lead impedance has three components:

1. The resistance of the *pacing lead* usually ranges between 6.0 and 150 ohms as measured *in vitro*.

2. The pure *tissue resistance* of approximately 200 to 500 ohms includes both normal and fibrotic myocardial tissue.

3. *Polarization resistance* is created by the alignment of a layer of opposite charges at the electrode-tissue interface during the pacemaker pulse (Fig. 17–3). This electrochemical potential opposes current flow

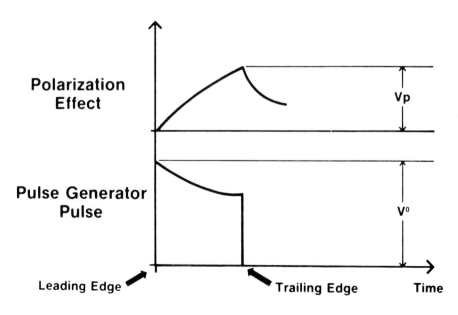

Fig. 17–3. Polarization voltage rises rapidly during initial portion of pacemaker pulse and reaches peak at trailing edge of pacing pulse. Polarization effect is then largely dissipated by diffusion before subsequent pacemaker pulse, usually within 200 msec.

and may represent from 15 to 35% or more of the total lead impedance. Polarization effect varies inversely with electrode surface area and directly with the output pulse width and current amplitude.

Normal lead impedance ranges between 250 and 1200 ohms* and usually decreases with electrode maturity. A loss of lead integrity should be seriously considered when a decrease of resistance below 250 ohms or an increase above 1200 ohms (dependent upon lead specifications) is demonstrable. As the output voltage of all pulse generators is usually designed between 5 and 6 volts, the current delivered into the pacing system may decline dramatically to a point of noncapture as high lead impedance occurs.

Cardiac Signal for Pacemaker Sensing

The sensing circuit of a ventricular demand pacemaker has been developed to respond selectively to the depolarization (QRS) potential in proximity to the pacing electrode and to reject undesirable signals such as T waves, myopotential artifacts, and electromagnetic interference. Maximal detection of the amplitude and frequency content of the ventricular depolarization wave signal or atrial depolarization wave signal, if an atrial demand pacemaker is used, is provided by a special design of the sensing circuitry. The spectrum of responses to QRS or P wave signals of most demand pacemakers is characterized by the amplitude-frequency sensing response curve in which the amplitude of the input signal is related to an appropriate frequency or time duration for that particular signal (Fig. 17–4).

QRS signals within the frequency range of 20 to 50 Hz usually require the least amplitude for detection (2 ± 0.5 mV) and correspond to the maximal sensitivity re-

sponse for most demand pacemakers. Electrical signals extraneous to the usual frequency spectra of the depolarization wave, such as skeletal muscle potential (above 70 Hz) and T wave (between 5 and 10 Hz), are selectively attenuated. These signals require considerably higher amplitude for detection and are usually rejected for pacemaker sensing. The detected cardiac signal is then used to inhibit or trigger pacemaker discharge in accordance with the sensing modality.

The cardiac signal available for sensing is best depicted by a properly recorded cardiac electrogram. The vertical deflection with the highest amplitude and optimal frequency content of the QRS waveform is almost always identified as the *intrinsic deflection* (ID). This rapid deflection appears as a vertical, nearly straight line segment and corresponds to activation of the myocardium surrounding the pacing electrode. The signal represented by the amplitude and frequency of the ID is usually maximally detected by the demand sensing circuit.

A statistically significant decrease of the rate of voltage change of the ID and a moderate decrease in its amplitude occur as fibrosis develops around the pacing electrode. Chronic pacing is therefore associated with a variable reduction in the cardiac signal available for sensing. The cardiac signal may become marginal or even subthreshold for pacemaker sensing as the electrode matures, particularly if the sensing measurement at primary implantation is close to 4 mV (see Chapter 18).

TESTING DURING PRIMARY PACEMAKER IMPLANTATION

Electrical testing is initiated during primary pacemaker implantation after the endocardial lead has been correctly positioned within the apex of the right ventricle under fluoroscopic control or an epicardial lead has been well secured into the

---

*An impedance of 1500 ohms is described for the Cordis ball-tip electrode.

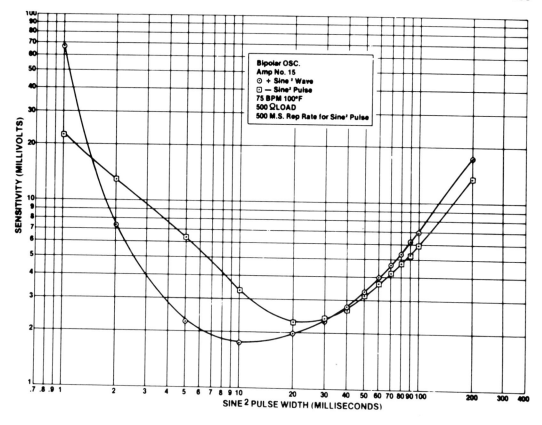

Fig. 17–4. Sensitivity characteristics of Medtronic Xyrel pulse generator (Model 5972) are depicted in amplitude-pulse width response curve, using sine² wave as arbitrary test signal. Signal of negative polarity (indicated by dotted box) in this model is maximally sensitive between 20 and 30 msec. A positive input signal (indicated by dotted circle) with pulse width of 20 msec or more, is of similar sensitivity but deviates from the negative signal below 20 msec.

myocardial wall during surgery. A PSA testing device that provides a constant-voltage or constant-current modality for stimulation and simultaneous digital display of the other measurement—current or voltage—is recommended. The instrument should also provide a testing mode for the principal functional parameters of the permanent pulse generator. The independent output pulse and the stimulus pulse duration of the testing device should correspond to those of the implanted pulse generator.

Pulse Generator Testing

The PSA has an electronic digital readout that can separately test the operational pa-rameters of the implantable pulse generator. The output pulse amplitude, pulse width, and discharge rate (pulse interval) of the pacemaker are measured with a PSA and compared to the specifications provided by the manufacturer. A pulse generator is considered defective if discrepant measurements are detected.

Stimulation Threshold Testing

The stimulation threshold of the implanted lead is measured with a sterile lead extension cable which connects the testing device to the electrode terminal of the lead. In the bipolar configuration, the negative connector of the test cable is attached to the cathodal electrode terminal that is usually the distal electrode of a pervenous lead, and the positive connector is attached to the anodal electrode terminal. In the unipolar mode, the negative connector of the test cable is attached to the patient's lead, and the positive connector to an indifferent electrode placed in moist subcutaneous tissue. The size of the indifferent electrode is important if accurate thresholds are to be obtained. An indifferent electrode plate of reduced surface area or one in contact with dry skin will augment impedance and thereby increase voltage threshold. An electrode plate with a surface area greater than 12 cm^2 usually provides an acceptable resistance. For this purpose we prefer an instrument such as the Goelet (bull dog) retractor. The choice of a large-sized indifferent electrode plate is important for consistent and accurate threshold measurements.

The output pulse, constant-voltage or constant-current, of the external testing device, set at the appropriate pulse width, is activated at a pacing rate 10 pulses/min. above the patient's spontaneous heart rate. The initial amplitude of the pulse is selected arbitrarily (about 3 V or 6 mA) and gradually decreased until complete capture is lost. Pacing threshold is indicated by the lowest amplitude that establishes consistent myocardial stimulation. Conversely, one may define the stimulation threshold by increasing the pacing stimulus amplitude until consistent capture is gained. A slightly lower pacing threshold will be obtained using a stimulus reduction approach because of stimulation hysteresis. The difference in stimulation thresholds of the two techniques is sufficiently small and clinically unimportant. Decreasing stimulus approach is favored because it provides continuous capture of the heart and safety for the patient who is pacemaker-dependent.

An acute stimulation threshold below 1.0 V for a constant-voltage pulse measured at the same pulse width as the implantable

unit or ideally 15% or less of the permanent pacemaker output voltage is recommended. For a constant current pulse, an acute stimulation threshold below 1.0 mA is recommended. A higher voltage or current threshold and a correspondingly calculated normal lead impedance is consistent with a poor electrode-tissue interface due to malposition or electrode contact with nonviable fibrotic tissue. In the constant voltage modality, an erratic current readout on the digital display in the presence of an intact lead will indicate an unstable endocardial electrode tip position.

Repositioning of the lead is indicated if pacing thresholds are unsatisfactory, and a new anatomic pacing site is selected that fulfills the recommended threshold requirements. In a bipolar system, the lead or electrode offering the best satisfactory stimulation threshold is selected as the cathodal or stimulation electrode.

The finding of a low satisfactory pacing threshold at primary pacemaker implantation represents the single most important electrical measurement reflective of an optimal electrode position. It also permits assessment of the output circuit "reserve" for successful long-term pacing.

Sensing Measurement

A satisfactory sensing measurement is another indispensable electrophysiologic pacemaker requisite supportive of good electrode position. The measurement of pacemaker sensing is established by using an appropriately selected PSA whose sensitivity calibration corresponds to that of the implantable pulse generator. The sensing circuit of this testing device detects the cardiac signal and generates an electronic digital readout in mV as a sensing measurement.

The lowest acceptable sensing measurement of a ventricular signal should be more than twice the nominal specified sensing threshold of the pulse generator or at least 5 mV. A good QRS signal is usually above 7 mV. A poor sensing measurement may indicate lead displacement, myocardial perforation, or an inadequate cardiac signal at the electrode site. When the sensing signal is less than satisfactory, lead reposition to another electrode site is indicated. Frequently a bipolar signal whose voltage amplitude is less than optimal may be converted to a unipolar signal of higher voltage.

The recording of a cardiac electrogram is also recommended during primary pacemaker implantation and reoperation, since it establishes a graphic display of the cardiac signal available for sensing. A QRS signal with appropriate amplitude-frequency characteristics is detected by the pacer sensing circuit, and satisfactory pacemaker sensing is therefore a direct function of the cardiac electrogram.

An electrographic cardiac signal is recorded in the polarity corresponding to the implantable lead system configuration, preferably with a physiologic oscilloscopic instrument of high impedance, high paper speed, and suitable frequency response (see Chapter 18).

The amplitude of the electrographic intrinsic deflection may be used as the sensing measurement when a PSA is not available. A peak-to-peak ID amplitude of at least 6 to 8 mV is recommended for acceptable pacemaker sensing. An ID of lesser amplitude should be considered unsatisfactory and consistent with a poor sensing signal. The presence of an ST segment elevation or a current of injury of at least 2 mV in height at the time of primary lead installation is also indicative of electrode contact with viable endocardium or myocardium and represents another criterion of satisfactory electrode position.

PULSE GENERATOR REPLACEMENT OR PACEMAKER TROUBLESHOOTING PROCEDURES

It is recommended that a constant-voltage pulse be used routinely for stimulation threshold measurements during pulse generator replacement or pacemaker troubleshooting procedures for the following reasons:

1. Most currently available permanent pulse generators have a constant-voltage output circuitry in which the leading edge of the voltage pulse remains constant with a lead resistance above 200 ohms. Current-limited pulse generators, on the other hand, generate a constant-current pulse only at a low lead resistance and function as a constant-voltage pulse at a higher lead impedance.

2. A safety margin is established between the voltage stimulation threshold and the implantable pulse generator output voltage. Chronic threshold variations and the expected rise in stimulation threshold with time make this assessment important, particularly for those patients who are pacemaker-dependent.

3. Voltage threshold is more useful in the evaluation of chronic lead integrity. A lead system of high resistance may have a normal or even low current threshold, but the voltage requirement will be abnormally high.

The highest acceptable chronic voltage threshold has been described as 3.0 to 3.5 V. The former is preferable, particularly for pacemaker-dependent patients, since it corresponds to a threshold of 60% of a 5 V pulse generator output and indicates a more favorable energy safety margin ratio of 3:1.

It is probably most judicious to consider a new lead system when the chronic threshold is above 3.0 V in a pacemaker-dependent patient or in other patients when an inordinate threshold elevation above 3.5 V occurs within 2 to 3 years following pacemaker implantation. A high output pulse generator can be implanted in patients with a marginally elevated voltage threshold.

The lead system must be replaced or repositioned if ventricular capture does not occur with a constant voltage threshold below 5 V, simultaneous high current, and normal lead impedance. This finding is consistent with a lead malposition (dislodgment or ventricular perforation), or an exit block due to excessive fibrotic reaction or nonviable tissue in contact with the pacing electrode. A bipolar pacing system can be converted to a unipolar configuration when exit block is present, if the previously available anodal electrode provides a satisfactory pacing threshold.

Pulse generator malfunction or poor lead-generator connection can be diagnosed when the stimulation threshold and lead impedance are normal, but pacing failure, either intermittent or continuous, is present. A reduced voltage output, rate decrease of 7 to 10% or more below the programmed fixed-rate of the pulse generator, and pulse width increase in certain units are consistent with battery depletion (Fig. 17–5). These functional characteristics of the pacemaker are measured with an appropriately selected PSA.

Correction of a poor lead connection will restore normal pacing when this problem is evident. Component or circuitry failure as a cause of pacemaker malfunction and noncapture is best determined by the manufacturer.

A diagnosis of lead fracture is tenable if the calculated lead impedance is increased above 1200 ohms as determined from Ohm's law as the ratio of average voltage to average current pulse during stimulation. An intermittent and partial lead fracture as the cause of pacing failure will show a high

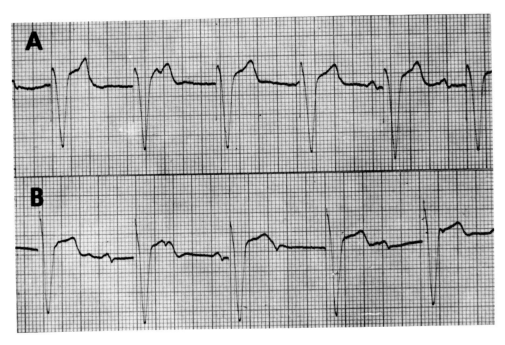

Fig. 17–5. A, Programmed basic pacing rate of 68/min (880 msec) at primary implantation of 4-cell mercury-zinc pulse generator with initial output of 5.2 V and pulse width of 0.5 msec. B, Pacemaker automatic interval of 1,040 msec (58 beats/min) recorded three years after implantation. Battery depletion was diagnosed, since this cycle length represented rate decrease of 15% compared to the programmed basic pacing rate. At reoperation, PSA measurement of pulse generator parameters showed pulse interval of 1,065 msec, voltage output of 2.5 V, pulse amplitude of 5.0 mA (at 500 ohm test load), and pulse width of 2.3 msec. Chronic stimulation threshold of ventricle was 2.4 V and simultaneous current readout 5.3 mA at 0.5 msec stimulus duration. Capture was maintained because of energy compensation provided by programmed increase in output pulse width to 2.3 msec.

voltage threshold and low to normal, but erratic, current reading in a high and rapidly changing lead impedance (Fig. 17–6). Intermittent loss of ventricular capture is associated with reduction of the stimulus pulse amplitude due to momentary separation of wire fragments and an excessive lead resistance. Complete lead fracture may rarely exhibit sensing function in the presence of an ineffective and attenuated stimulus pulse when a fluid conductive bridge is present between the separated ends.

A disruption of lead insulation is characterized by a normal voltage pulse, high current reading, and low calculated lead impedance, usually less than 250 ohms. The insulation break engenders a short circuit and alternative shunt of current flow into the tissues that reduces current density at the electrode site. This may also be associated with a change in the vectorial orientation and amplitude of the pacing spike.

A defective endocardial bipolar lead should be replaced, and a defective unipolar lead should be repaired or replaced. An epicardial bipolar lead system, on the other hand, can be unipolarized, if one lead is intact.

Sensing loss due to a meager or inadequate cardiac signal below the sensing threshold of the pulse generator requires electrode reposition or new lead installation to a site that allows a more satisfactory sensing signal. Selection of a pacemaker with a high sensitivity threshold is recommended if the chronic cardiac signal is marginal (1.5 to 3.0 mV) for pacemaker sensing.

Undersensing or failure of demand pacemaker inhibition may be due to pulse generator malfunction when the sensing measurement of the PSA is satisfactory and the recorded electrographic cardiac signal is adequate. These pacemaker malfunctions include circuitry and component failure, faulty magnetic reed switch, and leakage path between pacemaker terminals. The problem of oversensing due to inapparent and false signals is discussed in chapters 18 and 19.

OPTIMAL ELECTRODE SITE FOR PERMANENT EPICARDIAL PACING

An accurate prediction of an optimal epicardial pacing site cannot be determined by visual inspection of the heart. A healthy appearing myocardial site not infrequently

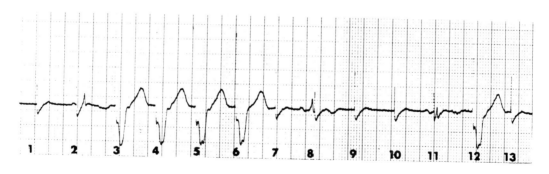

Fig. 17–6. Constant-voltage stimulation pulse of 5.0 V generated by PSA at rate of 105/min shows intermittent loss of capture (beats 1, 7, 9, 10, and 13), associated with decrease of the stimulus pulse amplitude. Digital readout of simultaneous current during constant-voltage pulse discharge was low and erratic; it ranged between 1.7 and 3.0 mA. Stimulation of ventricle (beats 3 to 6 and 12) occurred only when current pulse was 3.0 mA (highest stimulus artifact in ECG). Lead impedance was changing but variably high and ranged between 1600 and 3000 ohms. These findings are consistent with intermittent and partial lead fracture. (Beats 2, 8, and 11 are pseudofusion complexes.)

TABLE 17-1

Important Stimulation Parameters of Intraoperative Electrical Testing

PACING PROBLEM	CONSTANT VOLTAGE (V)		CONSTANT CURRENT (I)		LEAD IMPEDANCE 250–1200 ohms* (Normal)	SOLUTION
	V (V) Acute <1.0 (Normal) Chronic <3.0–3.5 (Normal)	I (mA)	I (mA) Acute <1.0 (Normal) Chronic <2.5–3.5 (Normal)	V (V)		
1. Malposition (dislodgment or perforation)	High	High	High	High	Normal	Reposition lead to another electrode site
2. Exit block	High	High	High	High	Normal	High output pacemaker Replace lead system Implant a new lead system
3. Faulty pulse generator	Normal	Normal	Normal	Normal	Normal	Replace pulse generator
4. Loose lead-permanent generator connection	Normal	Normal	Normal	Normal	Normal	Adjust lead connection
5. Unstable electrode position	Normal	Normal but erratic†	Normal	Normal but erratic‡	Normal	Reposition lead to a stable electrode site
6. Complete lead fracture						
a. without fluid conductive bridge	a. High	a. Zero	a. High	a. High	a. Infinity§	Repair or replace unipolar lead Unipolarize epicardial bipolar lead system
b. with fluid conductive bridge	b. High	b. Low	b. High	b. High	b. Very high§	Replace endocardial bipolar lead system
7. Partial lead fracture (apposed ends with momentary and intermittent separation)	High	Low and/or normal but erratic†	Normal or high	Normal and/or high but erratic‡	Unstable and changing but above 1200 ohms	Same as 6
8. Lead insulation break	Low	High	High	Low	Below 250 ohms	Same as 6

* Cordis ball-tip electrode has a lead impedance up to 1500 ohms.
† Sequential current changes more than 0.5 mA.
‡ Sequential voltage changes more than 0.5 V.
§ Lead impedance is calculable only with constant voltage testing device but is not measurable or accurate with constant current pulse output due to voltage limit of constant current PSA.

proves unsatisfactory for permanent pacing. The finding of disparate stimulation thresholds, particularly of the RV, underscores the importance of precise selection of the most suitable myocardial site, using the myocardial test electrode (MTE), prior to permanent lead implantation.

Myocardial Test Electrode (MTE)

The selection of a satisfactory electrode site prior to lead installation represents an important prerequisite for successful long-term cardiac pacing. The best permanent pacing site of either ventricle may be predetermined with a specially designed hand-held myocardial test electrode (Fig. 17–7). Preliminary electrophysiologic measurements obtained from this test probe, including the electrographic cardiac signal, closely predict the actual stimulation threshold and sensing value of the permanent electrode.

The myocardial test electrode (Medtronic

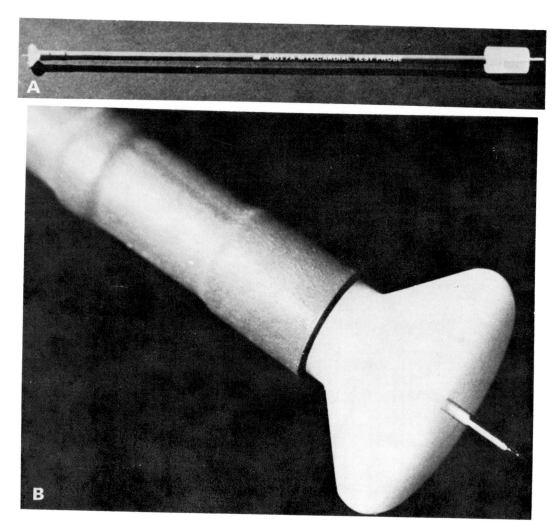

Fig. 17–7. A, Myocardial test electrode (Medtronic Model 6017A) is 25.4 cm in length. B, It terminates in platinum-iridium electrode needle with surface area of 5.3 mm². Depth of electrode needle penetration is 3.6 mm. Electrode characteristics approximate those of sutureless myocardial electrode (Medtronic Model 6917A).

Model 6017A) terminates in an exploring needle that approximates the penetration depth and electrode surface area of the sutureless myocardial lead (Medtronic Model 6917A). The terminal connector is attached to a PSA via a sterile lead extension cable. The MTE needle is inserted into a number of arbitrarily selected myocardial sites to determine the most suitable implantation site.

Myocardial testing sites are designated in our patients by a ventricular "map." For the exposed lower anterior wall of the right ventricle (RV), six areas are selected (Fig. 17–8). These areas are equally distributed between the atrioventricular (AV) and interventricular (IV) grooves and extend superiorly over two levels, 4 to 5 cm above the diaphragmatic margin. For the left ventricle (LV), three areas of the anterolateral wall extending from the apex to approximately 6 cm cephalad are delineated (Fig. 17–9).

The use of a ventricular "map" limits the number of test probe measurements and permits a simple and valuable preliminary electrophysiologic test technique for precise selection of the best epicardial pacing site. Most importantly, this technique reduces the risk of potential pacing failure by eliminating indiscriminate insertion of the electrode.

The optimal ventricular site ultimately selected for permanent electrode implantation should offer the lowest stimulation requirement and a high sensing measure-

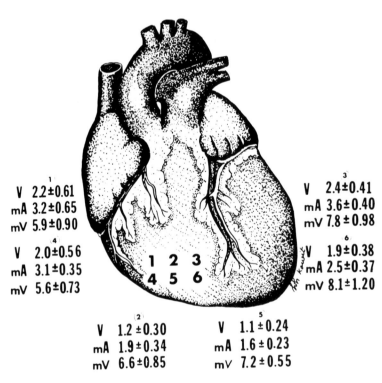

V   2.2±0.61
mA 3.2±0.65
mV 5.9±0.90

V   2.0±0.56
mA 3.1±0.35
mV 5.6±0.73

V   2.4±0.41
mA 3.6±0.40
mV 7.8±0.98

V   1.9±0.38
mA 2.5±0.37
mV 8.1±1.20

V   1.2±0.30
mA 1.9±0.34
mV 6.6±0.85

V   1.1±0.24
mA 1.6±0.23
mV 7.2±0.55

Fig. 17–8. Six myocardial testing areas of lower anterior wall of RV. Mean electrophysiologic measurements were obtained with the MTE from these six selected testing sites in 75 patients. Constant voltage pulse (pulse width of 0.5 msec) was used to determine stimulation threshold. Digital display of PSA indicated simultaneous current as function of resistance. Mean sensing measurements were determined from digital readout of PSA.

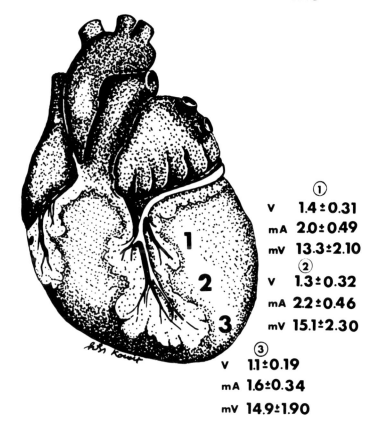

$$V \quad 1.4 \pm 0.31$$
$$mA \quad 2.0 \pm 0.49$$
$$mV \quad 13.3 \pm 2.10$$

②
$$V \quad 1.3 \pm 0.32$$
$$mA \quad 2.2 \pm 0.46$$
$$mV \quad 15.1 \pm 2.30$$

③
$$V \quad 1.1 \pm 0.19$$
$$mA \quad 1.6 \pm 0.34$$
$$mV \quad 14.9 \pm 1.90$$

Fig. 17–9. Three myocardial testing areas of anterolateral wall of LV. Each area is approximately 2 cm in diameter. Mean electrophysiologic measurements were obtained with MTE from these three selected testing sites in 38 patients.

ment. A site that provokes ectopic beats or bursts of ventricular tachycardia is considered unsatisfactory.

Electrophysiologic Measurements of Myocardial Sites Using MTE

Preliminary electrophysiologic studies in 113 patients using the MTE from a variety of epicardial sites of the right and left ventricles have led to important observations and specific conclusions relevant to permanent epicardial pacing.

Stimulation Threshold

1. The stimulation thresholds were relatively disparate for the six testing sites of the lower anterior wall of the RV but less disparate and more uniform for the three testing sites of the anterolateral wall of the LV.

2. The best average stimulation measurements were obtained from the lower central areas of the RV (areas 2 and 5). These areas offered an optimal permanent electrode site in more than 90% of our patients. The lower region of the anterolateral wall of the LV, area 3, was recognized as the best pacing site in 60% of our patients.

3. Area 5 of the RV yielded the most favorable average pacing threshold (1.2 V) for this chamber and was selected as the optimal site in 75% of the patients.

4. Right ventricular myocardial sites close to the AV groove (areas 1 and 4) and

IV groove (areas 3 and 6) offered unsatisfactory pacing thresholds, nearly 2V or higher. Only two areas, 4 and 6, were selected as optimal sites for permanent pacing in less than 10% of our patients.

Sensing Measurements

1. The average sensing measurements of the six testing areas of the RV ranged between 5.6 and 8.1 mV and, in general, were higher for sites closer to the IV septum.
2. The three left ventricular areas offered a mean sensing measurement that was less variable and was approximately twice that of the RV.

Electrophysiologic Measurements after Permanent Electrode Implantation

The available pacing sites of the anterolateral wall of the LV offer more consistent satisfactory measurements of stimulation than those of the RV. Myocardial sites outside the central areas of the RV are usually unfavorable and unreliable for permanent pacing.

The cardiac signal of the LV is twofold higher than that of the RV and distinctly advantageous when compared to all epicardial sites of the RV. The more consistently satisfactory pacing sites of the LV and its

superior cardiac signal lend strong support to the LV as the preferred cardiac chamber for permanent epicardial pacing.

Measurements obtained from a sutureless epicardial lead installed into selected optimal sites of the RV (75 patients) and of the LV (38 patients) are given in Table 17–2.

1. Average stimulation and sensing measurements after permanent epicardial lead implantation of either ventricle were approximately 10 to 15% better than the values derived from the MTE. The improved measurements were obtained approximately 5 minutes after epicardial lead installation and probably suggest a more stable electrode-myocardial interface.
2. The mean stimulation threshold of the LV (0.73 V) after epicardial electrode insertion was only slightly better than that of the RV (0.81 V).
3. The average sensing measurement of the LV (16.2 mV) is clearly superior to that of the RV (8.25 mV).

SELECTED READINGS

Barold, S.S., and Winner, J.A.: Techniques and significance of threshold measurement for cardiac pacing. Relationship to output circuit of cardiac pacemakers. Chest, *70*:760, 1976.

Coumel, P., Mugica, J., and Barold, S.S.: Demand pacemaker arrhythmias caused by intermittent incomplete electrode fracture. Diagnosis with testing magnet. Am. J. Cardiol., *36*:105, 1975.

Davies, J.G., and Sowton, E.: Electrical threshold of the human heart. Br. Heart J., *28*:231, 1966.

Dekker, E., Buller, J., and Van Erven, F.A.: Unipolar and bipolar stimulation thresholds of the human myocardium with chronically implanted pacemaker electrodes. Am. Heart J., *71*:671, 1966.

Furman, S.: Cardiac pacing and pacemakers. VI. Analysis of pacemaker malfunction. Am. Heart J., *94*:378, 1977.

Furman, S., and Escher, D.J.W.: Factors affecting electrical stimulation. *In* Principles and Techniques of Cardiac Pacing. New York, Harper & Row, Publishers, 1970.

Furman, S., Garvey, J., and Hurzeler, P.: Pulse duration variation and electrode size as factors in pacemaker longevity. J. Thorac. Cardiovasc. Surg., *69*:382, 1975.

Furman, S., Hurzeler, P., and DeCaprio, V.: Cardiac pacing and pacemakers. III. Sensing the cardiac electrogram. Am. Heart J., *93*:794, 1977.

TABLE 17–2

Measurement of Mean Voltage, Simultaneous Current Stimulation Threshold, and Sensing

	RV*	LV†
V	0.81 ± 0.21	0.73 ± 0.19
mA	1.30 ± 0.45	1.12 ± 0.35
mV	8.25 ± 2.60	16.20 ± 3.01

* 75 patients.
† 38 patients.

Furman, S., Hurzeler, P., and Mehra, R.: Cardiac pacing and pacemakers. IV. Threshold of cardiac stimulation. Am. Heart J., 94:115, 1977.

Furman, S., Parker, B., and Escher, D.J.W.: Decreasing electrode size and increasing efficiency of cardiac stimulation. J. Surg. Res., 11:105, 1971.

Greatbatch, W., et al.: Polarization phenomena relating to physiological electrodes. Ann. N.Y. Acad. Sci., 167:722, 1969.

Luceri, R.M., et al.: Threshold behavior of electrodes in long-term ventricular pacing. Am. J. Cardiol., 40:184, 1977.

Naclerio, E.A., and Varriale, P.: "Screw-in" electrode; new method for permanent ventricular pacing. N.Y. State J. Med., 74:2391, 1974.

Preston, T.A.: Chronic threshold measurement. Ann. Cardiol. Angeiol., 20:501, 1971.

Preston, T.A., and Barold, S.S.: Problems in measuring threshold for cardiac pacing. Recommendations for routine clinical measurement. Am. J. Cardiol., 40:658, 1977.

Preston, T.A., et al.: Changes in myocardial threshold: physiologic and pharmacologic factors in patients with implanted pacemakers. Am. Heart J., 74:235, 1967.

Preston, T.A., and Judge, R.D.: Alteration of pacemaker threshold by drugs and physiological factors. Ann. N.Y. Acad. Sci., 167:686, 1969.

Smith, D., McDonald, R., and Sloman, G.: Implanted cardiac pacemakers: experience with electronic testing. Cardiovasc. Res., 5:236, 1971.

Smyth, N.P.D., et al.: The significance of electrode surface area and stimulating thresholds in permanent cardiac pacing. J. Thorac. Cardiovasc. Surg., 71:559, 1976.

Thalen, H.T.: The artificial cardiac pacemaker. Am. Heart J., 81:583, 1971.

Tyers, G.F.O., Hughes, H.C., and Torman, H.A.: The advantages of transthoracic placement of permanent cardiac pacemaker electrodes. J. Thorac. Cardiovasc. Surg., 69:8, 1975.

Varriale, P., Naclerio, E.A., and Niznik, J.: Selection of site for permanent epicardial pacing using myocardial testing electrode. N.Y. State J. Med., 77:1272, 1977.

18

Electrographic Recordings in Cardiac Pacing

PHILIP VARRIALE
RAYMOND P. KWA
EMIL A. NACLERIO
JOSEF NIZNIK

An increased appreciation of the role of electrographic recordings of the heart as a valuable ancillary diagnostic technique in cardiac pacing has emerged in recent years. Clinically important information in a variety of pacing situations is derived from a properly recorded cardiac electrogram when used in conjunction with intraoperative electrical testing. This technique assists the physician in the selection of an optimal electrode site and in the evaluation of problems during pacemaker troubleshooting procedures. As a graphic display of the circumscribed electrical activity of the heart in contact with the pacing electrode, the cardiac electrogram is most useful as the best depiction of the cardiac signal available for pacemaker sensing.

Waveform and frequency characteristics of the ventricular or atrial signal are faithfully reproduced with the least distortion when electrograms are recorded with physiologic recording instruments under ideal conditions. The most appropriate analysis of these characteristics of the electrogram is provided with an oscilloscopic recorder of high input impedance, high paper speed (100 to 400 mm per second), and suitable frequency response (0.1 to 2500 Hz). The standard electrocardiograph has limited frequency response and paper speed for accurate measurement, but it may be used to record electrograms in other situations.

RECORDING TECHNIQUE

Electrograms are recorded in the appropriate polarity corresponding to the configuration of the lead system implanted. The unipolar electrogram is recorded by connecting the electrode terminal of the pacing lead to the precordial lead of the ECG machine and attaching the limb lead cable to the patient in the conventional manner. When an oscilloscopic instrument is used, the intracardiac cathodal electrode is con-

265

nected to the positive input of the recorder, and the negative input is connected to a subcutaneously placed indifferent plate electrode.

A bipolar electrogram is recorded by connecting the cathodal and anodal electrodes of the pacing lead to the left and right arm leads; the resultant electrogram is represented as lead 1. For oscilloscopic recording, the cathodal electrode is connected to the positive input and the anodal electrode to the negative input.

CHARACTERISTICS OF THE UNIPOLAR VENTRICULAR ELECTROGRAM (FIGS. 18–1 TO 18–3)

A unipolar electrographic recording of the endocardial surface or the epicardial wall of the ventricle, although influenced by the whole heart, reflects the predominant local electrical activity in contact with the pacing electrode.

The depolarization signal is best represented by a vertical, nearly straight line deflection described by Lewis and Wilson as the intrinsic deflection (ID). This important component of the QRS electrogram corresponds to the rapidly developed activation wave front in the cardiac muscle immediately beneath the electrode. Its amplitude and slope most consistently meet the essential requisites for pacemaker sensing.

Other components of the QRS waveform depict more slowly developed electrical activity that precedes and follows the intrinsic deflection. These components represent activation of more distant areas of the heart, including the contralateral ventricle.

Repolarization potentials are identified by an ST segment and a T wave. The acute electrogram is characterized by an elevated ST segment and becomes almost always isoelectric as the electrode matures.

The P wave is usually diminutive or absent and represents the far-field potential.

The configuration of the ventricular uni-

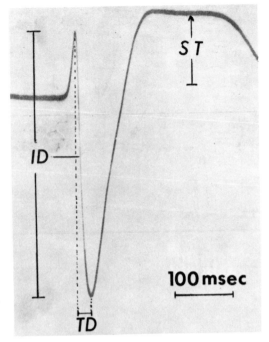

Fig. 18–1. Typical acute endocardial RV unipolar electrogram (EG). Intrinsic deflection (ID) is identified as vertical, nearly straight line deflection; its time duration (TD) is interval between peaks and measures 25 msec. (Paper speed = 200 mm/sec.)

polar electrogram is determined by the predominant polarity of the intrinsic deflection. For endocardial or epicardial right ventricular signals, the configuration is usually predominantly negative or, less often, predominantly positive or diphasic. The epicardial left ventricular electrogram is almost always predominantly positive or less frequently diphasic. A negative deflection is unusual and probably reflective of isolated myocardial damage or electrode position within the left ventricular cavity.

ANALYSIS OF THE INTRINSIC DEFLECTION

An analysis of the electrographic intrinsic deflection deserves special consideration

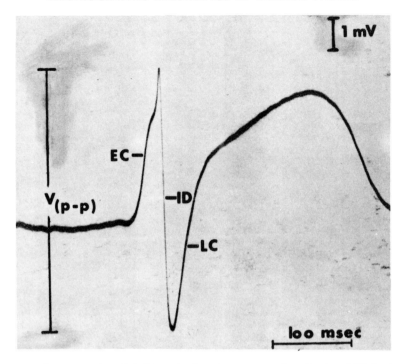

Fig. 18–2. Typical acute epicardial RV unipolar electrogram. Amplitude of ID is determined as peak-to-peak voltage in mV. ID is 8.5 mV. Early component (EC) and late component (LC) identify slowly developed waveforms that precede and follow ID. (Paper speed = 200 mm/sec.)

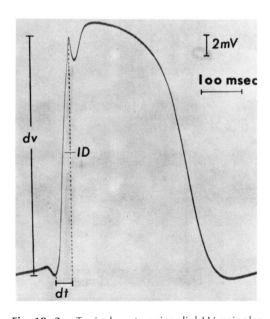

Fig. 18–3. Typical acute epicardial LV unipolar electrogram. EG is characterized by positive monophasic waveform. Slew rate of ID is defined as rate of voltage change (dv/dt) and measures 0.59 V/sec in this EG. (Paper speed = 200 mm/sec.)

because this discrete potential most consistently represents the ideal cardiac signal entering the sensing circuit of the pacemaker. The bandpass filter of the sensing amplifier responds selectively to certain characteristics of the ID that include (1) voltage amplitude, (2) time duration (frequency), and (3) rate of voltage change described mathematically as the dv/dt and termed the slew rate.

The amplitude of the intrinsic deflection is determined as the peak-to-peak voltage in mV and its time duration in msec as the interval between peaks. Expression of the ID signal within the "time domain" as opposed to the "frequency domain" is more clinically applicable to waveform analysis and is easily determined from electrographic recordings. The two domains are inversely proportional; that is, frequency equals 1/time and time equals 1/frequency. A signal characterized by a time duration of 20 msec has a corresponding frequency of 50 Hz.

The slew rate is another important parameter of the ID essential for pacemaker sensing; it is expressed as volts per second (V/sec). In addition to amplitude and frequency, the sensing circuit requires for detection a signal with a minimal slew rate of 0.3 to 0.5 V/sec.

An estimated slew rate of the intrinsic deflection is derived by simply dividing the amplitude by its time duration. In our study of 114 recorded acute ventricular unipolar electrograms, the calculated slew rate of the ID ranged between 0.3 and 1.6 V/sec with a mean of 0.62 V/sec.

Furman and co-workers described the rate of voltage change as a maximal slew rate using a special formula and found it to be 3 ± 1.5 V/sec for acute endocardial ventricular unipolar signals. The bandpass filter is designed to be more sensitive to the amplitude of a signal of high slew rate and conversely to attenuate signals of low slew rate. Slowly rising waveforms with low slew rate, such as repolarization potentials, are reduced and effectively excluded from pacemaker sensing.

CARDIAC SIGNAL AND PACEMAKER SENSING (FIGS. 18–4 TO 18–8)

The relationship between the cardiac signal as displayed by the electrogram and the sensing measurement generated by the sensing circuit of a PSA testing device whose sensitivity characteristics are similar to those of the implantable pulse generator is rather complex and not readily subject to precise determination. The following factors must be considered in the evaluation of pacemaker sensitivity toward an incoming cardiac signal: (1) sensing or source impedance, (2) input impedance of the sensing amplifier, (3) unique characteristics of the bandpass filter of the specific demand sensing circuit, and (4) amplitude, time duration (frequency), and slew rate of the cardiac signal.

The components of the sensing (source)

impedance include wire resistance, tissue resistance, and a more predominant component termed the polarization impedance. The latter component, which is usually about 2500 ohms or less, is related inversely to electrode surface area and directly to time duration of the signal. Sensing impedance as high as 5000 ohms may be encountered with small ball-tip electrodes.

The amplitude of the cardiac signal available for sensing is dependent on the ratio of the input impedance of the sensing amplifier (usually 20,000 ohms) to the sensing impedance. The influence of the latter on pacemaker sensing is apparent from the following example. A cardiac signal may be decreased as much as 20% when the sensing impedance approaches 5000 ohms in accordance with the formula $100/(F + 1)$, where F is the ratio of input impedance to sensing impedance. Cardiac signals are

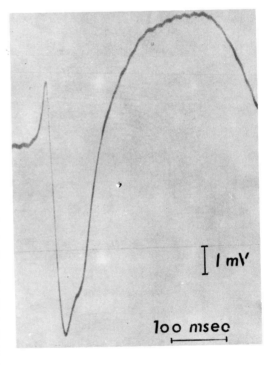

Fig. 18–4. PSA (Medtronic 5300) sensing measurement for acute endocardial RV unipolar signal was 9.5 mV. This matches amplitude (9.4 mV) of ID with time duration of 20 msec. (Paper speed = 200 mm/sec.)

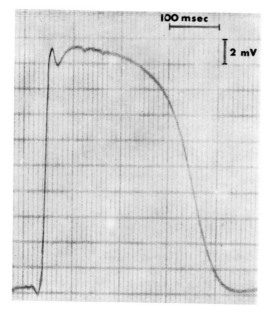

Fig. 18–5. EG ID of acute epicardial LV electrode site is inscribed in 25 msec with an amplitude of 19 mV. Pacemaker sensing measurement was 19 mV. (Paper speed = 200 mm/sec.)

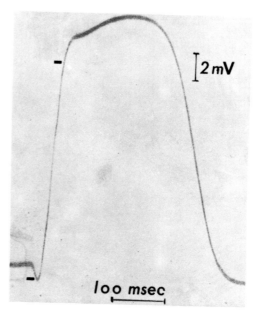

Fig. 18–7. Acute epicardial LV unipolar signal shows ID of 15.5 mV that was attenuated by sensing circuit to 11.3 mV, representing signal reduction of 27%. Signal time duration of 45 msec was probably responsible for this attenuation. (ID amplitude is indicated by the two markers. Paper speed = 200 mm/sec.)

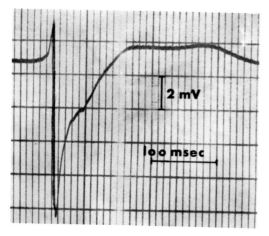

Fig. 18–6. Chronic endocardial RV unipolar signal showing an EG ID of 11.6 mV, inscribed in slightly less than 10 msec. Signals of this duration are usually attenuated in accordance with amplitude-frequency sensing response curve of testing device. ID signal was attenuated 28% by sensing circuit to produce sensing measurement of 8.3 mV. (Paper speed = 200 mm/sec.)

least attenuated when the ratio remains high because of low sensing impedance.

The bandpass filter of the demand sensing circuit will commonly detect cardiac signals with a frequency of 10 to 200 Hz. Required signal amplitudes for pacemaker sensing in this frequency range vary from 2 to over 10 mV. In general, amplifiers display maximal sensitivity to signals of 20 to 50 Hz. Most cardiac signals fall within this range regardless of whether the electrodes are unipolar or bipolar. The varied arbitrary test signals of different pacemaker manufacturers (sine^2, ½ sine, rectangular, square, triangular, or trapezoid waves) represent a single point approximation of the pacer sensing curve to verify sensing performance of a given pulse generator at the time of manufacture and are at best a rough approximation of the cardiac signal for sensing.

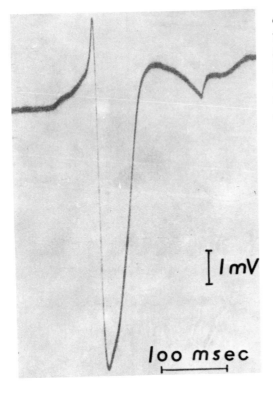

Fig. 18–8. Chronic RV unipolar EG with ID of 10.9 mV is inscribed in 20 msec. Sensing measurement of PSA was identical. (Paper speed = 200 mm/sec.)

of 66% to 126%) of the ID amplitude when this signal time duration ranged between 15 and 30 msec. PSA sensing measurements higher than the ID signal were found in 43% of the electrograms for this time duration; this finding correlated with a slightly higher slew rate. The average PSA sensing measurement was 83.5% (range of 61% to 114%) of the ID amplitude when the signals were less than 15 msec or greater than 30 msec. Although these findings are not applicable to the many types of available demand pacemakers, they offer insight and guidelines relative to proper sensing of cardiac activity as a function of the electrogram.

Compensation for signal attenuation by the pacemaker sensing circuit should be considered to ensure satisfactory pacemaker sensing when the electrographic cardiac signal is solely used as the sensing measurement. An electrode site should be selected that offers an electrographic ID of at least 6 to 8 mV and preferably with a time duration of 15 to 30 msec. This recommendation will minimize postoperative sensing problems.

We evaluated the relationship between the cardiac signal as displayed by the electrogram and pacemaker sensing as depicted digitally by a PSA (Medtronic Model 5300) from the same electrode site. Amplitude of the intrinsic deflection was considered to be the appropriate cardiac signal available for sensing. This study included 142 acute and chronic right and left ventricular unipolar electrograms. The characteristic responsible for the most consistent and reliable correlation between the amplitude of ID and PSA sensing measurement was the time duration of the ID signal. The recorded ID signals with a time duration of 15 to 30 msec were detected by the sensing circuit of the PSA with highest accuracy and least attenuation. On the average, the sensing measurement of the PSA was 98.8% (range

BIPOLAR VERSUS UNIPOLAR ELECTROGRAMS (FIGS. 18–9 AND 18–10)

Although the polarity of the recorded electrogram is determined in accordance with the configuration of the implanted permanent lead, it must be recognized that discrete differences exist between the unipolar and bipolar signals. The effect of an electrode position on pacemaker sensing may influence the selection of a lead configuration to achieve a satisfactory sensing signal.

A unipolar electrogram is recorded from an electrode system in which the cathodal pole is in contact with the heart and the anodal pole is placed in an extracardiac site. The cardiac signal is detected by the intracardiac electrode, and the anodal plate acts as a ground reference. The unipolar

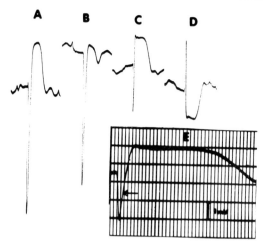

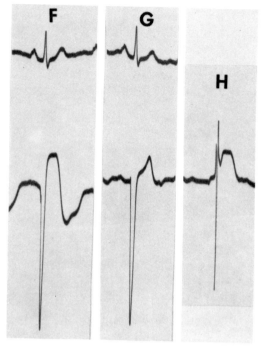

Fig. 18–9. Voltage signal of acute unipolar vs. acute bipolar EG from same endocardial RV electrode site. ID amplitudes of tip unipolar EG (A) and proximal unipolar EG (B) are the same (7.2 mV). Bipolar EGs taken in either polarity (C and D) show two sharp deflections that measure 2.7 and 4.0 mV, respectively. Sensing measurement of distal or proximal unipolar signal is 6.9 mV and clearly superior to that of bipolar signal which is 4.0 mV. Sensing measurement of bipolar signal is probably derived from second sharp deflection (indicated by arrow in E) that measures 4.0 mV. (Paper speed for A to D = 25 mm/sec and for E = 200 mm/sec.)

Fig. 18–10. Unipolar voltage signals (F and G) from either pole of the bipolar lead are identical to bipolar signal (H), and each has sensing measurement of 5.0 mV. (Paper speed = 25 mm/sec.)

signal is therefore determined by the potential difference between cardiac electrical activity and zero potential of the anode. The morphology and amplitude of the unipolar electrogram remain virtually unchanged regardless of the location of the indifferent electrode plate.

A unipolar system is more sensitive to external electrical signals particularly at lower frequencies. Little or no difference is noted in the bipolar or unipolar systems with electromagnetic energy of higher frequency, because the electrical energy is transmitted more directly to the pulse generator. An electrical signal emanating from skeletal myopotentials may induce electrical interference with the unipolar system; this problem appears to be unique to this electrode configuration.

In the bipolar system, both cathodal and anodal electrodes are intracardiac and the resultant electrogram is determined by the potential difference between the two electrode sites, each having a unipolar voltage. The bipolar signal is variably described and is dependent upon the orientation of the electrodes and the direction of the depolarization pathway. At one extreme the bipolar electrogram may be negligible or zero in voltage if the depolarization wave occurs perpendicular to the interelectrode axis and is equidistant from the electrodes. In this situation an identical depolarization signal will arrive simultaneously at both electrodes of the bipolar system and generate no potential difference. Conversely, an augmented bipolar signal greater than either unipolar signal may be described if the depolarization wave propagates parallel to the interelectrode axis. In this setting a

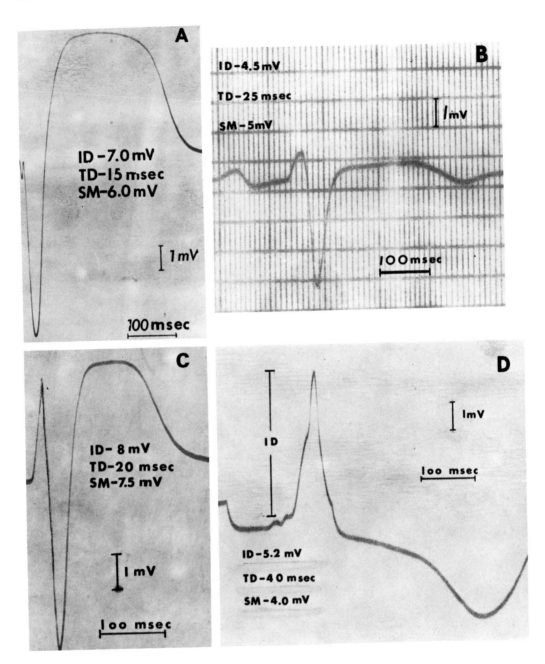

Fig. 18–11. EG recordings. A, Acute and, B, chronic epicardial RV unipolar signals from same electrode site. Sensing measurement (SM) initially was 6.0 mV and decreased 16.6% after 3 years of electrode maturity. By contrast, ID amplitude decreased 35%. (Paper speed = 200 mm/sec.) C, Acute and, D, chronic epicardial RV unipolar signals from same electrode site. QRS configuration changes from a predominantly negative waveform to a positive deflection after 2½ years. PSA sensing measurement decreased 46%, but ID amplitude decreased only 35%. (Paper speed = 200 mm/sec.)

phase difference in the arrival time of the depolarization wave at either pole produces a larger bipolar signal.

The unipolar cardiac signal available for sensing has been considered to be consistently superior to that derived from a bipolar modality. Furman and co-workers modified this view in their comparison of endocardial ventricular bipolar and tip unipolar signals. On the average the bipolar voltage signal was approximately the same as the unipolar signal, but showed greater variation. The bipolar voltage signal was greater than the corresponding tip unipolar signal in 43% of the electrograms studied. In 8%, the recorded bipolar signal was the same as the unipolar signal, and in 49%, the unipolar signal was greater.

Nonetheless, it is well-recognized that a suboptimal bipolar sensing signal may often be successfully changed to a more satisfactory signal by conversion to the unipolar configuration. On the other hand, the converse has not been demonstrated, that is, improvement of an inadequate unipolar signal by conversion to a bipolar system.

Furman et al. further demonstrated that the T wave voltage and ST elevation of the bipolar electrogram are approximately one third less than the corresponding unipolar measurements. If these physiologic signals are considered noise and undesirable for pacemaker sensing, a bipolar system then offers a superior ratio of depolarization signal to noise for proper sensing function.

CHRONIC ELECTROGRAM

The cardiac electrogram should be recorded at reoperation for pulse generator replacement or for pacing problems that necessitate surgical intervention to evaluate the cardiac signal for sensing. Fibrous tissue growth encapsulates the maturing electrode and increases the distance between the sensing electrode and electrically active myocardium. These factors evoke a moderate decrease in the amplitude of the intrinsic deflection and an even greater increase in its time duration (Fig. 18–11). In a study of chronic endocardial ventricular signals, the amplitude of the ID decreased approximately 10 to 15% and was associated with a statistically significant attenuation of the slew rate by approximately 40%.

A variable reduction of the amplitude and slew rate of the ID may be responsible for a marginal or subthreshold cardiac signal for pacemaker sensing (Fig. 18–12). This is

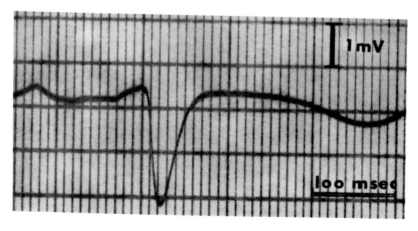

Fig. 18–12. Chronic endocardial RV unipolar EG from patient with intermittent sensing failure. ID measured 2.7 mV and time duration 20 msec. PSA sensing measurement was 3.0 mV. A pacemaker of higher sensitivity (sensitivity threshold = 1.8 mV) was implanted with restoration of normal sensing function. (Paper speed = 200 mm/sec.)

more likely to occur when the cardiac signal measured at primary implantation is within the lower limits of the acceptable range, that is, approximately 4 mV. In this circumstance, another electrode site that offers a more satisfactory signal for sensing must be sought or a pacemaker of higher sensitivity must be implanted.

The presence of an isoelectric ST segment is also characteristic of chronic electrograms and may be attributed to the formation of perielectrode fibrosis.

ATRIAL ELECTROGRAM

The recording of atrial electrograms from an endocardial or epicardial atrial lead is indispensable for pacing systems designed for atrial demand function. The unique characteristics of the amplitude-frequency response of an atrial sensing circuit differ significantly from those contained within a ventricular demand circuit. It is apparent that a testing device designed for the sensing measurement of the QRS signal cannot be substituted to obtain a suitable sensing measurement of the atrial signal.

The intrinsic deflection of the atrial signal is usually either biphasic or positive in waveform configuration. Amplitude of the atrial intrinsic deflection usually ranges between 0.5 and 6.0 mV with an average of 3.0 mV and an average ID signal time duration of 10 ± 5 msec (Fig. 18–13). Recorded atrial signals of 2 mV or higher are recommended because the sensitivity threshold of most atrial demand pacemakers is established between 0.75 and 1.50 mV.

REPOLARIZATION (ST SEGMENT) AND ELECTRODE POSITION

The presence of a variable elevation of the ST segment immediately following the intrinsic deflection is a normal phenomenon characterizing the acute ventricular electrogram. It reflects electrode contact with

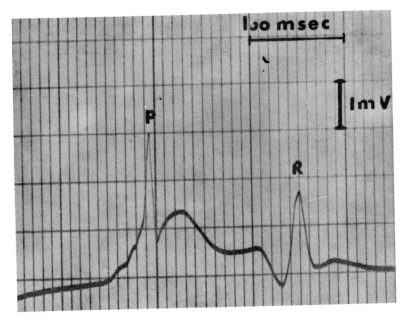

Fig. 18–13. Acute epicardial atrial unipolar EG (P) shows atrial ID of 2 mV and time duration of 10 msec. Ventricular depolarization (far-field activity) has smaller R wave potential (R). (Paper speed = 200 mm/sec.)

viable cardiac cells and represents another criterion of good electrode placement.

This repolarization abnormality or current of injury is generated by an electrophysiologic derangement of the focally damaged cell membranes induced by the myocardial trauma of electrode pressure or insertion. The ST segment returns to an isoelectric potential as the injured myocardial cells evolve into fibrotic tissue with electrode maturity. During placement of the primary lead, an electrode position offering minimal or no ST segment elevation is generally associated with an unsatisfactory stimulation threshold and frequently represents contact with nonviable or fibrotic cardiac tissue. ST segment elevation of at least 2 mV in height suggests satisfactory electrode placement, and further ST segment elevation is not usually associated with an improved stimulation threshold.

Excessive pressure of the lead against the endocardial right ventricular wall may wedge the electrode into an intramyocardial position or perforate the ventricular wall. In the former situation, sequential changes occur in the ventricular electrogram which is characterized by progressive ST segment elevation and reversal of the intrinsic deflection polarity depicted by a predominantly positive R wave configuration (Fig. 18–14). Withdrawal of the catheter will usually reduce the ST segment elevation to a lower height and return the intrinsic deflection to a predominantly negative polarity.

Myocardial perforation by an electrode is usually characterized by a return of the elevated ST segment to an isoelectric level and a variable QRS wave form corresponding to its abnormal site. Lead withdrawal from this extra-cardiac or intracavitary location to a proper electrode position will generate a ventricular electrogram of satisfactory configuration.

DEFECTIVE LEAD SYSTEMS

An electrogram usually cannot be recorded from a lead with discretely separated wire fragments from complete lead fracture. On the other hand, the electrogram of an electrode with intermittent and partial wire fracture may show severe alternating current interference or the presence of a false or contact signal that may be sensed by a demand pacemaker outside its refractory period (Fig. 18–15). A voltage signal with an amplitude ranging between 2 and 100 mV can be engendered by an abrupt change in lead resistance induced by momentary separation of the broken lead. These false or contact signals, not readily

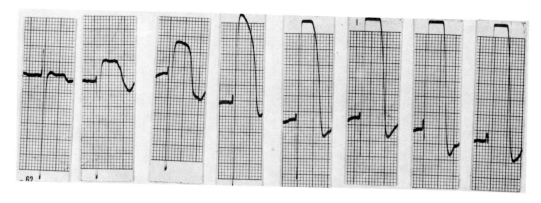

Fig. 18–14. Acute endocardial RV unipolar EG that undergoes sequential changes as result of increasing electrode pressure against endocardial wall. ID polarity becomes reversed as ST segment rises progressively.

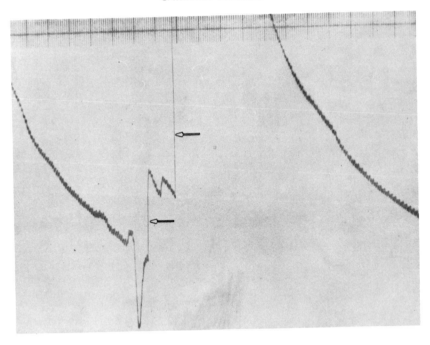

Fig. 18–15.   Direct EG recording from intermittent and partial lead fracture shows severe alternating current interference. Two voltage signals (indicated by arrows) are noted immediately after QRS and separated by 120 msec. Second voltage signal of higher magnitude produces amplifier saturation and "over shoot."

apparent in the surface ECG, are usually well demonstrated by the electrogram recorded from the fractured lead. These signals appear as bursts of fast signals or as isolated slow ones.

The cause of a chaotic pacemaker rhythm may then be related to oversensing when these false signals are identified in the electrogram. A defective fractured lead of an epicardial bipolar system may be identified by recording a unipolar electrogram from each lead. Conversion to a unipolar pacing system using the intact lead as the cathode is then indicated. An enlarged contact signal in the electrogram may be discerned by using a technique in which the defective lead is simultaneously paced and recorded.

A defective bipolar lead with an internal short circuit incident to insulation break will manifest a bipolar electrogram of zero potential. In this situation, identical unipolar electrograms are recorded from either pole of the lead. This defective bipolar lead

may also generate false voltage signals due to rapid changes in lead resistance.

UNSTABLE SENSING SIGNALS

The pacing system analyzer detects the appropriate cardiac signal and generates an electronic digital readout in mV as the sensing signal. Each QRS signal detected outside the refractory period of the testing device is electronically displayed as a specific measurement. Sequential digital readouts of the testing device that maintain a variation no greater than ± 15 to 20% of the average sensing measurement are usually considered stable measurements. Displayed signals of greater variation or erratic readings, either high or low, are considered unstable and have several causes.

1. *Premature ventricular extrasystoles or anomalous beats* typically interrupt stable R wave readings. The electrograms of

these signals may be characterized by an intrinsic deflection of variable amplitude and time duration, and the resultant sensed signal may be higher or lower than the normal cardiac signal in accordance with their characteristics (Fig. 18–16).

2. *Exaggerated respiration* engenders a moderate cyclic variation of the endocardial cardiac signal. The maximal attenuation of the ID amplitude during peak inspiration and maximal increase during peak expiration should not exceed 15% of the mean sensing measurement (Fig. 18–17). In some patients, deviations of greater magnitude may be noted, and they are responsible for intermittent sensing failure. This phenomenon is more apparent by recording the electrogram at low paper speed. A more secure electrode position should be established to eliminate exaggerated respiratory variation.

3. *Segmentation of the intrinsic deflection* refers to a severely distorted slope of the intrinsic deflection. It is characterized by gross notches or directional reverses during its entire inscription. A segmented ID may produce isolated segments of the ID of lesser amplitude and slew rate (Fig. 18–18). In this situation, only one segment may have sufficient characteristics for pacemaker sensing, and the sensing measurement corresponds to the amplitude of this isolated segment on the electrogram (Fig. 18–19).

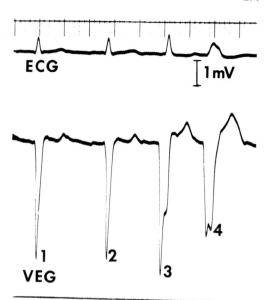

Fig. 18–16. PVC's often interrupt stable sensing measurements because of their varying amplitude and time duration. In this rhythm of atrial fibrillation, normally conducted beats (1 and 2) and fusion beat (3) produce higher digital readouts on PSA (approximately 6 mV) than the premature ventricular beat (4) whose sensing measurement is below 4 mV. ECG = electrocardiogram; VEG = ventricular electrogram.

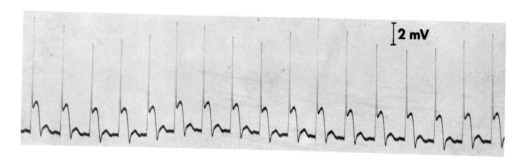

Fig. 18–17. Acute endocardial RV unipolar EG from patient showing slightly exaggerated respiratory variation. Maximal inspiratory and expiratory amplitudes of ID vary more than 15% of average sensing measurement that was 9.5 ± 1.6 mV.

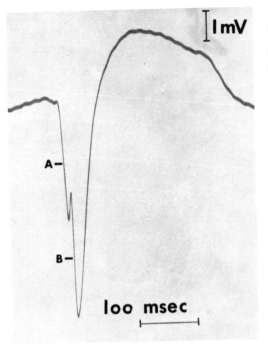

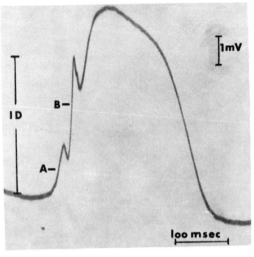

Fig. 18–19. Acute endocardial RV unipolar signal showing severe segmentation of ID into two unequal segments. PSA sensing measurement ranged between 3.0 and 3.9 mV and was most probably derived from segment B that measures 3.6 mV. Segment A is of insufficient amplitude (1.7 mV) and probably not detected by sensing circuit. (Paper speed = 200 mm/sec.)

Fig. 18–18. Acute endocardial RV unipolar signal shows significant segmentation of ID producing two segments (A and B) of equal amplitude (4.2 mV) and of equal time duration (20 msec). Since sensing measurement was 4.1 mV, either segment was sensed but not the entire ID. (Paper speed = 200 mm/sec.)

→

Fig. 18–20. Unstable sensing signal from chronic epicardial RV electrode site was obtained from electronic readout of PSA. This remarkable and anomalous EG shows positively oriented deflection of three unequal segments (A, B, and C). Sequential electronic readouts ranged from 2.5 to 5.5 mV. Unstable sensing signals may be attributed to sensing of one, or any combination of segments. ID of segment A is slightly more than 3 mV and that of segment B or C less than 2 mV. (Paper speed = 200 mm/sec.)

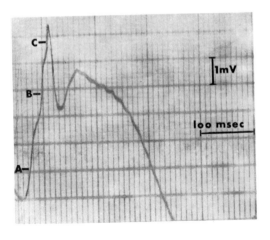

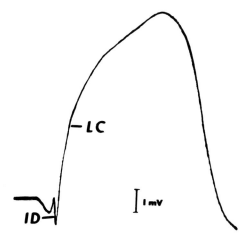

Fig. 18–21. Sensing measurement from acute epicardial RV electrode site was 5.0 mV. It is apparent that the cardiac signal available for sensing does not emanate from this ID of 1.2 mV. Rejection of this signal allows a late component (LC) of the QRS wave, augmented by the current of injury, to be sensed. (Paper speed = 200 mm/sec.)

No segment, one segment, or any combination of segments may be detected by the sensing circuit (Fig. 18–20). Sequential signals in this setting may generate a variable and unstable sensing measurement in accordance with the phenomenon of sensing reset* and be displayed by the PSA as an erratic electronic readout. Another electrode site that offers a more desirable QRS configuration characterized by an unmarred ID of satisfactory amplitude should be established.

SENSING NOT RELATED TO INTRINSIC DEFLECTION

Unusually, a component of the QRS wave other than the intrinsic deflection may provide the cardiac signal for pacemaker

sensing. This phenomenon appears to be more prevalent to the electrode site of an acute right ventricular electrogram.

The intrinsic deflection, although present, is rejected as a signal for pacemaker sensing because of a manifestly poor amplitude (1.0 to 2.5 mV) and slew rate (below 0.25 V/sec) or severe segmentation.

The signal for sensing in these anomalous wave configurations may correspond to a late deflection immediately following the true but inadequate intrinsic deflection (Figs. 18–21 to 18–23). This wave component, although less rapid in rise time than the intrinsic deflection, is often augmented in amplitude by the superimposed current of injury potential. Detection of this signal by a demand pacemaker may still occur because of its overall amplitude and frequency characteristics.

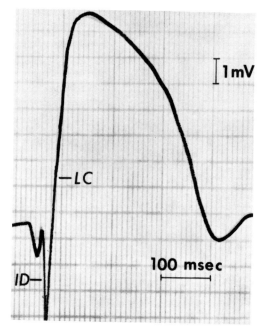

Fig. 18–22. PSA sensing measurement of EG unipolar signal of endocardial RV was 8.5 mV. ID is of insufficient amplitude (3.5 mV) to generate sensed signal. Sensing circuit was apparently reset to detect a late component deflection of adequate amplitude (10 mV) and time duration (30 msec). (Paper speed = 200 mm/sec.)

---

*The PSA (Medtronic Model 5300) detects either of two signal components that occur within a period of 30 msec outside its refractory period and generates an electronic readout for the larger signal.

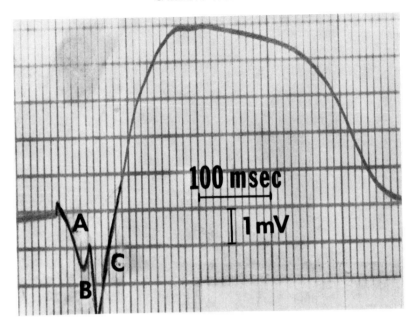

Fig. 18–23. ID (B) of this electrogram is of inadequate amplitude (2 mV) to be detected by sensing circuit. Sensing measurement of 3.5 mV was most likely derived from late component (C) of QRS wave whose amplitude was augmented by current of injury. (Paper speed = 200 mm/sec.)

The amplitude of this late deflection is prone to decrease as the current of injury becomes isoelectric with electrode maturity. The potential problem of sensing failure may materialize in the postimplantation period as the amplitude of this signal falls to a subthreshold level for pacemaker sensing. A ventricular electrogram characterized by this late deflection as a signal available for sensing should be considered unacceptable, and another electrode site associated with a satisfactory electrographic ID should be established.

The interpretation of pacemaker sensing not related to ID in these unusual situations is not apparent from the electronic readout of a PSA. This underscores one of the more useful and valuable contributions of recording cardiac electrograms during intraoperative electrical testing.

INTRACARDIAC LOCATION OF THE ELECTRODE (FIG. 18–24).

Unipolar electrographic recording may be used to identify the location of an electrode catheter within the heart or great veins. This technique is particularly applicable when a temporary pacing catheter is placed "blindly" under ECG control without fluoroscopy. The terminal end of the catheter is attached to the precordial lead of the well-grounded ECG machine, and an intracavity unipolar electrogram is obtained.

The amplitude of the P wave increases progressively as the pacing catheter approaches the right atrium, and the atrial deflection usually becomes larger than the QRS complex when the electrode tip enters the atrium. With sinus rhythm, a predomi-

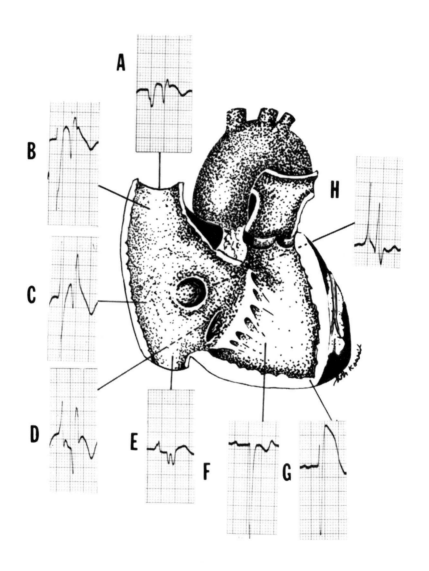

Fig. 18–24.   Position of electrode: A, superior vena cava close to right atrium (RA); B, upper RA; C, mid-RA; D, low RA; E, inferior vena cava close to RA; F, RV cavity; G, RV cavity with endocardial contact; H, coronary sinus.

nantly negative atrial potential usually characterizes the upper right atrium. A diphasic atrial signal is noted at the level of midatrium, and the low atrium usually generates a predominantly positive atrial complex.

The QRS amplitude increases greatly when the pacing lead enters the right ventricle, and the electrogram often exhibits a predominantly negative deflection (rS configuration). Intraventricular conduction abnormalities do not modify this basic electrographic morphology. The intrinsic deflection of the right ventricle usually measures 12 ± 5 mV. Endocardial contact is characterized by a variable elevation of the ST segment.

Prominent peaked atrial deflections, positive or diphasic, and often a predominantly positive R wave are noted when the pacing catheter enters the coronary sinus close to the epicardial surface of the left ventricle.

SELECTED READINGS

Barold, S.S., and Gaidula, J.J.: Demand pacemaker arrhythmias from intermittent internal short circuit in bipolar electrode. Chest, 63:165, 1973.

Barold, S.S., and Gaidula, J.J.: Failure of demand pacemaker from low voltage bipolar ventricular electrocardiograms. J.A.M.A., 215:923, 1971.

Coumel, P., Mugica, J., and Barold, S.S.: Demand pacemaker arrhythmias caused by intermittent incomplete electrode fracture. Diagnosis with testing magnet. Am. J. Cardiol., 36:105, 1975.

DeCaprio, V., Hurzeler, P., and Furman, S.: A comparison of unipolar and bipolar electrograms for cardiac pacemaker sensing. Circulation, 56:750, 1977.

DeCaprio, V., et al.: Respiratory cycle variations in pacer sensing signals. Med. Instru., 10:55, 1976.

Furman, S., and Fisher, J.D.: Cardiac pacing and pacemakers V. Technical aspects of implantation and equipment. Am. Heart J., 94:250, 1977.

Furman, S., Hurzeler, P., and DeCaprio, V.: The ventricular endocardial electrogram and pacemaker sensing. J. Thorac. Cardiovas. Surg., 73:258, 1977.

Furman, S., Hurzeler, P., and DeCaprio, V.: Cardiac pacing and pacemakers III. Sensing the cardiac electrogram. Am. Heart J., 93:794, 1977.

Gordon, A.J., Vagueino, M.C., and Barold, S.S.: Endocardial electrograms from pacemaker catheters. Circulation, 38:82, 1968.

Hughes, H.C., Brownless, R. R., and Tyers, G.F.: Failure of demand pacing with small surface area electrodes. Circulation, 54:128, 1976.

Lewis, T.: The mechanism and graphic registration of the heart beat. London, Shaw and Sons, Ltd., 1925.

Mugica, J., et al.: Methods for recording intermittent contact signals in demand pacemaker arrhythmias (11 cases). Pace, 1:222, 1978.

Myers, G. H., Kresh, Y.M., and Parsonnet, V.: Characteristics of intracardiac electrograms. Pace, 1:90, 1978.

Varriale, P., and Niznik, J.: Unipolar ventricular electrogram in the diagnosis of right ventricular ischemic injury. Pace, 1:335, 1978.

Waxman, M.B., et al.: Demand pacemaker malfunction due to abnormal sensing. Report of two cases. Circulation, 50:389, 1974.

Wilson, F.N: The distribution of the currents of action and of injury by heart muscle and other excitable tissue. In Selected Papers of Dr. Frank N. Wilson, Edited by F. Johnston and E. Lepeschkin. Ann Arbor, J.W. Edwards Publishing Co., 1954.

19

Pacemaker Electrocardiography

PHILIP VARRIALE
RAYMOND P. KWA

A conventional electrocardiographic recording represents the most frequently applied and valuable diagnostic tool in the evaluation of pacemaker function. The advent and rapid development of demand pacemakers of different electronic designs, varied pacing techniques, multiprogrammable pulse generators, and the multifarious abnormalities that often emerge have made pacemaker electrocardiography an increasingly difficult and complex discipline.

To be accurate and meaningful, the electrocardiographic interpretation requires specific knowledge of the electrical properties and operational characteristics of the individual pacemaker. In certain situations other diagnostic techniques, such as testing with a magnet or chest wall stimulation during an ECG recording, may furnish additional important diagnostic information in the appraisal of pacemaker function and in the analysis of pacemaker-related arrhythmias.

TERMS AND DEFINITIONS

The following terms and definitions relating to pacemaker functional characteristics merit consideration and must be understood by the physician concerned with the analysis and interpretation of the pacemaker electrocardiogram:

MODALITY OF PACING. There are three modes of pacing: asynchronous, inhibited, and triggered or synchronous.

Asynchronous Mode refers to the programmed pacing rate of a pulse generator that is not modified by spontaneous cardiac activity. The presence of an underlying cardiac rhythm will create competitive pacing.

Inhibited Mode refers to a demand or noncompetitive pulse generator that emits a stimulation pulse when the intrinsic cardiac activity falls below its programmed pacing rate or electronically determined time interval.

Triggered or Synchronous Mode also de-

283

picts a noncompetitive or demand pulse generator whose output pulse is responsive to the sensed electrical activity of the heart. For a *ventricular-triggered pacemaker* (VVT),* the stimulus is discharged within the detected QRS complex or refractory period of the heart initiated by this spontaneous beat, and cardiac stimulation is effective only when the rate of the sensed cardiac signal falls below the programmed pacing rate. An *atrial synchronized pacemaker* (VAT) establishes AV synchronous pacing. Detection of an atrial signal or P wave through one electrode triggers the pacemaker to discharge a stimulation pulse to the ventricle through a separate electrode after a predetermined electronic AV delay.

AUTOMATIC INTERVAL. The time interval in milliseconds (msec) between two consecutive pacemaker stimuli during continuous and uninterrupted cardiac pacing is the automatic interval. This interval will vary in accordance with the programmed pacing rate in pacemakers that offer rate programmability.

MAGNET OR TEST INTERVAL. This refers to the interval in msec between pacemaker pulses when a test magnet is applied over the pulse generator. Activation of a magnetic reed switch inhibits sensing function and generates a test interval or fixed-rate mode. In many pacemakers this test interval is approximately the same as the automatic interval; in others the magnet rate is distinctly higher. Fixed-rate pulse discharge induced by the application of a magnet is used as a test function to determine pacing capability and pacemaker battery depletion and for conversion of arrhythmias due to oversensing to fixed-rate pacing.

---

*Pacemaker nomenclature established by Inter-Society Commission for Heart Disease Resources in 1974 includes a three-letter identification code. The chamber paced, the chamber sensed, and the mode of response are represented by the first, second, and third letters. The following letter designations are used: V = ventricle; A = atrium; D = double chamber; I = Inhibited; T = triggered; and O = not applicable.

PACEMAKER REFRACTORY PERIOD. The period of the pacemaker timing cycle during which the sensing amplifier of the pulse generator becomes saturated and unresponsive to spontaneous or artificial electrical signals is the pacemaker refractory period. The refractory period is initiated by a pacemaker pulse or a sensed intracardiac electrical signal. In most pacemakers the paced and sensed refractory periods are the same and usually range from 200 to 400 msec.

The refractory period is designed to prevent pacemaker sensing of T waves or residual electrical field around the electrode such as polarization voltage or pulse after-potential.

RELATIVE REFRACTORY PERIOD. This period immediately follows the pacemaker refractory period and extends from several to 240 msec in duration. During this period the sensing amplifier coming out of saturation will respond to spontaneous or artificial signals by incomplete pacemaker recycling characterized by an inappropriately short escape interval. This phenomenon is termed partial pacemaker recycling (PPR) and appears to be related to a signal that is time- and not voltage-dependent.

ALERT PERIOD. The segment of the pacemaker timing cycle after the refractory period during which detection of cardiac or extracardiac electrical signals occurs is the alert period. These signals, spontaneous or artificial, are sensed and recycle the pacemaker to a new automatic or escape interval.

Continuous electromagnetic interference during the alert period will cause most demand pacemakers to revert to their programmed fixed rate modes. For the Cordis pulse generator, persistent electrical noise during the final one third of the refractory period (noise sampling period—Tn) will cause pacer discharge at completion of the timing cycle and subsequent reversion to fixed-rate pacing.

ESCAPE INTERVAL. The interval in msec between the onset of a normally generated cardiac signal that is sensed and the subsequent pacemaker stimulus is the escape interval. The electronic escape interval in most demand pacemakers is the same as the automatic interval. In a few pacemakers the escape interval is longer than the automatic interval and is termed positive hysteresis. This mechanism is designed to create more time for the emergence of intrinsic cardiac activity.

ATRIOVENTRICULAR SYNCHRONOUS PACEMAKERS

An atrial synchronous or AV synchronous pacemaker (VAT), initially introduced in 1963, is designed to discharge a stimulus pulse to the ventricle through one electrode after sensing atrial depolarization with another electrode. The ventricular electrode serves no sensing function and is triggered to discharge after a physiologic electronic AV delay, depending upon the heart rate (Fig. 19–1). The ventricular electrode reverts to fixed-rate pacing when the atrial rate falls below the escape rate of the pacemaker, and ventricular stimulation is rate-limited with rapid atrial rates in accordance with the pacer refractory period.

A more recent pacemaker unit (Medtronic Model 5993) incorporates a ventricular demand mode within the atrial synchronous pacemaker (VDT/I). This device

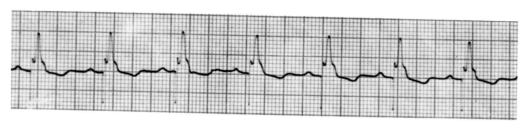

Fig. 19–1. Atrial synchronous pacemaker (VAT) triggers an effective ventricular stimulus after sensing atrial depolarization. Apparent AV delay is 0.20 msec.

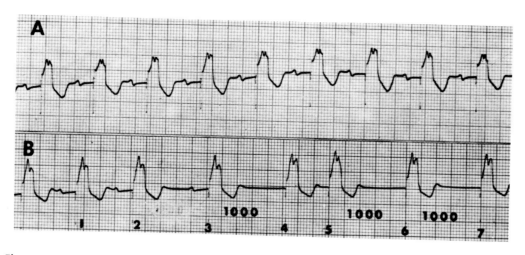

Fig. 19–2. Atrial synchronous ventricular inhibited pacemaker (VDT/I) in adult patient with complete AV block using epicardial leads attached to left atrium and left ventricle. A, Effective ventricular stimulus discharge occurs in synchrony with atrial rate above 60 beats/min. and with an AV delay of 240 msec. B, Ventricular demand pacing at escape interval of 1000 msec occurs when atrial rate falls below 60 beats/min.

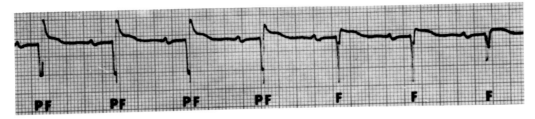

Fig. 19–3. Atrial synchronous pacemaker (VAT) in patient with restored AV conduction. An ineffective pacing stimulus is superimposed upon first four beats (pseudofusion beats—PF), since the programmed AV delay is longer than intrinsic PR interval. Fusion complexes (F) are apparent in beats 5 to 7 due to simultaneous activation from spontaneous and pacer pulses. Increased apparent AV interval of 280 msec may be due to delayed atrial sensing or early atrial synchronous pacemaker failure.

has an atrial sensing lead, a ventricular sensing-pacing lead and a common indifferent plate. The pacemaker triggers a stimulus pulse to the ventricle following a predetermined AV delay in synchrony with a normal intrinsic atrial rate (Fig. 19–2). Maximum ventricular pacing rate is limited to 120 beats/min. in accordance with a rate stablilization mode when an accelerated atrial rhythm appears. Ventricular demand pacing supervenes when the atrial rate falls below the pacer escape rate. Spontaneous ventricular activity outside the refractory period of this device is sensed and inhibits the pacemaker output pulse. The ventricular demand mode differentiates this unit from the conventional atrial synchronous pacemaker, since the latter is not noncompetitive with spontaneous ventricular activity.

An atrial synchronous pacemaker is non-competitive when AV conduction is intact and the PR interval is longer than the programmed AV delay. An ineffective pacemaker stimulus is superimposed upon the QRS complex within the refractory period of the heart when the electronic AV delay is longer than the intrinsic PR interval (Fig. 19–3). An atrial synchronized pacemaker can be associated with complex and bizarre ECG patterns when an atrial or ventricular ectopic beat, AV dissociation, retrograde atrial depolarization, or failure to sense atrial activity occurs.

ATRIAL OR CORONARY SINUS DEMAND PACEMAKERS

Atrial or coronary sinus demand pacing has been applied with increasing frequency to patients with intact AV conduction and

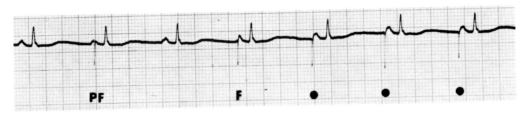

Fig. 19–4. Unipolar atrial demand pacemaker (AAI) in patient with sick sinus syndrome and intact AV conduction. Noncompetitive atrial pacing is established at automatic interval of 860 msec. Atrial fusion (F) and pseudofusion (PF) beats are present; they represent normal function and common ECG manifestation of demand pacemakers when intrinsic heart rate and pacer discharge are isorhythmic. Solid dots depict pure paced atrial beats.

severe bradycardia with or without tachyarrhythmia. Specially designed atrial electrodes can be introduced pervenously into the right atrial appendage or coronary sinus or attached to the atrial epicardium during thoracotomy to both pace and sense atrial electrical activity. An atrial demand pacemaker can provide inhibited (AAI) or triggered (AAT) atrial pacing.

Atrial fusion and pseudofusion beats appear not infrequently with atrial demand pacing and tend to occur when the pacing and spontaneous rates are closely linked (Fig. 19–4); this is a normal ECG manifestation common to all demand pacemaker modes. The ECG pattern of a fusion beat is characterized by a depolarization wave—P or QRS—that is simultaneously generated from the intrinsic cardiac impulse and the pacemaker stimulus. Fusion beats are usually of lesser width than the pure paced beat and may vary in ECG configuration contingent upon the relative contribution of the spontaneous and pacemaker impulses to the depolarization wave.

Pseudofusion beats appear electrocardiographically when a pacemaker artifact falls within the intrinsic QRS or P complex. The pacemaker stimulus is, of course, ineffective, since it occurs during the refractory period of the heart initiated by the spontaneous beat.

Atrial and coronary sinus demand pacemakers are designed with a long refractory period of 400 msec or slightly less to avoid sensing of the QRS signals and con-

sequent pacemaker recycling leading to inappropriate bradycardia. Atrial capture and sensing will be lost with an atrial or coronary sinus demand pacemaker when atrial fibrillation or flutter develops postoperatively for transient periods or at any time thereafter (Fig. 19–5). The complexes associated with atrial fibrillation or flutter are usually less than 1.0 mV, and "failure to sense" these signals converts the pacemaker to its fixed-rate pacing mode. In this circumstance, the atrial pacing stimuli are ineffective and innocuous, and proper pacing function will be manifest when a sinus mechanism and responsive atrium are restored. A variety of supraventricular arrhythmias, including atrial bigeminy, atrial fibrillation or flutter, or reentrant tachycardias, may be induced when an atrial demand pacemaker becomes competitive due to sensing malfunction.

ABNORMALITIES RELATED TO CAPTURE

Intermittent or total failure to pace, with or without detectable pacer stimuli, can occur at any time following pacemaker implantation. Numerous causes can account for capture abnormalities: problems related to the pulse generator, lead, electrode position, or myocardial responsiveness to stimulation.

Dislodgment of a pervenous lead from its initial endocardial position to a less satisfactory one (2 to 20% incidence), particu-

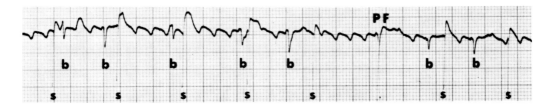

Fig. 19–5. Atrial demand pacemaker (AAI) that discharges continuously at automatic interval of 800 msec due to development of atrial flutter that appeared postoperatively for one day. Atrial flutter waves less than 1.0 mV are usually not sensed, and conducted intrinsic QRS beats (b) are irregular and unrelated to pacer pulses (s). This apparent lack of sensing is considered to be "pseudo-failure," since normal pacemaker function resumed after restoration of sinus activity.

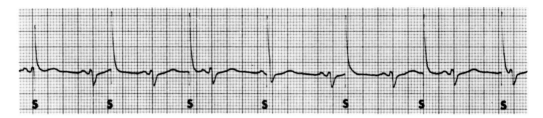

Fig. 19–6. Large unipolar pacemaker spikes (s) appear at programmed fixed rate of this pacemaker but fail to capture or sense. Intrinsic cardiac activity is dissociated from automatic discharge of pacemaker stimuli. Dislodgment of this endocardial lead was apparent on x-ray film, with the electrode being located within inflow tract of right ventricle.

larly during the first week following lead implantation, is a frequent cause of failure to capture. Pacemaker spikes of normal amplitude appear at the programmed pacing rate but fail to pace the heart intermittently or continuously. Lack of sensing may also be manifest with lead displacement (Fig. 19–6).

Failure to pace after lead implantation without evidence of electrode malposition (dislodgment or ventricular perforation) is termed exit block. Stimulation threshold, initially satisfactory, progressively rises above the pulse energy of the pacemaker because of perielectrode fibrosis consequent to ischemic damage or idiopathic fibrosis (Fig. 19–7).

In our experience true exit block is more commonly associated with epimyocardial electrode sites of the right or left ventricle than with endocardial lead implantation. When an excessive elevation of stimulation threshold with pacing failure occurs with endocardial leads, it is frequently due to electrode dislodgment, even if it is not radiologically apparent.

Myocardial perforation by a pacing electrode is another cause of failure to capture. A right bundle branch block pattern in V_1 of the ECG is manifest during intermittent capture if the transvenous electrode migrates to the left ventricular epicardial surface during stimulation (Fig. 19–8). Perforation of the right ventricular apex is also diagnosed radiologically by the presence of the electrode outside of the right ventricular cavity and within the clear space anterior to the heart. Associated clinical findings include diaphragmatic or intercostal muscle stimulation, pericardial rub, or a pacemaker

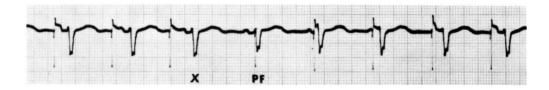

Fig. 19–7. Total failure to capture occurred in patient one year after left ventricular implantation of sutureless epicardial lead. Sensing function is intact when ventricular beat (X) emerges outside the pacer refractory period (320 msec). Pacemaker escape stimulus is superimposed upon following spontaneous QRS complex (pseudofusion beat—PF) and does not evoke ventricular stimulation. Pacemaker spikes of normal amplitude occur at programmed cycle length of 840 msec. At reoperation, electrode installation was intact and stimulation threshold of 5.5 V measured which was above pulse generator output. This is consistent with diagnosis of exit block subsequent to increased perielectrode fibrosis.

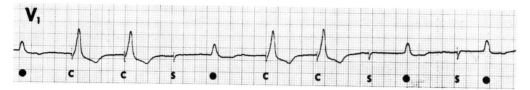

Fig. 19–8. Intermittent failure to capture developed incident to myocardial perforation by bipolar pacing lead. Captured beats (C) show RBBB pattern in lead V₁ secondary to epicardial LV stimulation. Recycling of pacer pulse (S) after spontaneous QRS complex (solid dot) indicates normal sensing function.

sound. Failure to pace as a result of perforation of the thin right ventricular wall by the sutureless electrode has also been described.

It is to be noted that the most common cause of RBBB pattern of paced ventricular beats during presumed right ventricular endocardial pacing is inadvertent placement of the electrode within the distal coronary venous system or its radicles and stimulation of the epicardial left ventricular surface (Fig. 19–9). Rarely, a pattern of RBBB or dominant R wave of the paced beat in V₁ can be seen from an apparently well-positioned pacing catheter in the right ventricular apex without perforation. Disappearance of the dominant R wave in V₁ is often apparent when this precordial lead is recorded at a lowered intercostal space.

Pacing failure without pacer stimuli is a frequent manifestation of complete lead fracture with widely separated wire fragments. Partial lead fracture is suggested when intermittent loss of stimulation is associated with intermittent attenuation of the stimulus pulse amplitude and normal pulse generator rate. The smaller pacemaker artifacts that fail to capture suggest momentary disruption of the pacing circuit due to intermittent separation between wire fragments and transient increase of lead resistance (Fig. 19–10). However, normal pacing may occur when the fractured conduction wire is well apposed.

Intermittent pacing loss also characterizes a lead insulation break and short circuit. This disruption of insulation produces an alternative path for current flow into the body tissue and reduces the current density necessary for stimulation at the electrode site.

Pacing failure may also be related to a

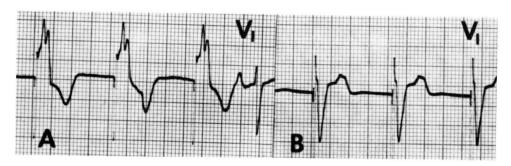

Fig. 19–9. Paced QRS complexes usually seen in V₁ of ECG. LBBB pattern (B) occurs with epicardial or endocardial right ventricular (RV) stimulation and RBBB pattern (A) with stimulation from an epicardial left ventricular (LV) electrode. RBBB pattern in V₁ may also be apparent with inadvertent electrode position within coronary venous system close to epicardial LV surface and rarely from lead in RV apex or from electrode perforation of interventricular septum.

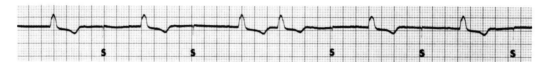

Fig. 19–10. Reduced unipolar stimuli (S) fail to capture ventricle. Sensing function is intact, since pacer spikes appear subsequent to spontaneous ventricular beats at regular escape interval of 840 msec. Wire conductor was separated by 3 mm on chest x-ray film close to its attachment to cephalic vein. Reduced current pulse secondary to complete lead fracture caused pacing failure, but sensing was maintained via fluid conductive bridge between wire segments.

deviance in pacemaker power source due to premature or end-of-life battery depletion. Power source depletion as a cause of this complication is inevitable for all pulse generators but less apparent today with the introduction of lithium or nuclear-powered pacemakers. These power sources provide a greater energy capacity and battery longevity than the conventional mercury-zinc cell; battery life is further extended in some pacemakers by programming the pulse generator to a lower output energy consistent with the stimulation requirement of the patient.

Other pulse generators are designed to provide energy compensation and longer pacemaker capture with time as the battery voltage declines. Energy available for stimulation is maintained relatively constant by a programmed increase in the output pulse width.

Absent pacemaker pulses and paced beats in the ECG characterize total battery failure or component malfunction. A pacemaker rate decrease of 7 to 10% or more below the programmed fixed rate is a firm indication of battery voltage depletion as a cause of pacing failure. The concept of rate slowing coincident to power source decline is applicable to all pulse generators. The programmed pacing rate is usually determined in the magnetic mode, as this test rate is constant for a specific pulse generator and can vary with the automatic interval to a slight extent. In certain pulse generators, the magnetic mode or test rate is distinctly faster than the basic pacing rate and decreases more rapidly with time than the normal pacing rate as battery voltage declines.

The output voltage decay of lithium or nuclear-powered pacemakers occurs more gradually and steadily with time, and early or slight pacing rate decreases are not readily detected by the standard ECG, since paper speed variations alone can produce a

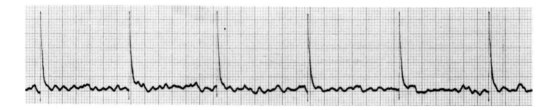

Fig. 19–11. Large unipolar pacing spikes are present at automatic interval of 1280 msec (47 beats/min). This represents rate decrease of 22% compared to initial programmed pacing rate of 60 beats/min and is firm indication of advanced battery depletion. Widely sloping decay curve of pacemaker artifact, 100 msec in duration, and atrial fibrillation obscure QRS complex immediately following pacer discharge. QRS complex was apparent in another lead showing smaller pacing spike and reduced decay curve artifact.

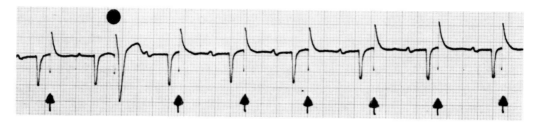

Fig. 19–12. Pacing function of demand pacemaker, inhibited by spontaneous cardiac activity, can be evaluated by application of magnet over pulse generator. This will induce fixed-rate pacemaker discharge, and pacer pulse captures the heart when it exceeds stimulation threshold of ventricle. One pacer pulse (solid dot) produces capture, since it occurs outside ventricular refractory period (280 msec). All other ineffective pulses (arrows) fall within ventricular refractory period and do not indicate pacing failure.

rate ± 5% of the true rate. A special monitoring device that permits an electronic digital readout in msec intervals or beats/min. is recommended and required.

The ECG will indicate pacemaker battery depletion or at least permit the physician to suspect this abnormal function as a cause of pacing failure when a sudden decrease in pacemaker rate greater than 10% of the programmed fixed rate occurs (Fig. 19–11).

The unipolar pacing stimulus as recorded in certain ECG leads may render analysis of pacing function difficult. This large unipolar pacing spike is followed by a widely sloping voltage decay curve artifact as wide as 280 msec that can obscure or distort the QRS complexes immediately following the pacing spike (Fig. 19–11). Additionally, this conspicuous deflection may simulate the current of injury characteristic of acute myocardial infarction or pericarditis. Saturation of the ECG input amplifier generates this decay curve artifact, and the amplifier response to this unipolar pacer spike does not represent the actual pacemaker pulse. Momentary insensitivity of the ECG amplifier to further electrical activity is manifest during a widely inscribed decay curve. Selection of a lead that is perpendicular to the vector of the decay curve will minimize this artifact and permit proper analysis of the paced QRS complex.

Myocardial stimulation by a pacemaker can be verified by two techniques when the demand pulse generator is inhibited by spontaneous cardiac activity. Carotid sinus pressure may induce significant slowing of the spontaneous cardiac rate to permit escape discharge of the pacemaker output pulse. This maneuver can be potentially hazardous to the patient when the pacemaker stimulus fails to capture and a period of induced ventricular standstill ensues. Pacing function is preferably tested by the application of a magnet over the implanted generator. The magnet activates a magnetic reed switch to inhibit sensing function, and a fixed-rate pacing mode is established (Fig. 19–12).

SENSING FUNCTION

The variety and complexity of situations related to sensing function, associated with modern demand pacemakers, have spawned diagnostic problems, often complex and intricate, that may be related to benign functional variations or serious malfunction of the pacing system. The ECG is extremely useful in the evaluation of sensing function and may offer a reasonably accurate diagnostic assessment, particularly when used in conjunction with other testing techniques, such as the magnetic mode or chest wall stimulation.

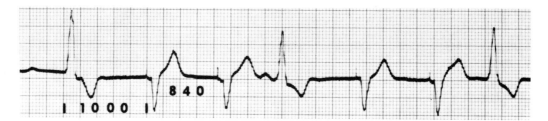

Fig. 19–13. Longer escape interval of 1000 msec than automatic interval of 840 msec is characteristic of positive hysteresis for this pacemaker. Erroneous interpretation of this mode has caused most pacemaker manufacturers to abandon this design.

Variations in the Escape Interval

An appraisal of sensing function is best initiated with an appreciation of the escape interval, as this concept has become the subject of considerable confusion and erroneous interpretation. The escape interval is defined as that period of time in msec between the onset of the normally generated cardiac signal that is sensed and the subsequent pacemaker stimulus pulse.

Long Escape Interval

Variations in the escape interval of demand pacemakers that are perceptively longer than the automatic interval are not uncommon. Often they are related to the normal functional characteristics of the demand pacemaker.

An escape interval longer than the automatic interval, termed positive hysteresis, was incorporated in a significant number of pulse generators (Fig. 19–13). Apparent malfunction of the demand pacemaker was often considered by many physicians who failed to recognize this normal functional operation of the pacemaker. Because of this problem, most pacemaker manufacturers abandoned the hysteresis mode and produced pacemakers with similar escape and automatic intervals.

A demand pacemaker discharges following a predetermined electronic escape interval, after sensing a spontaneous QRS

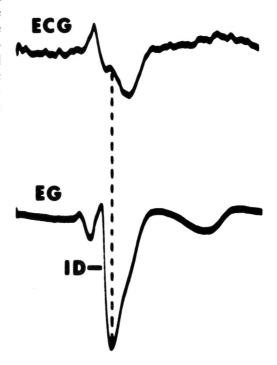

Fig. 19–14. Simultaneous ECG recording of a surface QRS complex characterized by RBBB and corresponding electrographic signal (EG) appearing at right ventricular apical electrode site. Time of sensing, 60 msec after onset of recorded surface QRS complex is represented by intrinsic deflection (ID) signal that measures 4 mV. Delayed time of sensing occurs when origin of an anomalous beat is within ventricle contralateral to sensing electrode site.

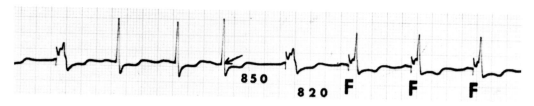

Fig. 19–15. Slightly prolonged escape interval of 850 msec is present after third spontaneous beat and differs from automatic interval of 820 msec. Sensing of this spontaneous QRS beat and demand pacemaker recycling occur 30 msec after inscription of surface QRS complex, indicated by arrow. Fusion beats (F) are also manifest.

beat or other electrographic signal. The electronic escape interval is identical to the automatic interval for most pulse generators. The apparent escape interval is measured from the onset of the recorded surface QRS complex, but the time of pacemaker sensing is related to the arrival of the corresponding electrographic cardiac signal at the sensing electrode site (Fig. 19–14). Recognition of this precise moment of sensing is not available by analysis of the QRS complex in the surface ECG. The time of sensing may be relatively early with a normally conducted QRS complex, or variably delayed for an aberrant or anomalous QRS configuration whose impulse origin or initial depolarization wavefront is further

removed from the electrode site. The apparent escape interval will of necessity be variably longer than the electronic escape interval and subject to greater variation with beats characterized by an intraventricular conduction disturbance (Fig. 19–15). This discrepancy in time between the apparent and electronic escape interval can be as much as 120 msec.

An apparent sensing failure by a demand pacemaker, for example, is often inferred when an apparently long escape interval or "late" pseudofusion beat appears coincident to certain ECG complexes depicted by an intraventricular conduction defect (Fig. 19–16). This phenomenon has been well documented when a ventricular sensing

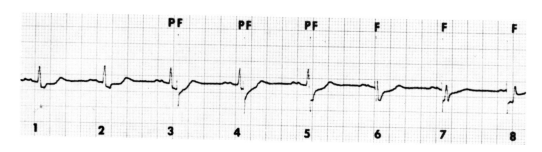

Fig. 19–16. Apparently long escape interval of 960 msec is present between onset of recorded surface QRS complex (beat 2) and subsequent pacemaker pulse that falls within terminal portion of QRS complex (beat 3) to produce a "late" pseudofusion (PF) beat. Difference between apparent escape interval and automatic interval (840 msec) is 120 msec and can be assigned to delayed arrival of electrographic cardiac signal of beat 2 at sensing electrode site. Continuous delayed sensing of intracardiac signal after completion of electronic escape interval generates "late" pseudofusion complexes for beats 4 and 5 and eventually fusion complexes (F) for beats 6 to 8. This ECG pattern represents benign functional variation and not sensing failure of demand pacemaker.

electrode detects electrographic signals corresponding to sinus beats with ipsilateral bundle branch block or ectopic extrasystoles arising from the contralateral ventricle. Although described for patients with left bundle branch block and a left ventricular epicardial electrode site, this apparent lack of sensing is usually more frequent in patients with right bundle branch block and a right ventricular electrode site.

Sufficiently delayed sensing of these spontaneous anomalous beats well after initial inscription of the recorded surface QRS complex will recycle the pacemaker and generate a stimulus discharge at an apparently long escape interval. Similarly, the electronic escape interval of a pacemaker can be completed and a pacemaker pulse emitted when the conducted or ectopic anomalous beat that occurs at a sufficiently long coupling interval generates a cardiac signal whose arrival time at the electrode site is delayed after the pacemaker has discharged. An ineffective pacemaker stimulus will be superimposed upon the terminal portion of the QRS complex as a "late" pseudofusion beat.

These observations correlate with the study of Castellanos and co-workers who studied the arrival time of excitation at selected ventricular sites during bundle branch block using intracardiac catheter electrodes. Excitation at the right ventricular apex occurred 50 to 60 msec after the onset of the recorded surface right bundle branch block beat in patients with sinus rhythm.

Apparently long escape intervals and "late" pseudofusion beats due to certain conducted or ectopic beats characterized by an intraventricular conduction defect should therefore be considered an innocent functional variation and not a malfunction of the demand pacemaker. Veritable failure to sense is diagnosed, however, when pacemaker pulses are discharged well beyond the surface QRS complex.

Short Escape Interval

Less frequently, escape intervals perceived as disproportionately short may occur and be consistent with the electronic design of the demand pacemaker. It is important to recognize that spontaneous cardiac signals, occurring within the refractory period of the demand pacemaker, will not be sensed and should not be considered a failure of sensing. Nonsensing of intrinsic cardiac beats is more frequent in pacemakers with longer refractory periods (Fig. 19–17). Knowledge of a pacemaker refractory period is therefore essential to determine whether a non-sensed spontaneous depolarization constitutes normal or abnormal sensing function.

An inappropriately short escape interval, termed partial pacemaker recycling (PPR), can arise from incomplete recycling of some demand ventricular inhibited pacemakers. This escape interval, shorter than the automatic interval, is usually induced by a premature ventricular beat that ap-

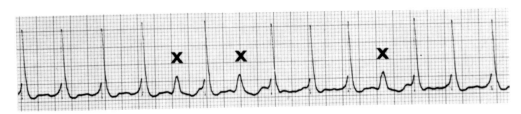

Fig. 19–17. Ventricular synchronous pacemaker with refractory period of 400 msec does not sense slightly earlier ventricular beats (X) that occur at coupling interval of 360 msec. Pacemaker senses other ventricular beats that occur beyond 400 msec by emitting ineffective stimulus within QRS complex.

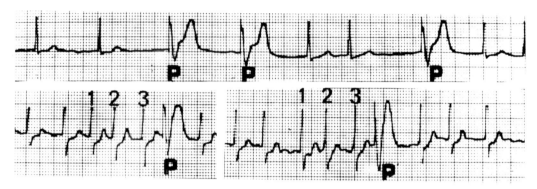

Fig. 19–18. Normal sensing function of QRS-inhibited pacemaker (Omni-Stanicor) that shows normal programmed escape interval of 1000 msec (upper strip). Beats (labeled 2) occurring in this setting of atrial fibrillation with rapid ventricular response (lower strip) are detected during noise sampling period (Tn) as an interference signal, and a pacer stimulus is discharged at completion of timing cycle in response to sensed beat (labeled 1). Noise sampling period of this pulse generator is another cause of apparent sensing malfunction. P indicates paced beat. (Reproduced with permission from Barold, S.S.: The noise sampling period: a new cause of apparent sensing malfunction of demand pacemakers. Pace 1:251, 1978.)

pears immediately after the refractory period. Sung and co-workers demonstrated partial pacemaker recycling in two pacemaker models (Intermedics C-Mos-1 and ARCO L1-2D) using chest wall stimulation and intracardiac programmed stimulation. Partial pacemaker recycling was induced when appropriately timed pulses were applied during a period extending from 110 to 240 msec following the absolute refractory period of the pacemaker. It appears to be related to signals that are time- and not voltage-dependent. A short escape interval incident to PPR should be considered a normal functional characteristic of demand inhibited pacemakers.

A short escape interval and subsequent reversion of a pulse generator to its fixed rate mode during rapid ventricular rates has been described by Barold and co-workers as another cause of apparent sensing malfunction of demand pacemakers. This phenomenon is a function of the noise sampling period (Tn) of the Cordis pulse generator. This period corresponds to the final one third of the pacemaker refractory period during which persistent electrical noise interference causes reversion of the

pacemaker to its fixed rate mode. The duration of the noise sampling period is linearly related to the programmed cycle length of the pacemaker and ranges between 75 msec for a rate of 100 pulses/min. and 125 msec for a rate of 60 pulses/min. A long noise sampling period may detect rapid tachycardias with short ventricular intervals as an interference signal and cause discharge of the pacemaker pulse at a short escape interval and subsequent fixed rate pacing (Fig. 19–18).

Abnormalities of Sensing Function

Undersensing

Sensing function abnormality of a demand pacemaker, termed undersensing, is a relatively common pacemaker complication readily detected by ECG recording. Undersensing as an expression of demand pacemaker malfunction is manifest when proper pacemaker inhibition fails intermittently or continuously in association with reversion to fixed-rate pacing for one or more timing

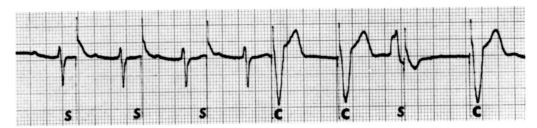

Fig. 19–19. Failure to sense spontaneous QRS complexes that occur beyond pacer refractory period and reversion to fixed-rate pacing mode are firm indication of undersensing. Ventricular capture (C) occurs only when stimulus pulse is beyond refractory period of heart. Ineffective stimuli are labeled S.

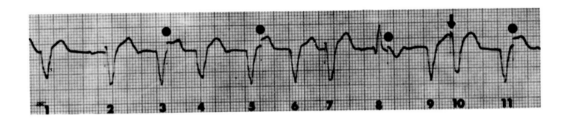

Fig. 19–20. Intermittent undersensing may produce asynchronous stimulus discharge and be potentially dangerous when pacemaker stimulus (arrow) falls within the vulnerable phase of T wave of spontaneous beat (beat 9). Repetitive ventricular response or even ventricular fibrillation may develop when myocardium is severely ischemic, hypokalemic, or toxic from antiarrhythmic drugs. Ventricular beats 1 and 4 are sensed and recycle the pacemaker. Ineffective stimuli are indicated with solid dots.

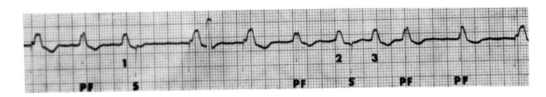

Fig. 19–21. Fixed-rate pulse output, at 800 msec interval, secondary to undersensing is present in patient with atrial fibrillation. Sensing measurement of cardiac signal during electrical testing at reoperation was 2.5 mV and slightly below sensing threshold for this pulse generator. Normal sensing function was restored after implantation of pacemaker of high sensitivity. Pseudofusion beats (PF) are present when pacemaker spike is superimposed upon intrinsic QRS complex. Pacer stimuli, outside refractory period of heart, capture the ventricle. Ineffective pulses are labeled S.

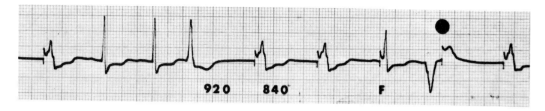

Fig. 19–22. Isolated sensing failure is denoted by pacer spike (solid dot) that occurs clearly beyond inscription of premature ventricular beat. Lack of sensing related to other PVC's of similar configuration and not with spontaneous ventricular beats was confirmed with long rhythm strip. PVC's, on occasion, may engender an inadequate cardiac signal whose characteristics (amplitude and frequency) for sensing are subthreshold. Slightly prolonged escape interval and fusion beat (F) are also present and consistent with normal pacemaker function.

cycles. Spontaneous QRS beats well beyond the refractory period of the pacemaker that are not sensed, are a firm indication of undersensing (Figs. 19–19 and 19–20).

Veritable undersensing is encountered in two situations. These include a cardiac signal of inadequate voltage and/or slew rate for pacemaker sensing at the sensing electrode site and a demand pacemaker malfunction. Electrode position, lead polarity, or myocardial factors may be responsible for the occurrence of an inadequate cardiac signal.

Loss of the intimate endocardial or epimyocardial position of a pacing electrode incident to lead malposition can create a reduced cardiac signal at the electrode site below the sensing threshold of the pulse generator. Similarly, a bipolar voltage signal, on occasion, is of diminished voltage amplitude when the corresponding unipolar signal is quite satisfactory for sensing.

The voltage of a cardiac signal that is marginal at primary implantation can be further reduced to an inadequate cardiac signal for pacemaker sensing, when excessive perielectrode fibrosis occurs secondary to ischemic damage or idiopathic fibrosis (Fig. 19–21). Sensing failure can therefore accompany exit block that is characterized by a failure to capture.

Not infrequently, undersensing of a demand pacemaker occurs only with certain premature ventricular beats and not with normally generated QRS complexes (Fig. 19–22). Analysis of the electrographic QRS signal corresponding to these PVCs will often show a signal of diminished voltage amplitude and/or slew rate. Additionally, the longer signal duration of the PVC increases sensing impedance of the electrode

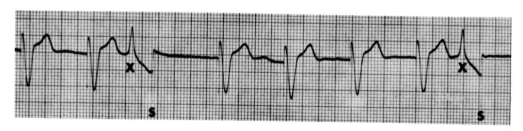

Fig. 19–23. Failure to sense ventricular beats (X) was related to faulty pulse generator and was due to internal high resistance short circuit that reduced pacer sensitivity characteristics. On bench testing, test signal required for inhibition was 15 mV. At reoperation, PSA sensing measurement of cardiac signal was 8.5 mV.

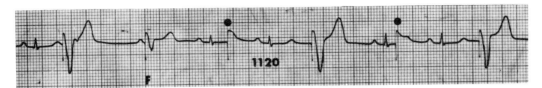

Fig. 19–24. Battery depletion in pulse generator produces consistent undersensing and decreased pacing rate discharge of 54 pulses/min. as compared to an initial programmed pacing rate of 60 pulses/min. Pacing function remains intact when pacer pulse falls beyond refractory period of heart. Rate decrease of most modern pulse generators usually occurs prior to loss of demand function. Solid dots denote ineffective pacer stimuli.

and further attenuates the available voltage signal for pacemaker sensing.

Cardiac signals below the pacemaker sensing threshold can also occur as a result of the myocardial response to ischemia, severe electrolyte imbalance, or antiarrhythmic drug administration. The latter two factors and their effects on the myocardium have been postulated but not clinically documented.

Undersensing due to pulse generator malfunction includes abnormalities of sensing circuitry or components that will cause reversion to fixed-rate pacing (Fig. 19–23). A faulty magnetic reed switch that remains permanently activated will also produce fixed-rate pacing and a total sensing failure. A leakage path between the pacemaker terminals will reduce the input impedance of the pulse generator and create considerable attenuation of the cardiac signal available for sensing. This pacemaker complication produces manifest sensing abnormalities prior to the loss of capture.

In certain pulse generators, now obsolete, the failure of demand function occurred with power source depletion prior to stimulus rate decrease or coincident with a perceptible rate decrease (Fig. 19–24).

Oversensing

Abnormal demand function due to oversensing is caused by the detection of undesirable and often inapparent signals that create pacemaker inhibition. This is characterized by intermittent and variable automatic or escape interval prolongation or by irregular, prolonged pauses terminated by a spontaneous beat. The irregular prolongation of the pacemaker timing cycle is usually less than two automatic cycles.

Extraneous or artificial voltage signals of sufficient magnitude can inhibit a demand pacemaker when they appear outside its refractory period and may arise from the following sources:

1. Physiologic electrical activity of the heart other than the appropriate QRS signal, such as the P or T wave voltage.
2. Extracardiac electrical activity generated by (a) polarization voltage or pacemaker afterpotential, (b) myopotentials arising in proximity to the pacing system, (c) false signals generated within a defective pacing system, and (d) extracorporeal electromagnetic interference.

Oversensing can create complex pacemaker-related arrhythmias, and an accurate diagnosis from the ECG recording may at best be inferential and not always persuasive. Proper appreciation of oversensing due to inapparent signals will often require intraoperative electrical testing, including an electrographic recording.

P wave sensing is rarely noted with a well-positioned ventricular lead but can be apparent, when the proximal electrode of an endocardial bipolar lead is displaced close to the tricuspid valve. Uncommonly, an epicardial lead installed close to the AV groove or an endocardial lead inadvertently placed within the coronary sinus system can also display P wave sensing.

T wave sensing due to a large and sharp electrographic voltage signal of sufficient slew rate can induce pacemaker inhibition and prolongation of the timing cycle. T wave sensing appears to be more conspicuously related to a paced ventricular beat than to a spontaneous beat. In accordance with this observation, Barold ascribes T wave sensing to the voltage contribution of the pacemaker polarization voltage or stimulus afterpotential which generates a larger T wave signal as an additive effect.

The polarization voltage is an electrochemical potential, represented by the accumulation of a layer of opposite charges at the electrode-tissue phase boundary during the stimulation pulse. Polarization voltage rises to a peak during the stimulus pulse and then decays by diffusion into the tissues, usually disappearing within 200 msec, before the subsequent pacemaker pulse. Polarization effect is inversely related to the electrode surface area and directly related to the pulse width.

A pacemaker of relatively short refractory period may sense a prolonged voltage decay waveform or pulse afterpotential and induce recycling from its own stimulus discharge. The emergence of a prolonged escape interval that is recycled by the pacemaker polarization effect and includes one refractory period and one automatic interval is designated "double reset." A constant regular prolongation of the escape interval that includes the pacemaker automatic interval and its refractory period can be related to sensing of an inapparent signal that occurs immediately outside the refractory period of the pacemaker; this ECG finding should arouse suspicion of oversensing secondary to T wave voltage and/or pacemaker polarization voltage (Fig. 19–25).

Oversensing due to pacemaker polarization effect, although rare, may continue to be a problem with pulse generators that offer a relatively short refractory period and longer stimulus pulse width of 1.5 msec or more, when used with an electrode of small surface area.

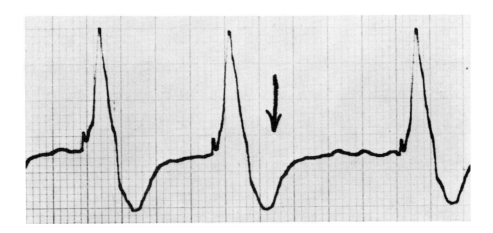

Fig. 19–25. Demand pacemaker inhibition and prolongation of escape interval to 1,100 msec (automatic interval = 760 msec) appear to be related to inapparent signal (arrow) within T wave inscription, and slightly outside pacer refractory period (350 msec). Oversensing secondary to large intracardiac T wave voltage and/or prolonged voltage decay of pacemaker afterpotential should be considered.

False Signals

Pacemaker inhibition characterized by variable prolongation of the timing cycle (the escape or automatic interval) or prolonged irregular pauses terminated by a spontaneous beat can occur when false signals are present and sensed outside the pacer refractory period. Sudden changes in the resistance within the pacing system can generate a voltage potential difference of sufficient magnitude at the electrode terminals to recycle the demand pacemaker.

Pacing lead fracture, complete or partial, characteristically produces spurious voltage signals between the cathode and anode. These signals are engendered by the "make and break" of intermittent and momentary separation of the well-apposed segments of the fractured lead (Fig. 19–26). This voltage transient is often not visible in the surface ECG but is usually apparent in an electrographic recording from the defective lead as a signal whose amplitude varies between 2 and 100 mV. These false or contact signals appear in the electrographic recording as a burst of fast signals or as isolated slow signals.

Random emergence of false signals outside the pacer refractory period will often induce a chaotic pacemaker arrhythmia. Rhythmic recycling of a demand pacemaker is apparent when these spurious signals emerge immediately after the refractory

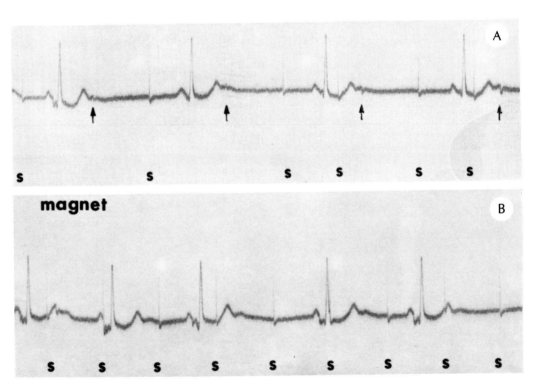

Fig. 19–26. A, Nonstimulating unipolar pacemaker pulses (S) are discharged irregularly due to intermittent sensing failure and rhythmic recycling by apparent voltage transient (arrow) that is evident in surface ECG 600 msec after each spontaneous beat. Genesis of these false voltage signals is related to mechanical systole that induces sudden resistance changes within pacing system incident to momentary separation of partially fractured lead wire. B, Application of a magnet over pulse generator converts irregular pulse cycle to fixed-rate pulse discharge (S) and eliminates oversensing due to these false signals.

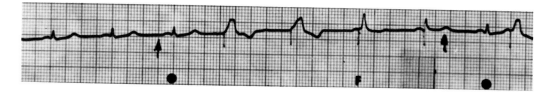

Fig. 19–27. Two spontaneous ventricular beats (solid dots) are not sensed and are followed by an inapparent short escape interval. Escape interval of these paced beats appears to be initiated by inapparent signal, presumably occurring at time indicated by arrow. Second dotted ventricular beat is truly not sensed, since it appears beyond pacer refractory period. At reoperation, a loose lead-generator connection was found and considered to be the cause of intermittent, random false voltage signals that recycled this demand pacemaker. Inconsistent sensing of spontaneous QRS beat was attributed to marginal cardiac signal that measured 2.6 mV. Sensing function was completely restored after implantation of pacemaker of high sensitivity and secured lead-generator connection.

period to produce an ECG pattern indiscernible from T wave or pacemaker afterpotential sensing.

Oversensing of false signals, associated with a pacemaker arrhythmia characterized by variable prolongation of the timing cycle or prolonged pause terminated by a spontaneous beat, is eliminated by magnetic induction to fixed-rate pacing.

A diagnosis of intermittent and partial lead fracture is suggested when attenuated pacemaker spikes appear during fixed-rate pacing induced by the testing magnet, and pauses of the pacemaker stimuli are separated by a multiple of the automatic interval. Variations in the amplitude of the pacemaker pulse during fixed-rate pacing are consistent with a sudden coincident increase in the pacing lead resistance due to

momentary separation of the wire or electrode. Absence of a pacemaker stimulus and a pause delimited by a multiple of the automatic interval suggest a pacemaker discharge into a transiently disruptive pacing system.

Other mechanisms within the pacing system responsible for the genesis of false signals capable of demand pacemaker inhibition includes the following:

1. Loose connection between the lead and pulse generator can induce intermittent and sudden changes of resistance within the pacing system (Figs. 19–27 and 19–28).

2. Intimate contact of an active pacemaker electrode with an adjacent inactive electrode can also create inter-

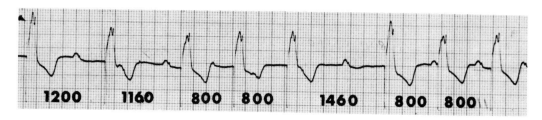

Fig. 19–28. Intermittent irregular prolongation of pacemaker automatic interval from 1160 to 1460 msec is present while basic automatic interval is 800 msec. Pacemaker is recycled by inapparent signals that randomly emerge outside pacer refractory period. Prolongation of pacemaker timing cycle is always less than two automatic intervals. This chaotic arrhythmia was converted to fixed-rate pacing by magnetic induction. Oversensing due to false voltage signals was found to be caused by a loose connection between lead terminal and pulse generator.

mittent voltage signals. The inactive electrode is often represented by a temporary pacing catheter that remains in juxtaposition to the permanent lead at the time of implantation and is withdrawn several days later.

3. Internal short circuit between bipolar electrodes due to an insulation break is extremely rare. Isolated disruption of insulation usually causes pacing failure by an external current shunt.

Inhibition of demand pacemakers by oversensing of nonpropagated, concealed ventricular extrasystoles, confined to the Purkinje system and myocardium immediately surrounding the sensing electrode, and not apparent in the surface ECG, was first suggested by Massumi in 1972. This unusual electrical phenomenon, not documented by a direct recording of the electrographic signal at the electrode site, has been considered by many as problematical and is currently rejected as a cause of oversensing. The characteristic ECG rhythm changes, presumably induced by these inapparent signals of cardiac origin, are more likely related to false signals arising within the pacing system.

Muscle Potential Interference

Demand pacemaker inhibition and unexplained pauses may also be encountered when sufficiently large voltage signals are generated during skeletal muscular activity in propinquity to the pacing system. Relatively strong contractions of the pectoralis major muscle in proximity to the pulse generator can create inhibiting myopotential signals with amplitudes of several millivolts (0.5 to 3 mV), and within a discrete frequency range, corresponding to the sensitivity characteristics of the pacemaker sensing amplifier circuit. Oversensing of skeletal muscle potentials leading to undetected and transient periods of nonpacing or

prolonged asystole appears to be peculiar to the unipolar modality of demand pacing. A limited rate increase will occur with unipolar synchronous pacemakers that respond to these myopotential signals. The Cordis pulse generator, which incorporates a noise sampling period during the final one third of its refractory period, is converted to its programmed fixed rate when continuous interference from muscle potential signals persists.

Unexplained pacemaker pauses due to diaphragmatic myopotentials have also been documented with demand pacemaker inhibition. Active contraction of the diaphragm during deep inspiration, coughing, straining, or Valsalva maneuver has been shown to generate myopotentials as high as 2 mV and transient pacemaker suppression of either unipolar or bipolar demand pacemakers. Oversensing of skeletal or diaphragmatic myopotentials with intermittent cessation of pacing or variable periods of pauses is readily converted to fixed-rate pacing by magnetic induction.

Electromagnetic Interference

Strong external electromagnetic fields will influence demand pacemakers and may engender interference with normal spontaneous pacing function. Devices such as an electrocautery (Fig. 19–29) and diathermy units, electric arc welder, radio and TV transmitters, radar, and automotive, aircraft, and marine ignition systems can emit sufficient pulsed energy to inhibit a pacemaker output stimulus. Unipolar demand pacemakers are more susceptible to inhibition by these external electrical fields because of the large dipole between electrodes. Strong continuous electrical interference is detected during the alert period of most pulse generators (or noise sampling period of Cordis pulse generator) and causes reversion to programmed fixed rate pacing.

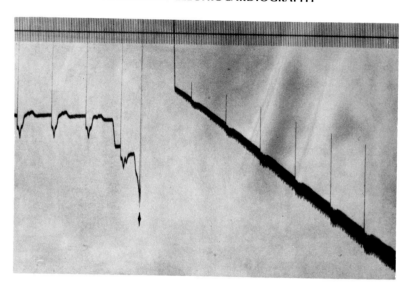

Fig. 19–29. Electrical field induced by electrocautery in proximity to pulse generator does not interfere with normal pacing function. ECG baseline is distorted with electrical noise, but pacemaker spikes continue to discharge and are apparently followed by distorted QRS complexes confirmed by palpation of arterial pulse. Recent improvements in pacemaker filtering design and special shielding provide increased protection against strong electrical fields engendered by many common sources of electromagnetic energy.

CHEST WALL STIMULATION

The sensing function of a demand pacemaker may be evaluated during paced rhythms by a relatively simple and safe technique, known as chest wall stimulation, using an underdrive procedure. External stimuli, insufficient in strength for myocardial stimulation, act as inhibiting signals to the demand sensing circuit when they occur outside its refractory period. These pulses are delivered from an external pacing device connected to ECG-type electrodes, placed on the outer chest wall in proximity to the electrode poles of the pacing system. Pulses from the external pacer at 4 mA or higher are emitted at a rate that will decrease the implantable pacemaker stimulus

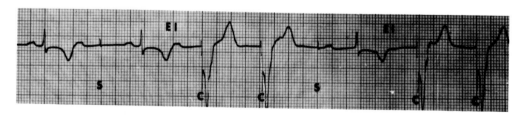

Fig. 19–30. External current pulses (S) are applied to outer chest wall at rate appropriately lower than pacemaker programmed fixed-rate. Output of implanted pulse generator is intermittently inhibited in response to external pulse. Spontaneous beats also emerge and are properly sensed with escape interval (EI) of 860 msec. Sensing function of pacemaker is therefore normal as designed. The underdrive procedure can be used to determine sensing capability of an implanted demand pacemaker that functions in its fixed-rate mode.

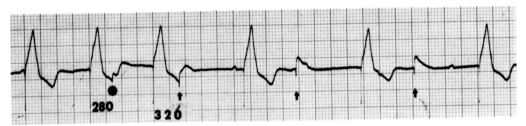

Fig. 19-31. External pulses are applied at varying coupling intervals to paced beats to determine pacemaker refractory period. External pulse (solid dot) occurring 280 msec after the second paced beat is not sensed. Second external pulse (first arrow) occurs 320 msec after third paced beat and recycles pulse generator to normal escape interval of 800 msec. Refractory period of this pacemaker is less than 320 msec and at least 280 msec.

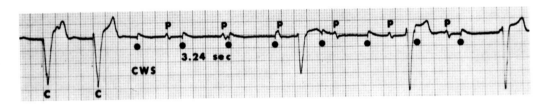

Fig. 19-32. Chest wall stimulation (CWS) at stimulus discharge rate (solid dot) appropriately higher than fast pacing rate inhibits demand pacemaker and induces asystolic period of 3.24 sec, followed by slow unstable ventricular rhythm. Underdrive procedure of CWS maintains pacing and is preferable in pacemaker-dependent patients who are subject to risk of asystole during overdrive or inhibitory chest wall stimulation.

discharge to almost half its programmed fixed rate. Emission of external pulse discharge should be adjusted so that it is sensed during the alert period of each alternate timing cycle.

The response of the permanent pacemaker to an intrinsic cardiac signal, if the latter emerges during underdrive, is then analyzed (Fig. 19-30). An inadequate cardiac signal for sensing at the electrode site is suggested if the implantable pacemaker senses the external pulse signals but not the spontaneous cardiac signals. The sensitivity threshold of a demand pacemaker should not be evaluated by this technique, since no relationship exists between the voltage amplitude of the cardiac signal and the amplitude of the external pulse.

External pulses that occur at varying coupling intervals to the paced beat will also permit determination of the pacemaker refractory period. This will confirm normal demand function when an early spontaneous beat is not sensed because of a long refractory period (Fig. 19-31). Inappropriately short escape intervals, consistent with partial pacemaker recycling by time-dependent external stimuli that fall within the relative refractory period of the pacemaker may also be established. These provide an explanation of this apparent abnormal sensing function during demand pacing.

Analysis of the underlying spontaneous electrical activity of the heart may be accomplished by utilizing chest wall stimulation to inhibit demand pacemakers that pace continuously. The external pulses are applied to the chest wall at an appropriately higher rate than the programmed rate of the permanent pacemaker to suppress its output pulse completely (Fig. 19-32). Elimination of the pacemaker rhythm may expose an underlying rhythm consistent with digitalis toxicity or indicative of pacemaker dependency.

SELECTED READINGS

Abernathy, W.S., and Crevey, B.J.: Right-bundle branch block during transvenous ventricular pacing. Am. Heart J., 90:774, 1975.

Barold, S.S., et al.: Inhibition of bipolar demand pacemaker by diaphragmatic myopotentials. Circulation, 56:679, 1977.

Barold, S.S., et al.: Evaluation of demand pacemakers by chest wall stimulation. Chest, 63:598, 1973.

Barold, S.S., and Gaidula, J.J.: Evaluation of normal and abnormal sensing functions of demand pacemakers. Am. J. Cardiol., 28:201, 1971.

Castellanos, A.J., et al.: A study of arrival of excitation of selected ventricular sites during human bundle branch block using close bipolar catheter electrodes. Chest, 63:208, 1973.

Coumel, P., Mugica, J., and Barold, S.S.: Demand pacemaker arrhythmias caused by intermittent incomplete electrode fracture. Diagnosis with testing magnet. Am. J. Cardiol., 36:105, 1975.

Falkoff, M., et al.: The noise sampling period: A new cause of apparent sensing malfunction of demand pacemakers. Pace, 1:250, 1978.

Furman, S.: Cardiac pacing and pacemakers. VI. Analysis of pacemaker malfunction. Am. Heart J., 94:378, 1977.

Furman, S.: Inhibition of a ventricular synchronous pacemaker. Am. Heart J., 93:581, 1977.

Furman, S., and Fisher, J.D.: Cardiac pacing and pacemakers. V. Technical aspects of implantation and equipment. Am. Heart J., 94:250, 1977.

Furman, S., Hurzeler, P., and DeCaprio, V.: Cardiac pacing and pacemakers. III. Sensing the cardiac electrogram. Am. Heart J., 93:794, 1977.

Furman, S., Parker, B., and Kranthamer, M.: The influence of electromagnetic environment on the performance of artificial cardiac pacemakers. Ann. Thorac. Surg., 6:90, 1968.

Green, G.D.: Assessment of cardiac pacemakers: Pacemaker frontal plane vectors. Am. Heart J., 81:1, 1971.

Kaster, J.A., Berkovits, B.V., and DeSanctis, R.W.: Variations in discharge rate of demand pacemakers not due to malfunction. Am. J. Cardiol., 25:344, 1970.

Kaul, T.K., and Bain, W.H.: Radiographic appearances of implanted transvenous endocardial pacing electrodes. Chest, 72:323, 1977.

Lasseter, K.C., Buchanan, J.W., and Yoshonis, K.F.: A mechanism for "false" inhibition of demand pacemakers. Circulation, 42:1093, 1970.

Leeds, C.J., Akhtar, M., and Damato, A.N.: Fluoroscope-generated electromagnetic interference in an external demand pacemaker. Circulation, 55:548, 1977.

Massumi, R.A., et al.: Apparent malfunction of demand pacemaker caused by nonpropagated (concealed) ventricular extrasystoles. Chest, 61:426, 1972.

Moss, A.J.: Therapeutic uses of permanent pervenous atrial pacemakers: A review. J. Electrocardiol., 8:373, 1975.

Mugica, J., et al.: Methods for recording intermittent contact signals in demand pacemaker arrhythmias (11 cases). Pace, 1:222, 1978.

Mymin, D., et al.: Inhibition of demand pacemakers by skeletal muscle potentials. J.A.M.A., 223:527, 1973.

Ohm, O.J., et al.: Interference effect of myopotentials on function of unipolar demand pacemakers. Br. Heart J., 36:77, 1974.

Parsonnet, V., Furman, S., and Smyth, N.P.D.: Report of the Inter-Society Commission for Heart Disease Resources. Implantable cardiac pacemakers: Status report and a resource guideline. Am. J. Cardiol., 34:487, 1974.

Piller, L.W., and Kennelly, B.M.: Myopotential inhibition of demand pacemakers. Chest, 66:418, 1974.

Sung, R.J., et al.: Partial pacemaker recycling of implanted QRS-inhibited pulse generators. Pace, 1:189, 1978.

Trevino, A.J., et al.: Chest-wall stimulation: A method of demand QRS-blocking pacemaker suppression in the study of arrhythmias. Am. Heart J., 81:20, 1971.

Vera, Z., et al.: Lack of sensing by demand pacemakers due to intraventricular conduction defects. Circulation, 51:815, 1975.

Waxman, M.B., et al.: Demand pacemaker malfunction due to abnormal sensing. Report of two cases. Circulation, 50:389, 1974.

Widmann, W.D., et al.: Suppression of demand pacemakers by inactive pacemaker electrodes. Circulation, 45:319, 1972.

20

Nursing Management of the Patient with a Pacemaker

ESTHER SHILLING

In recent years indications for the use of temporary and permanent pacemakers have broadened considerably because of developments in electrical control of cardiac activity. It has become increasingly clear, therefore, that time must be spent on educating the patient and his family in order to change a life-saving medical intervention to a reorientation to "living." For many patients, a failing heart represents the fading of life itself. What lies ahead is unknown and threatening, and the thought of a mechanical device regulating and controlling as vital an organ as the heart is terrifying. The nurse can help by making patient education a part of patient care because a well-informed patient is able to cope better with real or imagined problems.

Teaching can be accomplished through direct conversation, booklets, and visual aids (Table 20–1). Teaching is a nursing responsibility with a high priority in overall care of the patient. The circumstances surrounding initial pacemaker insertion, be it temporary, emergency, or elective permanent pacing, will dictate the amount of

TABLE 20–1

Teaching Methods

1. CONVERSATION
   a. Presenting factual information
   b. *Listening*
   c. Answering questions
2. VISUAL AIDS
   a. Booklets
   b. Pamphlets
   c. Flip charts
   d. Diagrams
   e. Film strips
   f. Models
3. ACTUAL PACEMAKERS AND LEADS

information discussed with the patient and his family preoperatively.

TEMPORARY PACING

Temporary pacing is usually an emergency or semiemergency procedure to

TABLE 20-2

Points to Include in a Brief Explanation of the Procedure for Temporary Pacemaker Insertion

Site of incision	Right or left external jugular, subclavian, antecubital, or femoral vein areas
Size of incision	None (if percutaneous) OR Small (2–4 cm)
Time	20–30 minutes, including positioning on the table and connecting to monitors
Pain and discomfort	Minimal; patient must lie still on a hard table; will be aware but sedated
Devices	A pacing wire will extrude through the incision site and be connected to an external pacemaker strapped to the anterior chest wall, arm, or thigh
Mobility after insertion	Controlled by technique or insertion of the catheter and by medical conditions
Monitors	As needed by medical condition
Benefits	Will control heart rate; allow time for unhurried decisions for subsequent therapy

control heart rate. The nurse must prepare the patient and his family quickly and adequately, despite the short time available. Good preoperative preparation enhances the patient's cooperation during the actual pacemaker insertion and assists the patient to cope with the inconveniences and mild discomforts after the procedure. A most important result of good preoperative preparation is a receptive and positive attitude toward permanent pacing should it be required.

A brief explanation of the procedure should include what is to be expected in terms of the time of the operation, the site and size of the incision, pain and discomfort, a description of the devices and monitors, and the benefits of therapy (Table 20–2).

The insertion of the temporary pacing catheter is optimally performed in an appropriately equipped cardiac catheterization laboratory, but in an emergency it can be performed at the bedside. *The simplicity of inserting the temporary transvenous wire categorizes the procedure as minor surgery, a point that should be emphasized during the preoperative preparation.*

If no nursing specialist such as a nurse clinician is available, professional registered nursing personnel with a basic nursing educational background should be capable of preparing the patient for temporary pacing and caring for the paced patient. Nursing responsibilities include both preoperative *emotional* and *physical* preparation. The consent to the operation must be signed by the patient or the next of kin. No preoperative sedation is required, although it may be prescribed by the physician. Proper safety precautions include the removal of artificial devices such as dentures, contact lenses, eyeglasses, and hearing aids. Time should be allocated for bladder and bowel elimination. Because the operation is done under local anesthesia, the patient need not be fasting if the operation is urgent. A history of drug allergy and daily routine medications should be obtained and charted. In the event the patient is allergic to a local anesthestic agent or is on anticoagulant medications, the physician must be informed immediately. Charting includes vital signs, time, observations of the patient's general condition, and any other pertinent information.

Pacing Modes

The pacing mode can be defined by identifying the heart chamber paced and sensed.[1] Several modes are commonly used.

Fixed-rate or asynchronous pacing (AOO, VOO) stimulates the chamber(s) at a constant rate. Competition between the pacemaker and natural cardiac activity may occur but is without hazard unless the threshold for ventricular fibrillation is low (e.g., after myocardial infarction or as a result of drug toxicity or electrolyte imbalance).

Ventricular inhibitory pacing (VVI) is the most frequently used external pacemaker mode. It is noncompetitive, uses the same electrode for both pacing and sensing, and is selected for 98% of all temporary pacing.

Atrial pacing (AAI) is applicable to sinus bradyarrhythmias in the absence of AV block. It is used with increased frequency (but still applies to only 1% of cases) at regular or overriding rates to stabilize rapid or irregular atrial or ventricular rhythms when atrioventricular conduction is intact, as it preserves atrioventricular synchrony and therefore enhances cardiac output. A special loop electrode for the atrium has been used for this purpose.

Atrioventricular sequential pacing (DVI) is a more complex method of restoring AV synchrony because two separate electrodes are needed. Both the atria and the ventricles are stimulated with a preset AV interval. This mode is used when normal AV conduction is absent. For temporary pacing, a specially designed multipolar catheter must be used. DVI pacing accounts for 1% of all temporary pacemaker therapy.

Understanding the External Pacemaker

The external pacemaker is usually powered by standard batteries that have a life expectancy of about two months. If there is no department of biomedical engineering, the nurse may be responsible for maintenance of the external pacemaker and must be familiar with the procedure to exchange the battery in the device. Each time the battery is replaced, the date should be indicated on a label fixed to the pacemaker. Fresh batteries and extra pacemakers should be readily available. Routine inspection and maintenance of the pacemaker are

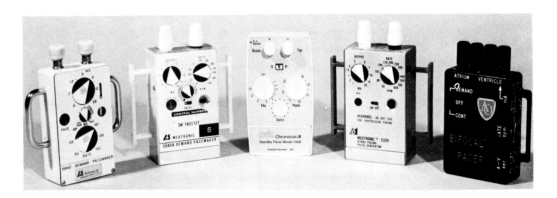

Fig. 20–1. Examples of external pacemakers: left to right, Medtronic, Model 5940; Medtronic, Model 5880A; Cordis, Model 156B; Medtronic, Model 5320 for atrial pacing only; American Optical extracorporeal pacer for AV sequential pacing.

essential. The pacemaker must be properly maintained. It should *not* be autoclaved or immersed in liquids; it can be gas sterilized *after* removal of blood or other particles by sponging carefully with water or alcohol.

There are several manufacturers of external pacemakers. Although the devices may look different, the control dials are essentially the same (Fig. 20–1).

There is an *on/off* switch. The operation of the control usually requires the use of both hands, in order to prevent accidental movement of the switch.

With the pacing catheter in the right ventricle the *mode of pacing* dial indicates fixed-rate pacing (VOO) or ventricular inhibitory pacing (VVI); the degree of sensing capability can be controlled with a *sensitivity* control. Should the pacing catheter be fixed in the right atrium, the mode of pacing then refers to the atrium (AOO, AAI).

The *output* dial indicates the strength of the stimulus (in milliamperes). The setting should be selected by the physician. A safe level is about two to three times threshold, which is the setting at which pacing is first achieved.

The *rate* dial indicates the number of times a minute the pacemaker will fire, with the range being 30 to 150 beats per minute. Most models have an indicating needle or light that demonstrates "pacing" or "sensing."

Each external pacemaker has a model and serial number which should be recorded to permit inventory control and rotation of devices. Ideally, the department responsible for initiating pacemaker therapy should maintain the inventory records. More than one department may be involved, such as the Cardiac Catheterization Laboratory, the Open Heart Pump Team, the Coronary Care Unit, the Intensive Care Unit, and the Emergency Room. Each unit should maintain individual records, but one central control unit should be responsible for overall inventory and maintenance.

Hospitals charge a daily rental fee for the use of the external pacemaker. Therefore, the nurse must record the date the device is disconnected and the temporary pacing catheter is removed from the patient.

Once the pacemaker has been removed, it should be cleaned and returned to the department responsible for its maintenance. The charge slip should be completed and forwarded to the proper accounting department.

ATRIAL PACEMAKER. A specifically designed external atrial pacemaker intended for atrial pacing only is available. *Ventricular pacing with the atrial pacemaker is contraindicated.*[2] The device is clearly identified with a bold type **warning** written on the faceplate. The control dials regulate the same parameters as those available with the ventricular external pacemaker, but the rate range is adjustable to 800 beats per minute.

AV SEQUENTIAL PACEMAKER. Another specific external pulse generator provides AV sequential pacing. This device is clearly identified by color (black) and printed information on the faceplate. The control dials for AV interval, rate in beats per minute, and current in milliamperes are located on the side of the unit. The *mode/on/off* switch is on the faceplate. There are four terminals, two positive (+) and two negative (−), for connection to the special electrode catheters.

SPECIAL CONSIDERATIONS. The external pacemaker should be separated from the skin surface by a piece of absorbent padding cut to size to protect the skin from pressure, to absorb sweat, and to provide comfort. The device may be held in place with a harness made of straps or bandage tied around the torso (Fig. 20–2), or strapped to the arm or thigh, depending on the site of insertion for the pacing catheter. The chest harness can be uncomfortable, especially for one who is obese or has pendulous breasts. Therefore, wrinkles or twists in the straps should be avoided, and the position should be checked periodically.

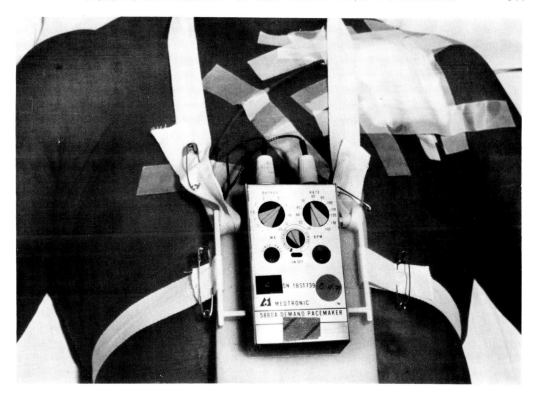

Fig. 20–2. Fixation of external pacemaker to anterior chest wall. Note padding under pacemaker.

Should the pacing catheter be unipolar it must be connected to the negative (−) terminal, and an additional wire (anode) from the (+) terminal must be sutured to the skin.

HAZARDS AND EFFECTS OF EXTERNAL ELECTRICAL FIELDS. The pacemaker electrode is a direct, low resistance current path to the myocardium, and even a minute amount of current can induce ventricular fibrillation. All hospital personnel involved in the care of patients with pacing catheters must be trained to prevent contact between catheter terminals and conductive surfaces. The following specific precautions must be taken:

1. Use only battery-operated pacemakers.

2. Use only *one* line-powered instrument connected to the patient at any given time, such as an electrocardiographic monitor or recorder. The patient should *not* be otherwise grounded (e.g., lying on a line-powered adjustable bed or on an x-ray table).

3. Catheter terminals should be handled carefully (Fig. 20–3). Never touch exposed terminals with a bare hand. Use gloves. Do not let the terminals contact liquids or conductive materials.

4. If the catheter is not connected to the pacemaker, the terminals should be insulated with rubber (a finger of a glove, for example), and fixed securely to the skin.

5. Make sure that the terminals are inserted into the pacemaker properly.

6. Minimize the use of adapters and extension cables because the added length and connections increase the risk of microshock and fibrillation.

7. Do *not* replace external pacemaker batteries while the pacemaker is in use on a patient.

External pacemakers operating in the

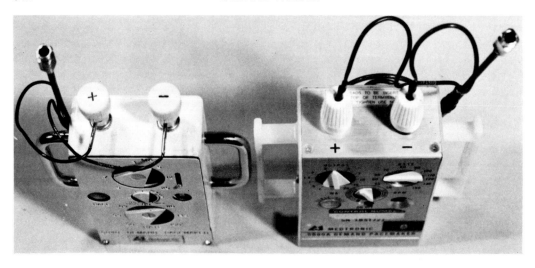

Fig. 20–3. Catheter terminal connections: anterior/posterior and superior.

fixed-rate mode are relatively immune to most sources of external electrical fields, but all sensing pacemakers designed to detect signals of a magnitude of only a few millivolts are inherently sensitive to external electrical fields, even though modern units prevent most external interference from affecting the unit's operation. Nevertheless, because strong interference may suppress the output of any pacemaker, electrocautery and electrocoagulating equipment should not be used near patients with external pacemakers, and electric razors should be used with care.

If the patient requires defibrillation, the pacemaker should be turned off and, if time allows, both wires should be disconnected from the terminals to prevent damage to the device (even though most external pacemakers are designed to withstand shocks up to 400 watt seconds).[3]

Postoperative Role of the Nurse

There are no rules about postoperative cardiac monitoring of temporary pacing because this depends upon the preexisting cardiac rhythm and the extent to which the patient is dependent upon the pacemaker. However, in most patients with temporary pacers, ECG monitoring is usually done. Upon return to the nursing unit, vital signs should be checked, the dressing should be inspected to detect bleeding or swelling, and the external pacemaker connections to the pacing catheter terminals should be examined to ensure that they are properly and securely connected. The pacemaker faceplate cover must be in place and kept on at all times except when the controls are adjusted. The patient should be made comfortable, observed for hiccoughs and chest wall or diaphragmatic stimulation, and given an analgesic if necessary.

Charting should include the date, time, site of catheter insertion, pacing mode, and the control settings for rate (in beats per minute) and output (in milliamperes). Any change in these settings must be charted. Any suspicion of abnormal function must be reported to the pacemaker physician immediately.

Of equal importance to physical care is supportive emotional care. Reassurance and reinforcement of preoperative information and clarification of the reason for the temporary pacemaker must be provided in simple, clear terms.

The temporary catheter is usually sutured to the skin with a silk suture. The catheter insertion site and surrounding area should be kept dry and clean and inspected regularly for signs of inflammation or infection. Antibiotic ointment should be applied to the skin perforation site every two to three days when long-term use is contemplated. If the antecubital vein has been used, an armboard may be used to prevent all but minimal arm movement. The elbow should be kept at the side because abduction may cause movement of the catheter tip.

The dressing covering a femoral insertion site may need more frequent reinforcement because its location makes it more prone to wetness. Care should be taken to prevent the cannulated leg from being flexed rapidly and sharply at the hip and thus causing the catheter to move within the heart.[4] Disoriented patients should be restrained to prevent accidental dislodgment of the electrode or disconnection of the pacemaker from the wire.

Evaluation Techniques

Because the most common problem associated with temporary pacing is failure to capture the heart, frequent cardiograms are indicated. Frontal and lateral chest roentgenograms after insertion confirm electrode position and serve as a reference in case of later difficulty. The physician will test the gain control periodically to assure that the setting remains sufficiently above threshold.

Specific Pacemaker Problems

If the pacemaker is not functioning properly, the cause of failure must be deter-

mined rapidly and corrected (Table 20–3). This is usually accomplished at the patient's bedside using the following assessment guides.

1. Is the pacemaker switch on?
2. Are the pacing controls set properly?
3. Do any pacemaker artifacts appear on the electrocardiogram?
4. Is there an appropriate response to each pacemaker stimulus?
5. Are the catheter terminals connected properly and tightly?
6. Are any portions of the exposed metal terminals of the pacing catheter touching each other?
7. Is the apical heart rate different from the pacemaker rate?
8. Does the patient's position affect pacemaker function?
9. Is stimulation of the diaphragm or chest wall present?
10. Is this stimulation related to the patient's position or to current output of the pacemaker?
11. Are there any sources of electromagnetic interference?

Loss of Pacemaker Artifact

If pacing has ceased and the pacemaker artifact on the electrocardiogram is absent but the pacemaker continues to discharge as shown by the indicator, the catheter terminals should be checked to establish that the connections are proper. If the device is *not* discharging and the switch is on, the battery may be depleted or the pacemaker is defective. Proper pacing can be restored by changing the external pacemaker.

If one of the two wires is broken, pacing may be restored by converting to a unipolar system, with the intact wire connected to the negative (−) pole. For electrical stimulation to occur, current must flow between two poles to create an electrical circuit. In a

TABLE 20–3

Common External Pacemaker Problems

SITUATION	PROBABLE CAUSE	CORRECT APPROACH
Loss of pacemaker artifact	Sensitivity too high	Reduce sensitivity
	Battery depletion	Change external pacemaker
	Loose, broken, or disconnected wires	Repair or replace pacing catheter
	Short circuit of wires	or ground wire
Failure to capture without loss of pacing artifact	Catheter malposition	Increase output; reposition patient; reposition catheter
	Battery depletion	Change external pacemaker
	Electrode insulation break	Increase output; repair insulation; change catheter
Rate malfunction	Faulty external pacemaker	Change external pacemaker
Loss of proper sensing	Catheter malposition	Reposition catheter
	Sensing too low	Increase sensitivity
	Faulty external pacemaker	Change external pacemaker
Oversensing	Sensitivity too high	Decrease sensitivity
	Interference	Eliminate electromagnetic interference
	Faulty external pacemaker	Change external pacemaker
Pacer-induced arrhythmias	Output setting too high	Decrease output
	Electromagnetic interference	Change mode or setting
	Altered threshold	Appropriate drugs
Stimulation of chest wall or diaphragm	Perforation	Reposition catheter
	Output too high	Reduce output
		Change patient's position

unipolar system, the negative (−) pole is within the heart; the positive (+) pole from the wire is sutured to the chest wall. In a bipolar system, the two poles are at the tip of the catheter.

Bipolar function can be restored if the break is accessible and can be repaired. Better contact for thin wires that are gripped poorly by some pacemaker terminals may be achieved by doubling the wire over metal, before insertion into the connector terminals. In the sensing mode, reduction of the sensitivity of the pacer may eliminate external signals, but the pacemaker will remain sensitive to cardiac signals.

Failure to Capture Without Loss of Pacing Artifact

If the pacemaker artifact is seen on the electrocardiogram, failure to capture may be due to malposition of the catheter, a break in the electrode insulation, malfunction of the pacemaker, sensing failure, or perforation of the right ventricular wall associated with stimulation of the chest wall or the diaphragm.

CATHETER MALPOSITION—THRESHOLD ELEVATION. Threshold elevation due to malposition of the electrode tip is the most common cause of pacing failure. An increase of the pacemaker output will usually solve this problem; if it does not, repositioning of the electrode is mandatory.

ELECTRODE INSULATION BREAK. Current diversion through a break in the electrode insulation reduces the current to the electrode tip and may cause pacing failure. Repair of the insulation break, increase of the current of the pacemaker, or change of the external device may restore proper pacing, but replacement of the wire will usually be required.

PACEMAKER MALFUNCTION: RUNAWAY/SLOW RATE. Malfunctions of the external pacemaker without loss of the stimulation artifact are usually rate-circuit related. Rate problems are corrected by changing the external pacemaker.

LOSS OF PROPER SENSING. Loss of the sensing response with reversion to fixed rate (AOO, VOO) pacing may occur because of a failing battery or a malfunctioning pacemaker, but is usually the result of an inadequate voltage signal to the sensing circuit due to electrode malposition or to abnormally small QRS signals. If this is accompanied by an elevation of the pacing threshold, the catheter should be repositioned. Other methods to restore proper sensing include increasing the sensitivity of the pacemaker or changing the external device.

Oversensing or sensing of unwanted signals (e.g., large T waves, extraneous electrical interference) will lead to improper pacing. Any electromagnetic interference must be eliminated. The sensitivity of the pacemaker must be decreased, or the pacemaker should be changed.

PACER-INDUCED ARRHYTHMIAS. The most dangerous rhythm disturbance, ventricular fibrillation, may be induced by cardiac stimulation during the vulnerable period of the heart (ascending limb and peak of the T wave), particularly in temporary pacing when the threshold for fibrillation may be lowered by digitalis toxicity or acute infarction, when the gain of the pacer has been set too high, or when spurious currents are introduced through the catheter. Other arrhythmias that may be induced include ventricular tachycardia, atrial fibrillation, and aberrant beats. In these instances specific management by the cardiologist is needed. It may include the use of drugs, change of pacing mode, or variation in pacing controls (sensing, rate, output) or a combination of these modalities.

PERFORATION, CHEST WALL TWITCHING, DIAPHRAGMATIC STIMULATION. Perforation of the right ventricular wall frequently results in loss of pacing and chest wall or diaphragmatic stimulation. Repositioning of the pacing catheter will restore proper pacing. When diaphragmatic stimulation or chest wall twitching is present but pacing of the heart is not interrupted, the output of the pacemaker should be reduced to eliminate the twitch but not enough to disrupt regular pacing. At times, the patient's position is a contributing factor, and repositioning the patient may be a temporary solution to the problem until the electrode can be relocated.

Surgical Complications

Surgical complications include infection, phlebitis of the vein of entrance, and pneumothorax or hemothorax. Fortunately, these problems are rare and usually avoidable. In infection and phlebitis the electrode must be replaced in a different site. Antibiotics are used in infection, but not phlebitis. Pneumothorax, especially when severe, may require insertion of a thoracotomy tube, but the electrode may usually be left in place. Rare complications include endocarditis (replacement and specific antibiotics mandatory), knotting of the catheter (may require complex extraction maneuvers or cardiotomy), air embolization during catheter insertion, and massive intracardiac thrombosis and pulmonary embolus (all very unusual and often fatal).

Other Medical Conditions

Coexisting medical conditions of all sorts further complicate the management of the pacemaker patient, and require even further care and cooperation of the nurse. These matters are obvious and require no specific comment here.

Cessation of Temporary Pacing

Temporary pacing will be discontinued when the acute condition has disappeared or, if not, when a permanent pacemaker is implanted. Just before disconnecting the external pacemaker, gradually decrease the pacing rate while monitoring the patient's heart rate by observing the electrocardiographic pattern displayed on the monitor or by palpating the radial pulse. Abrupt cessation of pacing may be followed by a period of asystole before a spontaneous rhythm resumes. How long the temporary electrode is to be left in place after resumption of normal pacing or after a permanent unit is inserted is a medical judgment. In general, it is safe to keep a noncomplicated wire in place a few extra days in case there is a recurrence of the original problem.

PERMANENT PACING

Once the physician has elected to implant a permanent pacemaker, consideration must be given to the following situations affecting the patient and his pending pacemaker implant: finances, job performance, electrical environment, other existing medical problems, physician coordination, rehabilitation anticipation, and follow-up (Table 20–4).

Financial Aspects

Pacemakers are costly, and there is no uniform third party insurance policy (Medicare, Blue Cross) for reimbursement. Permissible changes and methods of payment vary from state to state. Most hospitals require financial investigation before the operation. If the patient must pay for the pacemaker, hospitalization, and medical fees and family resources are exhausted or inadequate, attempts must be made to find financial assistance for the patient through social services and state or federal agencies. In New Jersey, the State Rehabilitation Commission is an excellent resource, servicing the "average" family when a member's illness will destroy the family's financial independence. The nurse can be

TABLE 20–4

Nonmedical Factors That Contribute to Pacemaker Selection

FACTOR	COMMENT
Cost	Self pay
	Maximum covered by insurance payment
	Maximum covered by social service agency
	Warranty in effect (pacemaker change only)
Pacer size	Patient's desires
	Body structure
Patient's stability	Reliable for long-term follow-up and continued contact with implanting physician necessary for protocol compliance in special situations (nuclear)
Mental competency	Necessary when *patient* has responsibility (rechargeable unit)
Job requirements	Electrical environment
	Body mechanics (lifting, bending)

helpful in disclosing such problems, in guiding the family to the proper agencies or services, and in seeing them through the entire procedure.

Occupation and Avocation

The surgeon must be aware of specific job requirements that may lead to later pacemaker problems so that, if alternatives are feasible, a more suitable operative technique may be selected. (For example, hunters or golfers may prefer a permanent implant on one side, or certain jobs may require use of one arm more than the other.) Should the patient be employed in an area where there is heavy duty electrical equipment or where there are strong radar or other magnetic fields, plans should be made to select an appropriate pacer and to prepare the patient for potential changes in occupation.

In most cases the patient should be able to resume whatever was normal and medically appropriate before the pacemaker implant. It is essential to emphasize this point. Unless the employment involves a potential hazard for the pacemaker system, the patient may usually return to pre-pacemaker employment. Unfortunately a few fields are closed to pacemaker wearers: interstate truck driving, participating in professional sports, and piloting a plane. The nurse should determine if the patient requires job training and refer him to the proper social agencies as soon as possible.

Preoperative Responsibilities

The potential pacemaker patient who has not had a temporary pacing and the attendant counsel will require all the support and advice discussed earlier. A patient with a temporary unit must be informed that the size of the device to be implanted is completely different from that of the external pacemaker. Even so, most patients are shocked by the size of an implantable pacemaker even though pacemakers have become much smaller. Therefore, it is sometimes better *not* to show an actual pacemaker to the patient until after it has been implanted. A simple explanation comparing the pacemaker size to a small pocket watch is more than adequate preoperatively.

Operative Site

The most common site for the pulse generator in transvenous pacing is below the clavicle in the right or left pectoral area. If possible, the pacemaker should be placed in a pocket on the nondominant side, but this decision is often dictated by the position of the temporary pacing catheter. Occasionally, the patient will have strong feelings about the position of the pacemaker and it then becomes necessary, for cosmetic reasons, to place the pulse generator in an unusual position, such as in the left retroperitoneal space, behind the rectus sheath, deep to the pectoralis major or minor, or behind the breast.

The operative technique selected by the surgeon will determine the site of the operation, type of anesthesia, operating time, postoperative mobility, pain, discomfort, and length of hospital stay. Following transvenous pacemaker implantation, usually done under local anesthesia in a catheterization laboratory or special procedure room, the patient usually returns to a nonmonitored area, is out of bed with assistance after 8 to 10 hours, is ambulatory thereafter, and is discharged on the third postoperative day.

Surgical techniques for implanting pacing electrodes directly into the myocardium are performed in the operating room under general anesthesia. The approaches include the subxyphoid, transmediastinal or transdiaphragmatic, or direct thoracotomy through the left fifth intercostal space. Several types of myocardial electrodes are used, most often the screw-in sutureless type. When thoracotomy is required, the chest is drained by an intercostal tube that is usually removed on the first postoperative day.

Regardless of surgical technique, special preoperative orders should include the following:

1. N.P.O. áfter 6:00 a.m.
2. Operative consent forms
3. Preparation of operative area
4. Antibiotics (optimal)
5. Sedation
6. Discontinuation of anticoagulant therapy (check with physician)
7. Prothrombin time or appropriate clotting profile

At our hospital we like to include mammography for patients in whom "long life" pacemakers will be used in order to detect impalpable breast tumors.

Immediate Postoperative Nursing Care

The patient should be made comfortable and connected to the monitor if applicable. Attention should be paid to vital signs, dressings for bleeding or swelling, drainage devices, and the physician's postoperative orders. Charting should include the preceding observations plus nursing evaluations about the patient's general condition. Complaints of pain in the operative site require administration of an analgesic.

Nursing Objectives and Responsibilities

The pacemaker nurse plays a vital role in patient care. The primary objectives of this role are to assist the medical teams to:

1. Teach the patient the medical and test facts about a pacemaker.
2. Teach the patient how to live with the pacemaker.
3. Develop the patient's confidence in the pacemaker and his new life style.
4. Encourage full rehabilitation.
5. Provide information and instructions to emphasize cooperation with follow-up programs.
6. Maintain pacemaker function and recognize pacemaker malfunction.
7. Prevent surgical complications.
8. Provide a safe hospital environment free of external electronic hazards.

The principles of care are both *clinical* and *technical*. Clinical care involves the medical supervision of the *whole* patient. Technical care is concerned with pacemaker function and prevention of complications specific to pacemaker therapy. Nursing observations must be based on knowledge of pacemaker function, modes, implantation techniques, and potential complications. Nursing skills are directed toward wound care, general physical and emotional care, prevention of problems related to surgical complications and pacemaker malfunction, and successful rehabilitation of the patient.

Wound Care

Generally the dressing covering the surgical site is removed on the first postoperative day unless there is an infected or draining wound. Occasionally the pacemaker pocket requires a suction drainage system because of excessive bleeding during the operation. Sutures are usually removed on the sixth or seventh day, but for the past few years surgeons in our hospital have switched entirely to subcuticular closure that requires no suture removal and provides a better short-term cosmetic result. No special wound care is required other than daily *gentle* washing to maintain cleanliness around the incision.

There may be an accumulation of blood in the pocket that will lead to edema of the operative site, skin tension, and pain. No treatment is required for minor collections which will reabsorb *slowly*. A large hematoma may require aspiration, but this is often ineffective until the clot has liquefied. Management of a hematoma will depend on its size. Generally, application of a warm compress (110°F) facilitates absorption and reduces discomfort. Occasionally, surgical evacuation of the hematoma is necessary.

Ecchymosis of the operative site is not uncommon, but sometimes discoloration may involve a large area from the axilla over the anterior chest wall. This discoloration is alarming to the patient, who must be reassured that it will eventually disappear completely and is not dangerous.

Prevention of Complications

In general, nursing intervention will be guided by the general physical condition and age of the patient, who more than likely will be over 70 years old when initially paced. During the first few weeks after transvenous pacer implantation a fall may dislodge the electrode. Therefore, the patient should be assisted getting in or out of bed and in the early attempts at ambulation.

Prophylactic antibiotic therapy is optional but frequently prescribed for 72 hours. Because pacemaker infections may lead to pacemaker extrusion or "catheter fever," conscientious observation and recording of the temperature is important, so that treatment may be started early.

Taking the pulse is a quick way to gain valuable information concerning pacemaker function, but the pulse must be counted for a *full minute* to assess the rate accurately. One must know the pacemaker mode and preset rate in order to interpret the pulse correctly. The most commonly implanted pacemaker is a VVI unit set at 70 beats per minute, with a tolerance of two or three beats per minute. This rate remains stable and does not vary unless some type of failure occurs.

Rates *faster* than the known rate of the pacer and fast irregular beats are usually due to spontaneous cardiac activity. In these instances it is not possible to know if the pacer is working without slowing the pulse to the preset pacer rate by carotid sinus pressure (to be done by the physician) or by observing the ECG while a magnet is placed over the pacer to convert it to a nonsensing mode (or in some units to speed it up to a faster rate). Rates *slower* than the pacer may be abnormal functions but are usually due to premature beats that *are not detected at the wrist*. Only an electrocardiogram can *document* pacemaker function and malfunction and should be immediately ordered once an abnormality is suspected.

Electrical stimulation of a noncardiac site, such as the phrenic nerve, diaphragm, or intercostal or pectoral muscles, may occur and will be seen as a rhythmic twitch of the upper abdomen or shoulder area. This is almost always caused by a technical problem (e.g., cardiac perforation, insulating screws missing) and will require operative intervention to correct.

The first step for the nurse is to recognize that a problem exists and to be aware of dire consequences of inadequate observations. Although most patients have adequate intrinsic cardiac activity to sustain life, sudden cessation of pacing may lead to asystole and death. Therefore, if pacemaker malfunction is suspected, have the patient remain in bed, offer an explanation of the situation in a calm and reassuring manner, notify the pacemaker physician, keep the patient fasting, and alert the catheterization laboratory so that the staff can rearrange the schedule as soon as the decision for surgical intervention is reached.

It is important to listen to the patient. What may sound like a minor complaint from a nonpaced patient may in fact represent a significant problem in the patient with a pacemaker. Complaints of dizziness or light-headedness, sudden onset of chest pain, or shortness of breath may indicate pacemaker malfunction.

Some of the routine postoperative orders are directed toward long-term follow-up care. These include electrocardiograms and posteroanterior and lateral chest roentgenograms within 48 hours. The "fixed rate" of the pacemaker, measured with an external magnet held over the implanted pacemaker, should be recorded on a digital counter either with a transtelephonic monitor or a special digital rate counter, both of which can be done at the bedside or with the patient directly connected to the test equipment in the pacemaker evaluation center. The recorded pacemaker pulse interval (in milliseconds) becomes the baseline value against which all subsequent data are compared during the life of the pacemaker. Such testing also serves as an introduction of pacemaker technical staff members to the patient and frequently stimulates conversation and interest about the pacemaker and about follow-up.

Predischarge Teaching

During the postoperative recovery period, the patient and his family must be provided with a variety of detailed pacemaker information:

Name of manufacturer
Mode of pacing
Function of pacemaker
Heart chamber(s) paced/sensed
Rate
Progammability features
Serial number
Identification card
Battery type (mercury zinc, lithium, nuclear, rechargeable)
Surgical technique, including types of suture for wound closure (absorbable or not; date for removal of sutures)
Expected pacemaker longevity
Connection of lead to pacemaker
Allowed activities
Restrictions
Electrical equipment, uses, precautions
Medical supervision
Pacemaker follow-up
Travel
Work
Specific situations
Sexual activity
Pacemaker related problems: symptoms; action to be taken
Social clubs
Dental care
Nonpacemaker-related illness

Existing medical problems
Wound care
Clothing

The nurse must be reassuring and sensitive to the patient's reactions in order to establish a trusting relationship that will enhance the patient's cooperation in the learning process. *Remember that teaching includes listening.* The patient and his family must be allowed time to ask questions. Pause frequently to allow the patient and family to absorb the information. Encourage questions by asking for them. The nurse must be unhurried, calm, interested, and concerned and must recognize when the patient is not learning. This may be indicated in a *covert* or *overt* manner. There may be obvious refusal to listen and perhaps the patient is not capable of learning. The covert reaction will be more difficult to detect but may be indicated by preoccupation with other tasks or problems or by claims of not feeling well enough yet. Such a reaction is often a form of denial that can usually be overcome by gently but firmly continuing the discussion, but at a somewhat slower pace.

Discussing the pacemaker with the patient and his family together often reduces anxiety. The nurse should address the family, at the patient's bedside, in a loud, clear voice. The patient will be listening and more than likely will become involved and stimulated to learn. Although an opportune time for reinforcement of information is while the patient and his family are together, the nurse must allow time for private conversations and instructions with the patient, and repeated visits may be necessary.

It is important to show the patient an actual model of the implanted pacemaker. Invite the patient to handle the device and also guide the patient's fingers gently over the implanted pacemaker, tracing its outline so that the hard subcutaneous object can be felt. This action will help to minimize the patient's concern about the unknown foreign body and enforce the reality of the pacemaker. Review the surgical procedure, explaining how the catheter was inserted and connected and how the pacemaker was positioned in a prepared "pocket." If nonabsorbable skin sutures were used for skin closure, be sure the patient has an appointment for suture removal. Encourage gentle movement of the arm on the affected side, reassuring the patient that any pain or discomfort with such activity will soon disappear.

Patients who can understand should be given information about pacing mode. One must explain exactly what *benefits should be derived from pacemaker therapy* and that the pacer is not designed to correct all their associated ailments and complaints. It is important to stress (but not guarantee) the reliability and durability of the pacemaker and to state that the pacer will restore normal activity compatible with age and medical condition. Any restrictions of activities will be explained by the private physician. Simply put, however, the patient can do what he feels well enough to do. An informed patient, adequately instructed, will not hesitate to ask questions about specific activities.

Some may participate in a variety of sports, such as bowling, golfing, hunting (as long as the rifle butt is *not* rested on the shoulder of the implanted side), fishing, walking, swimming, and running. The physician may restrict more strenuous activities such as tennis, basketball, cheer leading, and weight lifting. In making his decision he will take into consideration the site of the pacemaker and the technique of implantation, the amount of stress on the pacemaker wire, the consequences of sudden cessation of pacing, and the importance to the patient of the activity in question.

The pacemaker may give the patient new privileges as well as improve his performance of prior activities because of improved circulation to sustain bodily requirements for oxygen. Many pacemaker patients, despite advanced age, are vitally interested in sexual activity. The pacemaker often enhances sexual intercourse not only by reducing cardiac symptoms, but also by reducing the patient's preoccupation with fear that these symptoms will occur. The nonpaced sexual partner may have to initiate activity initially in order to reassure and encourage the paced partner that the surgery has not affected or reduced his sexuality or attractiveness. The patient may be concerned that the cosmetic results may be offensive to his partner; on the other hand, the nonpaced partner may be afraid of inflicting pain at the operative site or doing harm to the pacemaker system itself. Sexual activity will not adversely affect the pacemaker and may be resumed as soon as it is comfortable and desirable.

It is necessary to emphasize continued medical supervision by the primary physician who must supervise medical care, manage medications and diet, and advise on activities. Once the patient understands that the pacemaker is not a cure-all for every medical condition, the need for continued medical supervision becomes more obvious.

The patient should *carry* the pacemaker identification card. Because some people tuck important documents away for safekeeping, it is often necessary to stress that the card be carried at all times because it contains pertinent information about the patient, the pacemaker, and the physician.

Much has been said about electromagnetic interference (EMI) affecting pacemaker performance in previous years, but present engineering design modifications make pacemakers more resistant to such environments. Many authorities believe the dangers of EMI to be so minor that they do not find it necessary to discuss them in detail,[5] but precautions are necessary for sources of EMI that *may* inhibit an inhibitory pacemaker or trigger a triggered one. Pacemakers have been found unaffected by some household appliances, power tools, weapon detectors, and a long list of electronic equipment and gadgets.

Instruct the patient to inform the security guard at airport weapon detector areas that he has a pacemaker, not because the detector will affect the pacemaker, but the pacemaker may trigger the alarm. If any doubts exist, the patient must be directed to question the safety of specific electrical devices. Some devices are more likely to produce problems. A patient should stay at least *two feet* away from an operating microwave oven. Some, but not all, electric razors will affect the pacemaker. An electric razor should not be used *directly over the pacemaker*. Diathermy should *never* be used over the pacemaker patient. Myopotentials of pectoral muscle contractions can be shown to produce pacer inhibitions in up to 70% of patients, but true clinical manifestations are rarely seen.[6]

Dental care is safe, but the dentist should be advised to take the patient's pulse while using the equipment for the first time. Use of an ultrasonic cleaning device may be less safe, but this depends on the design of the device.[7] Prophylactic antibiotic therapy is indicated before and after extractions or other dental surgery.

Should the patient travel for extended periods, it is helpful to provide names and addresses of pacemaker physicians at his destinations in order to provide him continued emergency care and uninterrupted pacemaker surveillance.

Whenever possible, the medical department of the company where the patient is employed or the school nurse if the patient is a student should be provided with information about the patient's pacemaker and about potential problems peculiar to job- or school-related responsibilities. Instructions for action in the event a pacemaker problem occurs should be provided.

Both men and women may be concerned with the cosmetic effect of the surgery. Reassurance that the surgical trauma and discoloration will disappear is important. Provide guidance and make suggestions about undergarments and, if indicated, recommend custom-made garments which may fit more comfortably. Most women will benefit from wearing a brassiere while hospitalized and should be encouraged to do so, using a protective pad over the incision to prevent irritation from the brassiere strap.

The nurse may be asked to enter the parameter settings of an adjustable pacemaker on the identification card in the spaces provided for such data. If no space is provided, the nurse should record the necessary information on a small gummed label and affix it to the card.

Constant reassurance about pacemaker reliability is necessary. The pacemaker, like any electronic device, is subject to random failures of the electronic circuit, power source, and catheter, but pacemakers are extremely dependable. Nevertheless, the patient should be informed of the *remote* possibility of pacemaker failure, but one must stress that failure, even if sudden, will not be a disaster because some type of spontaneous heart action will return, and there will be time to seek help from the physician. Often the patient will have a phone transmitter, and the clinic performing the follow-up service can be contacted.

The nurse must devote considerable time to the discussion of pacemaker surveillance (follow-up) in order to impress upon the patient and his family that it is important for the patient's well-being. If a pacemaker clinic system is to be used, the patient should be told that 90% of problems can be detected before the patient will be aware of them. A complete description of the evaluation procedure will allay anxiety associated with follow-up procedures. If possible, the nurse should refer to brochures, pictures, and other visual aids to demonstrate that pacemaker evaluation does *not* cause pain or discomfort. It is also helpful to arrange a visit from another patient with a pacemaker who has made an excellent adjustment. Who can better say to a new pacemaker wearer, "What are you concerned about? Look at me, I have a pacemaker."

In the event pacemaker surveillance con-sists of transtelephonic monitoring only, simple clear instructions must be provided. The patient should make several calls himself until he feels comfortable about using the equipment. The effect of the magnet on the pacemaker must be explained in order to prevent abuse of its application. If the patient lives alone and is not capable of performing the test, it will be possible to get assistance from other services or from family or friends to help the patient on monitoring days.

Pacemaker follow-up eliminates the need for the patient to count his own pulse daily, a practice that we do not advise. Unfortunately, not every patient has access to an organized follow-up program, and in that case teaching the patient and his family how to take and count the pulse may be required. (There are also self-test devices that the patient may purchase if this is the only method of follow-up that is feasible.) The following steps should be included: (1) Explain why taking the pulse is important. The patient must understand that the pulse is a reflection of both heart action and pacemaker activity. (2) Demonstrate the technique for counting the pulse. (3) Have the patient return the demonstration. (4) Provide an acceptable pulse rate range. (5) Instruct the patient to contact his physician in the event a different pulse rate is counted.

To prevent prolonged hospitalization, post-discharge needs should be assessed early to allow referrals to social service, community nursing service, or homemaker service or placement in an extended care facility or nursing home. The nurse should know the requirements for such referrals and utilize assistance programs when necessary.

Barring complications the recovery period for pacemaker surgery is short. Most patients feel better quickly and have an improved sense of well-being. They are usually appreciative and grateful for the efforts of the health team and look to the nurse for continued support and friendship.

It has been said, "I have a new birthday . . . a new lease on life." The patient with a pacemaker has a real "zest for life." When the pacemaker patient says, "I'm all charged up," indeed, it is a true statement.

REFERENCES

1. Parsonnet, V., Furman, S., and Smyth, N.P.D.: Implantable Cardiac Pacemakers: Status Report and Resource Guideline. Pacemaker Study Group (ICHD). Circ., 50-A21-35 (#4), October 1974.
2. Medtronic, Inc.: Model 5320 External Atrial Pacing Physician Manual. September 1974.
3. Winslow, E., and Marino, L.: Temporary cardiac pacemaker. Am. J. Nurs., 75:586, 1975.
4. Furman, S., and Escher, D.: Principles and Techniques of Cardiac Pacing. New York, Harper and Row, 1970.
5. Bacharach, B., Chung, E., and Morris, J.: Your Pacemaker Patient. Minneapolis, Medtronic, Inc., 1975, p. 8.
6. Parsonnet, V.: Pacemaker Implantation. Blades' Surgical Diseases of the Chest, 4th edition. Edited by D. Effler. St. Louis, C.V. Mosby, 1978.
7. Simon, A., et al.: The individual with a pacemaker in the dental environment. J. Am. Dent. Assoc., 91:1224, 1975.

SELECTED READINGS

Bain, B.: Pacemakers and people who need them. Am. J. Nurs., 71:1582, 1971.
Barold, S.: Modern concepts of cardiac pacing. Heart Lung, 2:238, 1973.
Barstow, R.: Nursing care of patients with pacemakers. Cardiovasc. Nurs. 8:#2, March-April, 1972.
Berkovits, B.: An Ideal Pacemaker: Cardiac Pacing. Proceedings Vth International Symposium on Cardiac Pacing, Tokyo, 1976. Edited by Y. Wantanabe. Amsterdam, Excerpta Medica, 1977, pp. 592–595.
Bilitch, M., Furman, S., and Morris, J.: So your patient has a pacemaker. Patient Care, 72:10, 1972.
Brogan, M.: Nursing care of the patient experiencing cardiac surgery for coronary artery disease. Nurs. Clin. North Am. 7:#3, 1972.

Care of the Pacemaker and the Pacemaker Patient: Health Devices, 92, February, 1974.
Chung, E.: Artificial Pacemakers. Quick Reference to Cardiovascular Diseases. Philadelphia, J.B. Lippincott Co., 1977.
Davis, M.: Socioemotional component of coronary care. Am. J. Nurs., 72:705, 1976.
Deberry, P., Jefferies, L., and Light, M.: Teaching cardiac patients to manage medications. Am. J. Nurs., 75:2191, 1975.
Escher, D.: Medical aspects of artificial pacing of the heart. Cardiovas. Nurs., 8:#1, 1972.
Forbes, D.: Coming at staff nurses: Early post-op heart patients. RN Magazine, 39:59, 1976.
Fuhrer, L., and Bernstein, R.: Making patient education a part of patient care. Am. J. Nurs., 76:1798, 1976.
Germain, C.: Helping your patient with an implanted pacemaker. RN Magazine, 37:30, 1974.
Gill, C., et al.: An Overview of Pacing. Medtronic Currents, The Cardiovascular System as it Relates to Heart Pacing. Minneapolis, Medtronic, Inc. 1973.
Glenn, F.: The elderly as surgical patients. RN Magazine, 37:60, 1974.
Harmer, B., and Henderson, V.: Textbook of the Principles and Practice of Nursing, 5th edition. New York, The Macmillan Co., 1955.
Hudak, C., Gallo, B., and Lohr, T.: Critical Care Nursing. New York, J.B. Lippincott Co., 1973, p. 55.
Hunn, V.: Cardiac pacemaker. Am. J. Nurs., 69:749, 1969.
Kos, B., and Culbert, P.: Teaching patients about pacemakers. Am. J. Nurs., 71:523, 1971.
Kos, B., and Culbert, P.: Teaching the patient with a pacemaker. Cardiovasc. Nurs., 6:#6, November-December 1970.
Laird, M.: Techniques for teaching pre- and postoperative patients. Am. J. Nurs., 75:1338, 1975.
Medtronic, Inc.: Model 5880A External Demand Pacemaker Physician Manual, 1971.
Myers, B.: Sutures and wound healing. Am. J. Nurs., 71:1725, 1971.
Nordling, N.: Electromagnetic and electrostatic interference in electronic cardiac pacing. Impulse, 9:20, 1978.
Parsonnet, V.: Innovation in Implantable Pacemakers—1975. Electrochemical Bioscience and Bioengineering.
Rockwell, S.: Electricity: it doesn't need to be a problem. RN Magazine, 35:35, 1972.
Williams, C.: The CCU nurse has a pacemaker. Am. J. Nurs., 72:900, 1972.
Williams, C.: That patient with a pacemaker—There's lots you can do. RN Magazine, 71:21, 1971.

21

Pacemaker Interference

KENNETH W. EXWORTHY

The last decade has seen dramatic increases in the number of pacemakers implanted. Since pacemakers have electronic circuitry, they are susceptible to electromagnetic interference (EMI). Concerns about this fact are frequently expressed by many patients and their physicians in letters and telephone calls to pacemaker manufacturers.

No fatalities due to interference have been reported. The situations in which interference has been noted have not had serious consequences.

There is an increasing use of electrical devices of every description in the home, clinic, and in industry. Newer pacemakers generally are less susceptible to interference than their predecessors, but are being implanted for an ever increasing variety of reasons in an ever younger population. Exposure to potential electromagnetic interference is, therefore, increasing rapidly. To prevent EMI from becoming a serious clinical problem for the patient with a pacemaker, physicians, manufacturers, and government regulatory agencies must continue their vigilance.

It is the intent of this chapter to provide information needed to maintain this vigilance. Background is provided to allay the patient's concerns and to pinpoint problem areas in the patient's home or working environment. Questions about these special situations can then be referred to the pacemaker manufacturer for specific information.

ENVIRONMENT

For most of history the only electromagnetic interference (EMI) sources were natural. Such phenomena as lightning, the slow changes of the earth's magnetic field, and sunspots may have been noticed, but had little effect in the business of men. In the last several decades, however, man has learned to produce powerful electric and magnetic fields. He has studied their effects and used them in the design of much of the machinery we now take for granted. The gasoline internal combustion engine relies on an electric ignition system; electric motors of various types power innumerable appliances, tools, and machinery; electric current is used in electric stoves, arc welding, and induction furnaces. Another effect of moving electric charges is to produce electromagnetic radiation of electric power. This effect has nothing to do with the ionizing radiation of x-rays and radioactive sources. Electromagnetic radiation is used in the design of radio and television transmission systems and microwave ovens. The same electronic concepts used in the development of electric pacemakers are used in a myriad of electronic instrumentation and computers.

Not all electronic devices do a good job of containing the fields they produce (poor shielding); others affect the power supply system (poor filtering). Some use electricity in such a way that interference is virtually guaranteed (electrosurgery). The numbers of these intentional and incidental radiators in the environment is increasing at a rapid pace. Efficiency in the use of energy becomes translated into "switching" power supplies that produce more interference than their "linear" predecessors. According to *Electronic Design*, RFI (radio frequency interference) and EMI (electromagnetic interference) are rapidly racing out of control. Millions of citizen's band (CB) radios have been licensed in the last few years. Industry works to reduce cost per item by increasing the power levels of electrically operated production machinery.

To counter this situation in the United States the Federal Communications Commission (FCC) has put stringent new limits on a variety of electrical devices. The Federal Drug Administration (FDA) has proposed specifications limiting susceptibility and emission levels of implantable pacemakers and all other devices used in medical facilities. The need for regulations indicates clearly that interference of one electric device with another is a regularly occurring fact of modern life. It must be dealt with in a clinical environment and in other environments. Patients with external

pacemakers rely on the compatibility of that device with the hospital environment. Patients with implanted pacemakers must be aware of EMI in their work and home environments.

AWARENESS

Virtually any electrical device has the potential for interference with other devices. This interference may take forms all the way from indicator problems to "shut-off." An extreme example was the household of a few years ago which had few branch circuits. The (then) newer, high wattage appliances could easily "interfere" with the operation of other devices by blowing a fuse common to both. This problem was solved by isolation; the high wattage devices were assigned a circuit of their own which reduces interference in most modern installations.

In the modern hospital or clinic, however, interference problems usually cannot be solved so easily. Various instruments must be designed to work in harmony, since failure or degradation of function may be hard to recognize. The first line of defense is awareness. Personnel must realize, for instance, that the crackling heard when "static" discharges form under a bed cover is akin to lightning flashes in a storm and to a pacemaker output. All are pulses of electric current.

Other such realizations follow naturally. Devices operating from a common power system may be affected if the power system is defective. Also, because of their common power source, they may affect each other. Devices which switch on and off steadily have the capability, in many situations, of producing a magnetic pulse each time. High power devices of whatever form have great potential for being sources of interference. Many low power devices have great potential for being susceptible. The human body can carry small currents of electricity below the threshold of feeling which nevertheless

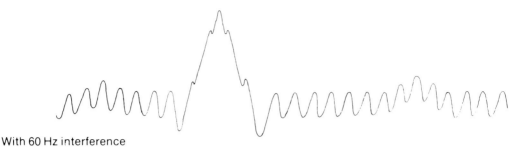

With 60 Hz interference

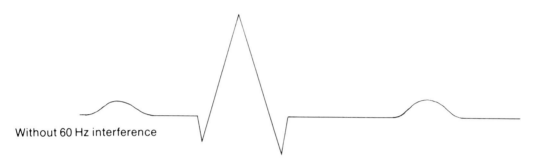

Without 60 Hz interference

Fig. 21–1. Illustrative ECG tracings.

may cause interference with delicate instrumentation (Fig. 21–1).

The pacemaker user must be especially aware of electrically operated devices in his environment. It is useful to realize the difference between microwave cooking, induction heating cooking, and resistance heating. It may be of some importance to know that diesel engines do not have electric pulse ignition, that induction motors are basically different from universal motors, and that amplitude modulated transmission is a far more likely interference source than frequency modulated.

Various types of electrosurgical tools have great interference potential. They produce radiation, typically can be directly coupled to other devices, and may affect the power system.

ELECTRICAL CONCEPTS

The basic concepts of pacemaker electrical interferences are easily grasped. The major point is that a voltage large enough to disrupt circuit operation must be produced somewhere in the pacemaker circuit. *Voltage*, therefore, must be understood. Voltage is electrical pressure. It is analogous to hydraulic (fluid) pressure. Pressure differences across any conducting medium will force a current to flow in the medium. Consider a drip coffee pot. Fluid pressure is produced when water is poured into the reservoir. This pressure forces water to flow through the coffee grounds which in this example (fluid) are conductive media. The rate of flow (current) is proportional to the resistance of the grounds and the height (pressure) of the reservoir. In electrical terms, current produced by a voltage source (pressure source) is equal to that source voltage divided by the media resistance. This is a statement of what is known to be Ohm's law:

$$I \text{ (terminal} = V \text{ (source } \div R \text{ (media}$$
$$\text{current)} \quad \text{voltage)} \quad \text{resistance)}$$

Aquarium with battery and probes.

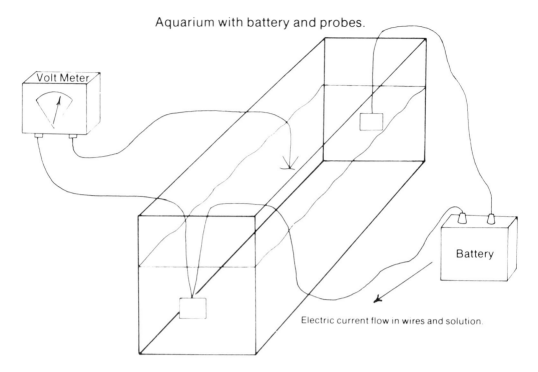

Fig. 21–2. Aquarium with battery and probes.

The more voltage, the larger the current; the larger the resistance, the smaller the current.

As a "paper" experiment, visualize connection of a battery across a continuous conducting medium such as a tank of saline solution (Fig. 21–2). The electrodes are at either end of the tank. Current flows because the saline solution is an electrical conductor. Now probe into the saline solution with a device that measures differences of voltage (a voltmeter). If one terminal of the voltmeter is connected to one battery electrode and the other terminal to the probing electrode, it will be found that all gradations of voltage appear in the tank up to the battery voltage.

Why is this? Well, just as the terminal current produces a voltage drop equal to source voltage across the whole media resistance, so does this current produce smaller voltages across parts of the media

resistance. Ohm's law still applies and may be stated in a new, equivalent way:

$$V \text{ (measured} = I \text{ (circuit} \times R \text{ (resistance)}$$
$$\text{voltage)} \quad \text{current)} \quad \text{of circuit measured)}$$

Voltages can be produced in the body in a similar fashion. Consider a man standing erect with a battery connected, one terminal to his head, the second to his feet (Fig. 21–3). Current flows in his body and voltages are produced by the resistance of his body. If we connect our measuring device from foot to knee, for example, a certain voltage will be measured. As we probe higher up on his body (in the direction of his head), larger voltages will be measured. We can draw lines on his body where the voltage has a constant value. These are lines of equipotential. If now we connect the voltmeter from one equipotential line to the

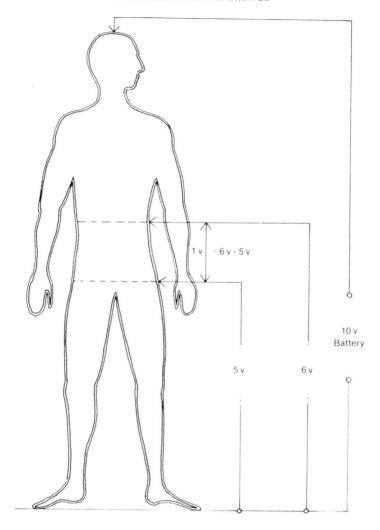

Fig. 21–3. Voltages produced in the body.

next, we find that the voltage measured is the difference between the two values on the lines. A pacemaker sensing circuit is just such a measuring device and will sense these voltage differences. This is the mechanism for conducted interference. Although we have used a battery (steady voltage) for our example, low frequency alternating voltages (such as exist in commercial power systems) produce equivalent effects.

The next basic concept to investigate is coupling. How is a voltage produced in the body by external sources? There are three ways. The first is by conduction. We have explored this type of coupling in our discussion of voltage. This coupling is by direct contact such as handling live electric circuits.

Other coupling mechanisms are electric and magnetic fields. In order to become an interference source these fields must produce voltage in the pacemaker circuitry. How does this happen? Consider first a loop of wire with a nearby permanent magnet. If we connect a voltmeter to the ends of the wire loop, we will notice that the meter

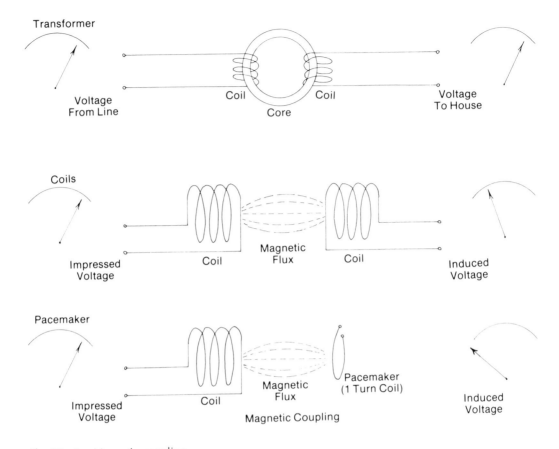

Fig. 21–4. Magnetic coupling.

will indicate a voltage whenever the magnet is in motion. By experimenting we can find that the voltage produced is proportional to the number of turns, speed of the magnet, strength of the magnet, and the coil area. The magnet produces what is called magnetic flux. When this flux "links" the coil and is *changing*, a voltage is induced in the coil. This principle is used in the magnetos of lawnmower and snowmobile ignition systems, for example, to produce the high voltage spark at the spark plug. A coil carrying electric current will produce magnetic flux just like the magnet and can be used like a magnet. If such a coil is brought near a second coil, flux will link the second coil (Fig. 21–4). The flux may be changed either by a change in current in the first coil or by a relative movement. Either will

cause a voltage to be induced in the second coil. Examples of the useful application of these principles are seen around us everyday. The operation of transformers, for instance, relies on changing current in one coil (primary) to produce changing flux in an iron core which is used to link the flux with another coil (secondary). Because of the proportionality of voltage and turns in the coils, dangerous high voltages (used for efficient transmission) can be "transformed" into the relatively safe low voltage used in our homes. The operation of generators relies on the action of rotating one coil carrying current inside a second coil. A voltage is induced in the second coil. Such generators and transformers form the basis of our entire electric power system.

The implanted pacemaker and its lead

form a single-turn coil with net area determined by details of the implant site. Changing, low frequency magnetic fields induce a voltage in this loop which the pacemaker will sense. Since higher frequency fields may link directly to small loops in the pacemaker electronics, microwave fields may also affect pacemaker operation.

The third type of coupling is by electric fields. We are all familiar with some of the manifestations of electric fields. Hairs standing-on-end when near a "charged" nylon blouse, dust sticking to a plastic object, and clinging of clothing all demonstrate their presence. What is happening here? Such effects are seen when electric charged particles are in excess supply on one object. This condition may be produced by friction of air or other objects. There are two types of charged particles in matter, those termed "positive" and others termed "negative." Whether the positive or negative charges are in excess supply determines the net polarity of the object. When a charged object is brought near another, particles of opposite polarity are attracted to the surface of the other object. The attractive force is what causes clinging.

The rearrangement of charged particles on each of the objects constitutes an electric current. The effect can be quite pronounced if a grounded conducting object is brought near a wire carrying a high level alternating voltage. *Alternating* means that the wire polarity reverses at a regular frequency determined by the rotation speed of a generator—usually 60 cycles per second in the United States. Charges in the wire change polarity as the voltage alternates. Opposite charges are induced in the grounded object, giving rise to an alternating current in the ground circuit as the polarity of the wire alternates. This current flows *without any conductive connection*. The current magnitude depends on the strength of the field expressed as a ratio of voltage to separation distance, the size of the objects, and the frequency of alternation. This effect is used in capacitors which

are essential parts of all radios and other electronic equipment.

Low frequency alternating electric fields can induce currents in the body. These currents pass through the conductive body tissue to produce effects similar to those noted for conductive coupling.

High frequency alternating electric fields induce voltages on conducting wires in the pacemaker electronics directly and produce effects similar to those of the high frequency magnetic fields. It is instructive to note that the radiation of radio waves involves power carried in space by alternating and interrelated electric and magnetic fields. In any situation involving high frequencies both the electric and magnetic field interference potentials must be taken into account.

PACEMAKER RESPONSE

The pacemaker response to particular types of interference depends on details of its circuitry and lead system. Asynchronous or fixed-rate pulse generators have no sensing circuitry and are therefore generally immune to low-level interference. Very high-level inputs, such as nearby application of electrosurgical coagulating currents, should be avoided because they may couple enough energy to affect the asynchronous oscillator directly.

Ventricular inhibited and other types of demand pacemakers have a sensitive amplifier designed to respond to signals generated by the heart when it contracts. Interference voltages that mimic the signal produced during a heart beat and occur at rates up to the inhibition-reversion changeover frequency are likely to inhibit this type of pacemaker. If signals appear at a higher rate, another circuit recognizes them to be interference and reverts the pacemaker to a fixed rate. Depending on the type of pacemaker, this reversion rate may be lower, the same, or higher than the set pacing rate. The inhibition-reversion changeover frequency varies over wide limits depending on model and intended use. It is nearly always in the range between 7 and 50 cycles per second (hertz). External pulse generators are designed with and without reversion circuitry. Refer to the manufacturer's literature to determine which is being used in your clinic if a question arises.

Pacemaker response to EMI is related to the type of coupling. The effects on external and implanted pacemakers will depend upon the circuitry of the pacemaker, the waveform of the interfering current, and the frequency of the magnetic, electric, and radiated fields.

Conducted Interference

As previously described, conducted interference enters the body by direct contact between the skin and live conductors. The interference current produces voltage drops across the body's conductive tissue. In this way, a voltage drop is impressed across the pacemaker's sensing electrodes. Whether a change in pacemaker output occurs in response to this stimulus depends on details of the pacemaker circuitry and the waveform of the interfering current. *Waveform* is a term used to describe the variations with time of the electric voltage on a conductor.

The voltage across a battery does not change appreciably with time. It is therefore called steady or direct voltage. If impressed on a conducting medium, this voltage will give rise to a direct current (DC). Other sources of direct current are electronic DC power supplies, automotive *generators*, and photovoltaic solar cells.

The voltage in a household receptacle changes smoothly with time, assuming positive and negative values alternately 60 times per second. This is called alternating voltage. Its waveform is sinusoidal (varying in time according to values predicted by the mathematical sine function). When impressed on a conductor, it produces alternating current (AC). Alternating voltages may be of any frequency from low (such as household voltage) through medium frequencies (such as generated by electrosurgical generators), to microwaves and higher. The current producing tissue heating in microwave diathermy alternates 2.45 *billion* times per second.

A third type of waveform combines some of the characteristics of both direct and alternating voltages. This is called a pulse waveform. It may have a variety of forms, but the one most likely to cause pacemaker interference mimics the heart QRS pulse as displayed on an ECG tracing. This pulse turns "on" smoothly, rises to a peak and returns to "off" in about 25 milliseconds. It is then off for about 800 milliseconds. Pulse waveforms are common in computers, radars, morse code (CW) radio transmission, electric fences, and automobile ignitions.

Direct currents in the body produce sensation when current level is changed by skin movement relative to the electrodes. In these circumstances shock is similar to that produced by alternating currents. A direct current which is turned on and off becomes a pulse current.

Alternating currents in the body produce physiologic effects depending on the amplitude and frequency. At low frequencies, alternating current causes muscle contraction. As frequency increases, nerves are unable to respond and the current passes unnoticed. At power frequency (60 cycles per second) the passage of about 250 microamperes through the body can just be felt. As current increases, the sensations of shock become stronger, and at about 6 milliamperes muscles contract so strongly that a conductor cannot be let go.

Pulse currents produce physiologic effects depending on repetition rate and waveform. Pulse currents introduced into the nervous system are the basis for the various pain blocking and muscle stimulating devices in common usage today. The pacemaker output is a pulse of current which stimulates heart tissue and produces a contraction.

Direct currents in the body have no effect on a pacemaker that has filtering circuits to remove steady voltages. They allow the sensing function to operate unimpaired.

Pacemaker response to alternating voltages varies from inhibition at frequencies below the inhibition/reversion cutoff to reversion at higher frequencies. The pacemaker may be sensitive to alternating currents in the range 30 to 60 cycles per second and usually will revert with a few millivolts across the sensing electrodes. This voltage can be produced in the body by currents as low as 40 microamperes for a unipolar implant with the lead in the direction of the current. This current is below the threshold of sensation. With a bipolar implant, currents in this frequency range will be felt if they are large enough to affect the pacemaker. Similar response may be expected of an external pacemaker (remember that no reversion capability may be available). Pacemaker sensitivity to alternating voltages usually decreases as frequency increases.

Pulse currents may mimic the heart R wave and be sensed by the pacemaker at millivolt levels. Sensed pulse currents with low repetition rates will produce inhibition of demand pacemakers. As the rate is increased, the pacemaker will return to operation in the reversion mode. Pulses of radiofrequency current (produced by turning a transmitter on and off) may be rectified in the pacemaker and have an effect similar to that of the low frequency pulses.

A patient may encounter sources for conducted alternating and pulse currents in many situations. In the clinic there may be improper grounding of various monitoring instruments and/or equipment. Frequency of this current would be 60 cycles per second, causing reversion if an effect is noted. Handling exposed lead ends or an external pacemaker terminal while in contact with other equipment may also introduce power frequency currents. Electro-

surgical techniques and defibrillation introduce currents of large magnitude into the body. Most demand pacemakers will be inhibited by electrosurgical currents and it is recommended generally that the electrosurgical device be used sparingly and that the patient's cardiac output be monitored. Manufacturer's literature should be consulted if there is a question about how near electrodes can be to the pacing system. If possible, place the indifferent plate in such a position that current from the cutting electrode does not pass directly by the pacemaker.

Away from the clinical environment the patient has many other possible contacts with conducted interference. Handling live signal generator wiring, touching the antenna, feedwire, or other unshielded parts of a radio transmitter, changing welding electrodes, defective power tools and appliances all carry the risk of conducted current. Effects depend on the frequency and magnitude of the current. For specific information concerning hobby or work situations it is best to consult the pacemaker manufacturer. He will know the response of the particular pacemaker model to the interference in question and the liklihood of a problem.

Note that the most likely interference possibility is reversion of unipolar pacemakers due to power frequency currents. All powerline connected devices used by or on pacemaker patients should be checked for proper powerline isolation (either insulation integrity or grounding). Clinic and home wiring systems should be checked for conformance to wiring codes. Bipolar pacers are less sensitive than unipolar pacers. Properly designed, new, cord-operated portable appliances can display leakage levels as high as 0.5 milliamperes (ANSI standard for tolerable leakage level). This means there may be small or nonexistent margins between normal and reversion operation of a unipolar pacemaker while handling such devices.

The use of pulse-producing nerve

stimulators should be evaluated carefully, since these devices definitely have the capability of affecting a demand pacemaker. Current paths should be kept away from the pacemaker and confined as much as possible.

Low Frequency Magnetic Fields

Magnetic field intensity is measured in units called gauss. Static magnetic fields are produced by direct currents and by permanent magnets. Flux density of about 20 to 30 gauss will activate the reed switch of many pacemakers. This activation usually results in asynchronous operation. The patient's environment may contain magnets or coils with this capability. Some refrigerator doors, mechanics' magnets, electric cables carrying over 10,000 amperes (common in electrolytic reduction plants), lifting electromagnets, and magneto magnets all have this strength.

Dynamic fields are produced by coils and wires carrying alternating currents. The effect such a field may have depends on the effective area the lead contacts in the body. Again, unipolar implants are most sensitive. Bipolar endocardial pacemakers are less sensitive than are unipolar devices, and paired myocardial leads are intermediate in sensitivity. Power frequency (60 cycles per second) fields of one half gauss will revert a sensitive implant. One half gauss will be produced in the proximity of a conductor carrying 250 amperes (similar to that of industrial alternating welding currents). When a single conductor is placed in a loop (a common practice of overhead welders), one meter in diameter will produce one half gauss with only 40 amperes; interference is a virtual certainty with even low current hobby welders if such a loop is around the pacemaker. This field strength decreases quickly with distance, however, and at a meter from such a loop the field is reduced by a factor of 10. The patient should be aware of any isolated high current conduc-

tors in his environment. Such industrial machinery as arc furnaces, resistance heaters, low frequency induction furnaces, and spot welders should be avoided.

Medium frequency, high-level fields produced by ultrasonic exciters, induction heaters, and some theft detectors are open to suspicion. Consult the manufacturer for specific information in this area.

External pulse generators connected in the usual bipolar configuration are not affected by the low magnetic field levels produced by clinical equipment.

Low Frequency Electric Fields

Electric fields are measured in units of volts per meter. A static electric field causes no current flow and has no effect on an implanted pulse generator. Static charges build up on insulating materials and discharge in pulses of electric current. These discharges may affect an external pacemaker, and it is prudent to avoid materials causing such discharges in the clinic. Breakdown field levels such as these are very high (hundreds of thousands of volts per meter) and cause noticeable physical effects.

Alternating fields at power frequencies can be much smaller and still affect a pacemaker. The body currents induced in a person by a field of about 3400 volts per meter will be sufficient to cause reversion of a sensitive unipolar implant. The internal mechanism is the same as described under conducted interference. Bipolar implants of less sensitive pacemakers can raise this level to hundreds of kilovolts per meter. Of some consequence also is the fact that large ungrounded conducting objects (such as a car or truck) will have more current induced by the alternating field, and touching such an object may raise body current tenfold. Fields large enough to cause reversion in such a situation exist under virtually all distribution and transmission lines. As with common appliances there may be little margin between normal and reversion operation.

There are few sources of electric fields at medium frequencies with the possible exception of some industrial ultrasonic equipment. Questions in this area again should be referred to the manufacturer of the pacemaker.

High Frequency Radiated Fields

At high frequencies, magnetic and electric fields become closely coupled and can be used to transmit power through space. Interference effects can be produced by either magnetic or electric field components. The dimensions of efficient radiating and receiving conductors become smaller until in the microwave range, antennas are of the same approximate size as a pacemaking system.

The body acts as an energy absorber in this frequency range. The 2450 megahertz frequency of microwave diathermy and ovens was chosen because of efficient en-

ergy transfer to meat. The consequence of energy absorption in heat and flesh irradiated by 10 milliwatts per square centimeter results in an approximate doubling of the heat load which eventually will produce tissue damage. This has been selected as the biologic hazard power level and is equivalent to 193 volts per meter in free space. A worst case test of 200 volts per meter at 450 megahertz has been proposed by the FDA.

Most modern implantable pacemakers function normally in microwave fields of this magnitude. Some will operate inside a 500 watt microwave oven while it is cooking.

Interference sources are multiplying rapidly in the very high frequency (TV) range (Table 21–1). Mobile transmitters of 100 to 200 watts are in common usage. Fields around vehicles can reach very high values. Citizen's band transmitters number in the millions. Although the legal 5 watt, 27 megahertz output produces minimal fields unlikely to produce interference, many illegal rigs up to 200 watts exist. Again, most

TABLE 21–1

Examples of Sources of Pacemaker Interference

COUPLING	LOW FREQUENCY	MODERATE FREQUENCY	HIGH FREQUENCY
Conduction	Appliances Power wiring Nerve stimulators	Radio antenna Feedwire Electric Experimenting Electrosurgery	Radio antenna
Magnetic	Welding Hi-current conductors Induction furnaces	Induction furnaces and heaters Ultrasonic exciters	
Electric	Powerlines Static pulses	Few sources	
Radiated Electromagnetic		Ham radio transmission CB	Microwave oven TV Transmission 2-Way radio Radar FM

modern pacemakers are immune to interference in this range.

Many amateur radio operators transmit on the frequencies of 1.8, 3.5, 7.0, 14, 21, and 28 megahertz. They are allowed peak power output of 2 kilowatts. This power level can produce dangerous fields near the antennas. All equipment should be carefully shielded and grounded. Most modern pacemakers, but definitely not all, are immune to interference in this range. If a question appears, consult the pacemaker manufacturer.

External pacemakers are used in a less stringent environment. Likely radiation levels established by the McDonnell-Douglas Company in a study conducted for the FDA have resulted in proposed specifications for all devices used in a medical facility. Levels are in the range of 2 to 7 volts per meter from 10 kilohertz to 1000 megahertz. Some of the newer external pacemakers are not affected at these levels, but older models may be.

In summary, large improvements have been made in modern pacemakers. Most such pacemakers are immune to many common sources of interference. However, new electric devices appear almost daily making continuing user awareness and manufacturer vigilance mandatory if the present excellent record is to be maintained. Examples of sources of interference are presented in Table 21–1.

SELECTED READINGS

AAMI PM Std. FDA Contract #223-74-5083, August, 1975.

Adams, J.W., et al.: Near field electric field strength levels of EM environments applicable to automotive systems. 1977 IEEE International Symposium on EMC Record.

Bronaugh, E.L., et al.: Electromagnetic emissions from typical citizens band mobile radio installations in three sizes of vehicles. 1977 IEEE Symposium on EMC Record.

Federal Drug Administration: Electromagnetic Compatibility Standard for Medical Devices, MDS-201-0004.

McDermott, J.: News. Electronic Design, 24:18, 1976.

Smyth, N.P.D., et al.: The pacemaker patient and the electromagnetic environment. J.A.M.A., 236:227, 1974.

22

Cardiac Pacemaker Follow-Up

DRYDEN MORSE
GERALD M. LEMOLE
ALLAN ZINBERG
THEODORE STERN

The installation of a permanent pacemaker in a patient is only the beginning. Whether the pacemaker is working properly, whether it is suitable for the particular pacemaker patient, and, if it is programmable, whether it is properly adjusted are questions for follow-up evaluation. Another phase of the physician/patient relationship involves the replacement of the pacemaker when the battery wears out or the readjustment or replacement of the electrode if it comes out of the heart or breaks. In addition, the pacemaker patient who is a cardiac patient may have dysrhythmias such as tachycardia, coupling, or extrasystoles.

Although 85% of pacemaker patients are over the age of 65, and 55% of patients live for an additional five years following pacemaker insertion, approximately 25% of these patients will live ten years. Women with pacemakers live slightly longer than men. An occasional younger patient with a pacemaker because of congenital heart block will have the same life expectancy as a person without a pacemaker. Patients in these groups will certainly outlast their batteries and require monitoring to detect impending battery exhaustion to avoid clinical syncope, collapse, and death.

Pacemaker follow-up is necessary to check not only the condition of the pacemaker battery but also other failures of the system which may be divided into three areas. In approximately 20% of patients following implant, the threshold may rise to a level that makes the pacemaker ineffective. This may be due to scarring around the electrode tip incident to direct current leakage from the pacer, to actual motion between the transvenous electrode and the endocardium, or to similar changes in an epicardial lead.

Secondly, the lead itself may become corroded or have a break in its insulation. The wire inside the pacemaker lead may break due to the motion of the clavicle or to the patient's fiddling with the pacemaker.

A third cause of pacemaker system failure is sudden failure of the electronics in the pacemaker. This has occurred commonly in early mercury zinc-oxide powered pacers and does happen even in the hermetically sealed lithium pacemaker, although less frequently. In summary, the appraisal of the pacemaker system includes not only the pacemaker battery but the whole pacing system, the heart's reaction to it, and detection of non-related arrhythmias.

Patients now have pacemakers implanted predominately for conditions other than complete heart block, which was the primary indication for pacemakers when they were first implanted. Sick sinus syndrome, incomplete AV block, bradycardia with congestive heart failure, and tachycardia syndrome are a few of the other indications for which pacemakers are now used. Pacemaker patients are peculiarly prone to arrhythmias. We detected significant arrhythmias in 18% of 8000 patients during a three-year period. The most common were multiple tachycardias, extrasystoles, coupling on the paced beats, and the onset of atrial fibrillation. When necessary, the administration of drugs and/or reprogramming (when possible) of the pacemaker rate may overcome some of the more serious problems.

TELEPHONIC MONITORING

Most of the pacemaker manufacturers will now furnish a telephone transmitter of the ECG variety with the pacemaker. The physician can then ask the patient to call (1) a commercial pacemaker surveillance company, (2) the pacemaker manufacturer, or (3) his own office if he has a receiver to check the pacemaker at regular intervals over the phone. The patient can also call whenever he experiences syncope or palpitations or feels the pacemaker is not working properly. Some of the transmitters detect pulse width over the phone, and some can detect whether there is capture by sensing the pulse from a finger plethysmograph (Fig. 22–1).

The possession of a transmitter gives pacemaker patients a feeling of security rather than of apprehension as was feared when these units were first distributed. There is a unit the patient can use himself to detect the pacemaker's rate. This unit is probably rarely appropriate, since only a few patients are equipped mentally to differentiate between their own beats and paced beats.

In all telephonic electrocardiographic monitoring it is important that the American Heart Association standards for ECG wave shape and frequency response of the transmitter be maintained as far as possible. Some present telephonic follow-up electrocardiographic equipment does not meet these or other standards, and determination of capture can be uncertain, especially in bipolar pacing systems.

The purpose of a telephonic monitoring system is to determine (1) capture, (2) proper sensing, (3) pacing rate, and (4) the presence or absence of pacer rhythm and arrhythmias. The physician must be aware that an arrhythmia, apparent on a telephonic recording, is not always amenable to precise identification. It is also obvious that a telephonic monitoring system does not allow diagnostic and therapeutic techniques such as carotid pressure or pacer overdrive with an external pacer.

Telephone monitoring is not a complete diagnostic system. Most telephone monitoring systems result in a single lead electrocardiogram being taken over the telephone (Fig. 22–2). If there is a suspected abnormality, it is essential that the patient be seen in a clinic, physician's office, or a hospital in order to arrive at a proper diagnosis. All the monitoring system can do is to observe that there is some abnormality which on a "one lead electrocardiogram" seems to require further investigation. The diagnosis may be made when the patient is physically present in the hospital or physician's office with facilities for a complete

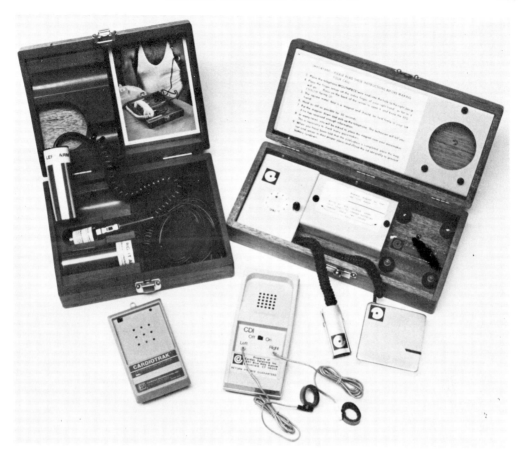

Fig. 22—1. Transtelephonic transmitters. Clockwise, beginning top left: Arco ECG receiver (placement of electrodes under arms is shown in inset); former Cardiac Datacorp Transmitter which gave pacer artifact, interval, and capture through a finger plethysmograph; new Cardiac Datacorp (CDI) unit which transmits ECG; Cardiotrak ECG unit manufactured by Instromedics and distributed with the pacer by Cardiac Pacemakers Inc. Other similar models exist.

history or examination and multiple lead electrocardiograms.

Modern pacemakers manifest a slow discharge rate at the end of their pacer life. Before the rate of some lithium units slows, there is also an earlier increase of the pulse width of the pacemaker artifact with battery depletion. In mercury cell powered units, the pacemaker rate slows 10% from its original rate during a period from two to six weeks before it will fail. During this time the patient should be admitted to the hospital for implantation of a new pulse generator. Little to no experi-

ence has been gathered regarding the failure mode of lithium batteries as yet.

Use of a pacemaker surveillance system has reduced the incidence of emergency readmissions for pacemaker failure to as low as 2% in our experience. If a pacemaker surveillance system is used at, for instance, weekly intervals, it is likely that it will also detect electrode problems before they become a catastrophe. Most electrode breaks occur with the ends of the wires still in contact or near contact so that intermittent "capture" continues.

Close follow-up is indicated after pace-

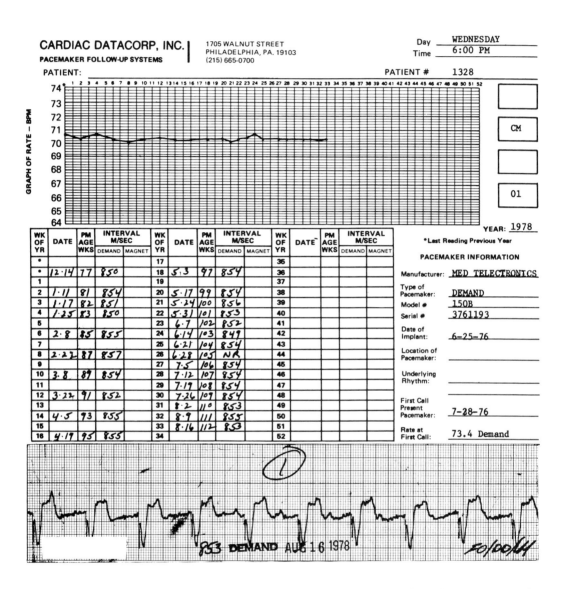

Fig. 22–2. Commercial transtelephonic follow-up chart of patient with a demand ventricular pacemaker initially implanted June 25, 1976. The demand pacing rate and interval in msec are recorded from the electronic readout of the receiver at selected call-in intervals 77 to 112 weeks postimplantation. The mounted ECG rhythm strip recorded at the last monitored follow-up (August 16, 1978) is provided with the pacemaker record to the physician of reference after each telephonic follow-up.

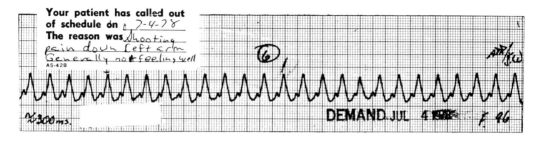

Fig. 22–3. Serial #5P25348. Date of Implant 2-28-76. First Call Present PM 6-1-78. Rate of First Call 71.3BPM. *Interpretation and Conclusion:* ECG tracing shows regular tachycardia at 190BPM.

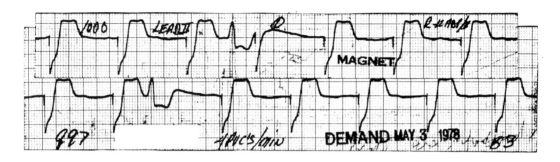

Fig. 22–4. *Cordis* Demand Omni Stanicor Serial # 162C43372. Date of Implant 4-18-77. First Call Present PM 7-20-77. First Call Rate 70.6BPM with magnet. *Interpretation:* In the *magnet* mode the pacer becomes fixed rate and the PVC does not reset the timing cycle. In the *demand* mode, the PVC is properly sensed and the next paced beat is appropriately delayed. *Conclusion:* Normal pacing function.

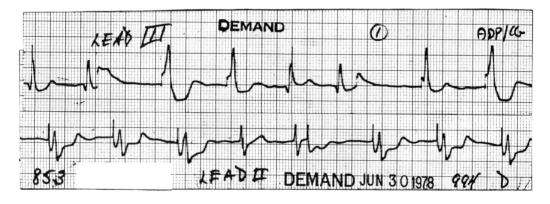

Fig. 22–5. Medtronic 5954 Serial # 6F02279. Date of Implant 2-2-77. First Call Present PM 7-8-77. First Call Rate 70.4BPM Demand. *Interpretation:* Throughout the tracing there is spontaneous ventricular activity which the pacemaker fails to sense and consequently fires inappropriately as after the second and sixth complexes. *Conclusion:* Loss of sensing.

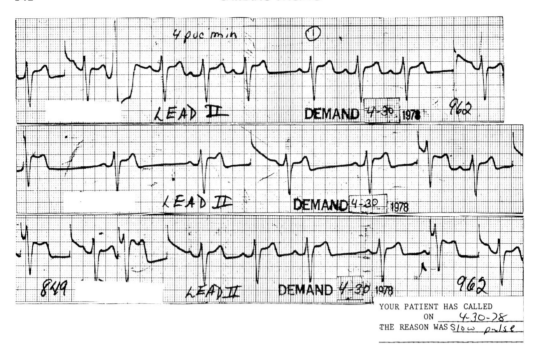

Fig. 22–6. Medtronic 5951 Serial # 5407415. Date of Implant 9-15-75. First Call Present PM 12-7-77.
Rate of First Call 70.9BPM. *Interpretation:* Each of the leads shows pacing spikes with failure to
capture. Sensing is irregular. *Conclusion:* Loss of sensing and capture.

maker implantation. Early dislodgment of the electrodes is sufficiently frequent for Mantini and others to recommend weekly checks for the first month. In Germany during the first 50 days following implant an increase in threshold is the most common cause of pacemaker failure, but the incidence decreases after this period. Furman reports that electrode problems occurred in 9.5% of all his implants.

Since battery decay or exhaustion occurs as a less frequent problem, it is no longer the main purpose of telephone monitoring. Analysis of recent data shows that sensing problems, electronic failures, and arrhythmias are proportionately on the increase (Figs. 22–3, 22–4, 22–5, 22–6).

Schedules of Telephonic Follow-Up

Until now the schedule frequency for telephonic follow-up of pacemaker patients has been determined by a combination of reviewed failure data and clinical judgment. The original Medicare schedule for follow-up after implant is Schedule A (Table 22–1).

Schedules based on the amount of risk acceptable (risk/benefit ratio) have been derived by statistical analysis of a large body of data (Table 22–2). Clinical needs determine the schedules to detect existing or impending malfunction before it becomes hazardous to the patient. No system is infallible, but experience indicates that the probability of not detecting a malfunction will be only 0.5% if the present Medicare schedule is used, provided the frequency of calls is increased during the first six weeks.

All pacemakers may have battery failure. The newer lithium battery systems appear to offer significantly improved longevity, but our present experience is insufficient to determine the battery failure mode of the lithium units. Therefore, the schedule for

TABLE 22–1

Schedules for Pacemaker Follow-up

PACEMAKER	MONTHS AFTER IMPLANT	FREQUENCY
CARDIAC DATACORP		
Schedule A	1–6	Bimonthly
	7–15	Monthly
	16–18	Biweekly
	19–failure	Weekly
Schedule B	1–6	Bimonthly
	7–18	Monthly
	19–22	Biweekly
	23–failure	Weekly
Schedule C	0–12	Bimonthly
	13–18	Monthly
	19–30	Biweekly
	31–failure	Weekly
Schedule D*	0–1	Weekly
	2–failure	Monthly
MEDTRONIC TELETRACE		
Mercury-zinc	1–6	Bimonthly
	7–15	Monthly
	16–18	Biweekly
	18–battery depletion	Weekly
Lithium or Nuclear	0–1	Weekly
	2–36	Monthly
	36–battery depletion	To be determined

* Recommended by HEW Ad Hoc Medical Committee specifically for lithium power sources, April 19, 1979.

lithium units is based upon the incidence of non-battery failures in the first five years past implant. As this experience develops further, the schedule will be modified. The schedule in Table 22–3 is suggested for follow-up of lithium units after first implant to provide 0.5% risk. The schedule should not be less frequent than every two months for several reasons:

1. The transmitter's batteries can deplete, or other transmitter failures can occur. Therefore the monitoring system must be checked.
2. Patients will forget how to use the system or even forget where they put their transmitters. (If the patient is on a two-month schedule, it is wise to ask him to check the transmitter on at least a monthly schedule.)

A "failure" at our telephone follow-up center is more correctly described as an incident detected during a telephone test which suggests pacemaker system malfunction and triggers the notification of the patient's physician. The precise cause of the malfunction may not be verified until later. We now urge that patients receive transmitters at the time of pacemaker implant so that telephonic follow-up can begin immediately after discharge. Most of the data in Table 22–2 was obtained using Schedule A.

TABLE 22–2

Pacemaker Cumulative Survival Summary[1]
                                   All Pacers

MONTHS SURVIVED	TOTAL AT START OF MONTH	FAILED or "PULLED" DURING MONTH[2]	REMOVED FROM RISK[3]	CUM % OK BEG
0–5	18,313	184	1,915	100.00
6–11	16,214	386	2,725	98.93
12–17	13,103	511	2,452	96.34
18–23	10,140	1,055	2,001	92.17
24–29	7,084	1,729	1,507	81.30
30–35	3,848	1,109	890	58.69
36–41	1,849	630	541	39.22
42–47	709	212	212	23.22
48–53	244	52	52	14.52
54–59	75	15	15	10.55
60–65	13	3	3	6.39
66–72	3	1	1	4.48
73	1	1	1	2.99
		5,888[4]	12,425	

[1] This table was extracted from a lengthy month-by-month computer readout. This abbreviation allows concise presentation of representative data.

[2] Failed: component failure, rate decline (presumed battery depletion), loss of capture, erratic rate change, broken electrode, high pacer ratio, no evidence of pacer activity, rate decline and loss of sensing, rate decline and loss of capture.

[3] Removed from Risk: deceased, cancelled from service, still functioning (but only up to this month).

[4] Thus 5,888 pacers were removed for all "failure" causes; battery failure, electrode failure, electronic failure, erosion, infection etc., and 12,425 pacers either are still functioning, or the patients died or were cancelled from the service.

For each month after implant the Proportion Failing was converted to a "time between failure" expressed in weeks at a given probability level. For example, in the nineteenth month after implant of a mercury-zinc powered pacer, there is a 1% probability of abnormal function during an interval between calls of 4 weeks and a 0.5% probability during an interval of 2 weeks. It is thus possible to construct a calling schedule at a given risk level based on month-by-month analysis of time between failure.

Calculations indicate that our old Schedule A represents approximately a 0.5% risk level and Schedule B about 1%. Since these schedules are based on the clinical experience and choices of many physicians, it is likely that 0.5% to 1% represents acceptable risk levels for calling schedules.

Recall

A telephone follow-up system is peculiarly indicated to register changes in patients' addresses and to keep contact with them. When a recall occurs, if each telephone registry has a record of the model number of each patient's pacemaker, it can send to the physician(s) of reference with each report of a telephone call the fact that this pacemaker is the subject of a recall.

TABLE 22-3

Schedule for Pacemaker Follow-up Based on Risk

PACEMAKER	RISK	MONTHS AFTER IMPLANT	FREQUENCY
Mercury-zinc	0.5%	1–6	Bimonthly*
		7–15	Monthly
		16–19	Biweekly
		20→	Weekly
	1.0%	1–15	Bimonthly
		16–19	Monthly
		20–23	Biweekly
		24→	Weekly
Lithium	0.5%	0–1	Weekly*
		2–23	Monthly
		24→	Biweekly
	1.0%	0–1	Weekly
		2→	Monthly

* Initially, monitoring every week for the first 6 weeks is recommended for original pacemaker implants.

The patient's physician can then decide what action is required: e.g., more frequent monitoring, replacement of the pacemaker at this time, or testing of the patient's underlying rhythm by overdriving. (A decision can be based on the patient's demonstrated degree of pacer dependency).

PACEMAKER CLINICS

In the past, pacemaker clinics have been widely utilized to follow large groups of pacer patients in a uniform manner. Electrocardiograms and radiographs are supplemented by analysis of the pacemaker's electronic output on an oscilloscope. Today many follow-up systems obtain merely the pacer rate by an electronic interval counter and take an ECG. This may be supplemented by measurement of the pulse duration of the pacemaker spike. Most pulse generator and lead failures can be detected by these methods without the additional expense and inconvenience of the electronic spike analysis. The latter, how-

ever, may be diagnostic in patients with early lead fracture.

The rationale for the measurement of pacer pulse duration is that in the lithium unit of at least one manufacturer (Medtronic's Xyrel) the rate is held constant and the pulse width increases as the voltage of pacemaker batteries becomes exhausted. Finally the rate decreases as an end-of-life signal. Monitoring pulse duration in patients with pacemakers in which this parameter is programmable (Arco, C.P.I., Cordis, Intermedics, ESB Medcor) is important in determining pacer longevity and proper action when failure is due to threshold rise.

Annual or biannual examination of the *patient* and the pacemaker are important for several reasons. Radiographs should be taken at least every two years to ensure that the pacemaker in the patient indeed is the pacemaker registered in the clinical records. Otherwise unexpected difficulties with connections such as a bayonet (Biotronik) connection may transform a simple change into a replacement of a whole system, or the fact a pacemaker is programmable may be missed. Parsonnet has listed the advantages of a clinic as (1) direct contact with the patient (interview, examination, instruction, reassurance), (2) accuracy of diagnosis (multilead ECG, radiograph), and (3) direct interventions, reprogramming, and overdriving.

At the clinic, pacemakers of the ventricular-inhibited variety, i.e., VVI, can be inhibited by an external pacemaker to determine the underlying rhythm of the patient. This will indicate if the patient is totally pacemaker-dependent. A more vigorous action, in both follow-up and early replacement, should be undertaken when the patient's pacemaker is a model that has had a number of premature failures.

Finally, the pacemaker area can be examined for any tendency of the pulse generator or lead to erode through the skin. If erosion is about to occur, placement of the pulse generator in a new area or underneath the muscle may be critical to avoid infection when skin erosion becomes complete, and replacement of the entire pacing system may be necessary.

PROGRAMMABLE PACEMAKERS

At this time we are witnessing an upsurge in the use of programmable pacemakers (Table 22–4). Programmable units are used because they allow a lowering of the rate to 60 or less and may make it possible for the patient's own rhythm to prevail with consequent saving of the batteries and better cardiac output from the atrial contribution. Decrease in the output of the pacemaker to a safe level above the stimulation threshold causes a second saving of the pacemaker batteries which will again result in greater pacemaker longevity. In one programmable unit (Cardiac Pacemakers, Inc. Microlith P) pulse width is adjusted to conserve battery energy and measurement of it is necessary, especially at implant, to ensure a safe margin above the energy threshold for effective pacing.

When programmable pacemakers are in wide use, a major function of the clinic will be their control (some are complex in function; see Table 22–4). They should be programmed to near threshold, but at a safe margin above it. Programmable pacemakers permit the adjustment of the *rate* either downward to allow normal sinus rhythm to appear or upward to overcome extrasystoles. Checking to see if normal sinus rhythm will appear with the pacemaker set down to 60 is an important part of pacer follow-up.

COSTS

Monitoring is now becoming less frequent, less costly, and more widespread. Some of the pacemaker manufacturers such as Cordis, Edwards, Intermedics, Medtronic, and Telectronic will furnish free follow-up surveillance. Medicare will pay for telephonic follow-up in patients over 65, both for patients' safety and for continuation of pacemaker implants for a maximum period between insertions.

Total replacement of a lithium pacemaker with a programmable unit costs approximately $4000. The less often this occurs the better. It should be observed that Cordis and Medtronic, for instance, warrant some of their lithium pacemakers for replacement for life. Cordis will also pay up to $5000 towards hospital and physician's fees, above the allowance made by third party carriers, when some of their lithium pacemakers require replacement because of battery depletion (at any time) or component malfunction. Other companies have similar warranties, differing in details.

RECOMMENDED SCHEDULE

We recommend no one schedule for the systematic follow-up of all pacemakers or

TABLE 22–4

Programmable Pacemakers—1978 (Many models and other companies omitted)

MODEL	SOURCE OF ENERGY	CAPACITY AH	CURRENT CONSUMPTION μA	RATE BPM	PROGRAMMED FUNCTION		
					OUTPUT CURRENT	PULSE DURATION (msec)	SENSING
CPI* Microlith (505)	Li Iodine	3.3	36	Beat by beat 30 to 119	NO	0.05 to 1.9	NO
CORDIS 190 A7 Exten. Range	Li Cu Sulf	1.8	20	60 to 100 6 choices	2 4 6 9 MA	Depends on rate	NO
EDWARDS 215, 21U	Li Ag Chr	1.2	16.5	60 to 100 8 choices	NO	NO	NO
INTERMEDICS 251	Li Iodine	1.2	9.6	60 to 120 7 choices	NO	NO	NO
MEDCOR Lithicon 370F	Li Iodine	1.7	—	50 to 100 4 choices	NO	0.4 or .08	1.0 mV 2.5 mV
MEDTRONIC Xyrel VP 5995 5994	Li Iodine	1.4 1.4	11 15	30 to 100 8 choices	NO	NO	NO
BYREL (bifocal 5992)		1.4	18 to 49	63 to 109 5 choices	NO	NO	NO
INTERMEDICS† 253 Cyberlith	Li Iodine	2.2	9.6	30 to 120 15 choices	NO	0.15 to 2.29 15 choices	0.6 to 2.8 7 choices

Adapted from B. Dodinot, MD. (Stimucoeur) Hiver, 1977.
* Cardiac Pacemakers, Inc.
† Also has telemetry and mode programming.

all patients. Instead we suggest a rationale based on two information sets. The first is the patient's requirements as related to arrhythmias, pacer dependency, distance from medical facilities, and his other diseases (besides his status as a patient who has a pacemaker implanted). The second basis for the schedule relates to the risk factors for failure in similar cases with the particular type of pacemaker and electrode system.

STATISTICAL ANALYSIS

A further statistical remark should be made: Actuarial analysis of the results of pacemakers followed by telephone systems will give an apparent greater longevity of 30 to 50% when compared to a method that analyzes all removed pacemakers for how long they have been in.

For instance, analysis of all mercury-powered pacemakers removed in the past gave a mean life of 19 months, in 1969, which gradually rose to 25 months, in 1978. Analysis by the actuarial method shows a median life over 30 months for the same pacers. This *median* presentation does not represent the true picture of pacemaker performance. The *mean* does describe performance.

A second critical observation in comparing statistics is the requirement to state whether the pacemakers that are removed from analysis for various reasons are included in the result or not.

In summary *follow-up is more than just a pacemaker telephone transmitter unit.* Other essential ingredients are knowledge, concern, experience, and responsibility on the part of those who are carrying out the follow-up.

SELECTED READINGS

Bayliss, C.E., Beanlands, D.S., and Baird, R.J.: The pacemaker twiddler's syndrome. Can. Med. Assoc. J., *99*:371, 1968.

Bette, L., et al.: Results of permanent cardiac stimulation therapy. In Advances in Pacemaker Technology. Edited by M. Schaldach and S. Furman. New York, Springer-Verlag, 1975.

Dreifus, L.S., et al.: The advantages of demand over fixed rate pacing. Dis. Chest, *54*:6, 1969.

Edhag, O.: Long Term Cardiac Pacing. A Monograph of the Karolinska Institute, Stockholm, Sweden, 1969, p. 67.

Furman, S.: Cardiac pacing and pacemakers. VIII. The pacemaker follow-up clinic. Am. Heart J., *94*:795, 1977.

Furman, S.: The future utility of transtelephone pacemaker monitoring (Editorial). J. Electrocardiol. *9*:199, 1976.

Hartzler, G.O., et al.: The hemodynamic benefits of atrioventricular sequential pacing after cardiac surgery. Am. J. Cardiol., *40*:232, 1977.

Mantini, E.L., et al.: A recommended protocol for pacemaker follow-up: Analysis of 1,705 implanted pacemakers. Ann. Thorac. Surg., *24*:62, 1977.

Morse, D.P.: Discussion of "Pacemaker Recall", MacGregor, A., J. Thorac. Cardiovasc. Surg., *5*:665, 1977.

Morse, D.P., et al.: Preliminary experience with the use of a programmable pacemaker. Chest, *67*:544, 1975.

Morse, D.P., et al.: External radiomagnetic control of pacer rate and power. Chest, *64*:403, 1973.

Parsonnet, V.: Survey of pacing in the United States in 1975. *In* The Pacemaker and Valve Identification Guide. Edited by D. Morse and R. Steiner. New York, Medical Examination Publishing Company, 1978, pp. 1–8.

Parsonnet, V., et al.: An appraisal of pacemaker follow-up techniques. *In* Boston Colloquium on Cardiac Pacing. Edited by J.W. Harthorne and H.J. Th. Thalen. The Hague, Martinus Nijhoff Med. Div., 1977, pp. 147–158.

Rettig, G., et al.: Results of long term follow-up in pacemaker patients. Curr. Concepts Pacing, p. 16, Nov.-Dec. 1977.

23

A Multiparameter Telemetry System for Cardiac Pacemakers

G. FRANK O. TYERS
ROBERT R. BROWNLEE

Pacemaker follow-up programs have three primary functions: to decrease emergency pacemaker replacements, to maximize mean pacemaker implant duration for a given model, and to reassure the patient and the physician. The ideal program should be cost- as well as care-effective; that is, it should cost less than the savings generated by reduction of emergency and prophylactic replacement reoperations.

All nonrechargeable cardiac pacemaker power sources have a finite but variable functional life. Factors affecting pacemaker longevity include the initial capacity of the power source (cell or battery), the shelf storage energy loss (circuit and power source self discharge), electrode stimulation energy requirements, stimulation rate, the percentage of time the pacemaker is inhibited, and random electronic component anomalies or failures. The wide variability in pacemaker longevity has made it necessary either to replace all pacemakers prophylactically a relatively short time following implantation, based on worst case assumptions, or to institute a patient follow-up program that allows prediction of impending power source depletion and other failure modes before they occur. Notification of the follow-up physician and the patient and subsequent replacement of the pacemaker with only a small fraction of its functional life remaining can be obtained in a high percentage of cases.

The improved power sources, electronics, and hermetic encapsulation now available from the majority of pacemaker manufacturers make the 10-year pacemaker a possibility. This has led some physicians to question the need for continuing even current pacemaker follow-up programs. Random malfunctions of electrodes and electronic components, however, continue to occur, and even though premature failure of current lithium, nuclear, and rechargeable power cells is rare, these systems will eventually exhaust their energy supplies.

Under special high drain circumstances this can occur in a relatively short time, even with the best available commercial cells. For example, programmable output pacemakers utilizing solid state lithium-iodine power cells could theoretically last for over 20 years when programmed to their lowest output energy at nominal stimulation rates but could conceivably last less than 3 years when programmed to their widest pulse width or highest stimulus current or voltage and high stimulation rates. Similarly, electrodes with small surface areas generally have a high impedance resulting in conservation of power source energy, whereas electrodes with large surface areas or lead insulation defects can result in low resistance passage of extra or excess energy from the pacemaker and therefrom early or premature depletion of the pacemaker power source. Further, although the 702E solid state lithium iodine battery used in the original relatively large lithium pacemakers has a 90% probability of achieving a 10-year pacing life, all of the currently available lithium pacemakers contain newer, smaller versions of the same cells or one of a variety of lithium anode-nonhalogen cathode cells about which relatively little is known regarding their capacity to sustain a pacemaker for 10 years.[1] Recently, the capacity of some early halogen and nonhalogen lithium cells has been downgraded.

Compared to premature replacement of an earlier epoxy-potted mercury-zinc battery powered pacemaker which might have cost the patient a few extra months of pacing service, too early "prophylactic" replacement of a lithium-powered generator may waste years of functional pacer life and thousands of dollars for unnecessary hospitalization. To maximize pacemaker patient safety and confidence and minimize health care costs will require more accurate follow-up over longer periods with the improved pacemakers now available. It cannot be assumed that the current pacing systems will outlive their hosts, as the survival rates of patients, 1, 5 and 10 years

following pacemaker implantation were 88, 61, and 49%, respectively, in a recent large series.[2] Fortunately, unlike the situation a few years ago when most units were powered by the shorter-lived mercury-zinc batteries, a majority of physicians no longer make it a practice to prophylactically replace pacemakers after a specified period. In a recent survey, two thirds of the physicians polled indicated that each patient was monitored individually and the pacemaker was not replaced until the first sign of malfunction or impending battery depletion.[3] In another recent survey, over 85% of responding physicians stated that the time of pacemaker replacement was dictated by monitoring results. Common monitoring methods, including pulse rate monitoring, pulse extension monitoring, and wave form analysis referred to in these surveys, have been discussed in other chapters of this book. However, the limitations of current follow-up systems will be briefly reviewed to provide a better understanding of and an introduction to our new multiparameter telemetry system.

CONVENTIONAL PACEMAKER FOLLOW-UP SYSTEM

By far the most commonly used established method of pacemaker follow-up is the periodic determination of pacemaker rate to assess battery condition. Most mercury-zinc battery-powered pacemakers of the prelithium era still have several weeks of effective life left when their rates slow relatively suddenly by 5 to 8 pulses per minute, generally indicative of depletion of a single cell out of a four- or five-cell battery. Weekly monitoring allows prediction of impending total battery exhaustion and the need for elective pacemaker replacement. Except for moisture-related excess current drain, it is unlikely that all cells in a battery pack will be depleted simultaneously.[4] In that respect multiple cell systems provide a safety margin near end of the pacemaker's life, even though general reliability may be reduced. Unfortunately a standard rate decrease indicator has not been adopted by all manufacturers, and apart from unit variations within a given series from a particular manufacturer, whole series of pacemakers have experienced rate drifts, either upwards or downwards, prior to end of life, complicating accurate prediction of impending battery failure by the rate change method.[5] Even today, an occasional unit will suddenly increase its stimulation rate at some time following implantation (Fig. 23–1).

The introduction of rate and pulse width

programmable pacemakers coupled with occasional accidental programming without the intent of the patient or physician (phantom programming) have further reduced the value of rate change and pulse extension methods for predicting impending battery failure. In two of our patients, phantom programming to a rate of 65 was induced by the magnet in the Cardiac Data Corp. patient telephone monitor. We replaced one of these pacemakers for the common indication of a rate decrease before hearing the first report on phantom programming.[6] When phantom programming of the second unit occurred, we understood the problem

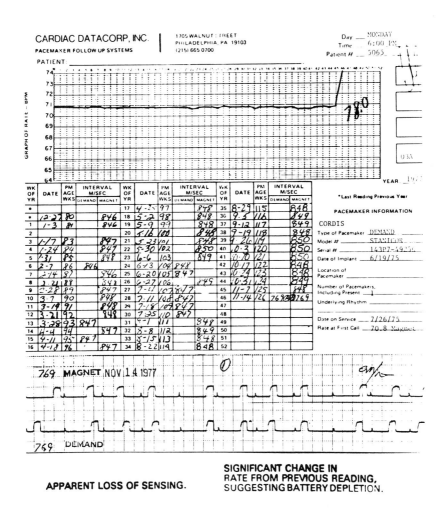

SIGNIFICANT CHANGE IN
RATE FROM PREVIOUS READING,
SUGGESTING BATTERY DEPLETION.

APPARENT LOSS OF SENSING.

Fig. 23–1. Sudden pacemaker rate increase following 29 months of implantation. Another unit in our series also exhibited this behavior.

and simply programmed the pacemaker back to its standard rate and confirmed the accuracy of other rates to preclude battery depletion.

Whether performed in a physician's office, a clinic, or by transtelephonic transmission, waveform analysis and pulse width techniques also depend primarily on pacemaker stimulation rate decrease or pulse-to-pulse interval increase, as indirect evidence of declining pacemaker battery or cell voltage. The major limitation with the established techniques of pacemaker follow-up is the data transmission rate which is limited to approximately 60 to 120 pulses per minute, i.e., 1 to 2 cycles per second (1 to 2 Hz). Thus the present stimulation rate-dependent pacemaker follow-up techniques do not allow direct assessment of the power source voltage in conjunction with monitoring of cell impedance, electrode stimulation impedance, refractory interval, or hermetic integrity of the pacemaker capsule. These and additional parameters can all be assessed directly with a higher frequency, stimulation rate-independent, telemetry monitoring system.[7]

TELEMETRY SYSTEM FOR DIRECT PACEMAKER MONITORING

Telemetry is a common engineering term applied to a variety of techniques to remotely monitor the function of devices or processes. The best publicized telemetry monitoring systems have been in space probes and include long-range biotelemetry of astronauts. Radio telemetry is not new, even in pacemakers. The pacemaker stimulation pulse output in all pacemakers transmits a radio frequency signal from the lead. This signal can be received transcutaneously on a simple pocket-sized transistor radio. This allows simple assessment of pacemaker rate and thereby a crude determination of battery voltage. However, when data are telemetered at frequencies of 1 to 2 Hz, a severe restriction is placed on the number of functions that can be simultaneously transmitted.

A feature unique to the telemetry pacemaker system we have developed is an independent multiparameter transmitter contained within the implanted pacemaker and operating at a much higher frequency than the pacemaker stimulation rate. The telemetry data pulse transmission rate chosen falls in the range of 300 to 600 Hz (i.e., 18,000 to 36,000 pulses per minute). Thus, as the pacemaker battery or cell voltage drops, rather than looking for an end-of-life rate drop of a few pulses per minute, the telemetry system provides for the relatively easy detection of a decrease of thousands of cycles per minute. The higher frequency additionally provides a convenient data carrier that allows simultaneous transmission of the condition of multiple pacemaker functions through use of short-term, transient frequency changes that appear as FM (frequency modulated) pulses relative to the average background frequency.

It may be easiest for the nonengineer to conceptualize the telemetry system as an electronic window into the pacemaker that simultaneously assesses multiple electronic functions in a manner not entirely dissimilar to an electronic automobile engine analyzer. Thus, multiple vital pacemaker functions can be examined without interfering with electrocardiographic and other physiologic data. Parameters that have to date been utilized in clinical follow-up programs include direct monitoring of cell voltage, ECG-independent stimulation rate, hermetic encapsulation integrity, electrode stimulation impedance, power cell impedance, refractory interval duration, and a sense event indicator. An indicator of optimal location of the magnet and telemetry probe, which assists the patient in correct positioning of the magnet for pacemaker conversion to the fixed rate mode, as required for standard rate change follow-up, is also part of the telemetry system.

Technique

It might logically be assumed that a transmitter capable of sending multiparameter data would add significantly to the size and complexity of the implanted pacemaker. However, the transmission system contained within the implant consists of only a low-powered, 10-microwatt, 3-transistor computer transmitter coupled to an electromagnetic transmission coil. Transmission distance is 2½ inches (without telephone linkup). Transmission and energy consumption take place only when the transmitter is activated by a magnet-controlled reed switch. In most applications this occurs simultaneously with magnet activation of the fixed rate mode for standard rate change monitoring. In Figure 23–2, the telemetry subcarrier band of frequencies

chosen for the initial telemetry pacemakers is illustrated, as well as the position of the international music standard note A, above middle C, which is 440 Hz. Thus the frequencies activated in the external receiver by the telemetry system are in the audible range of tones commonly encountered in daily living. The simplest form of monitor for an implanted telemetry pacemaker would include only a standard pacemaker magnet to turn on the implanted monitoring system and an inexpensive pocket transistor radio to pick up the transmission from the pacer. A tuning fork is tapped or a pitch pipe is blown to determine the location of international music standard note A. The basic status of the implant can be determined by listening to the tone coming from the radio. Any tone of higher pitch than A indicates normal function of the

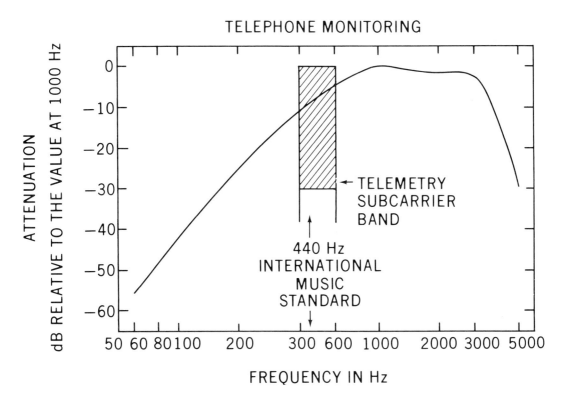

TELEPHONE MONITORING

Fig. 23–2. Range of frequencies from 300 to 600 Hz used in the multiparameter telemetry pacemaker monitoring system. For comparison, ECG transtelephonic transmission is done in the range of 1500 Hz—the high-pitched squeal heard when activating an ECG transmitter.

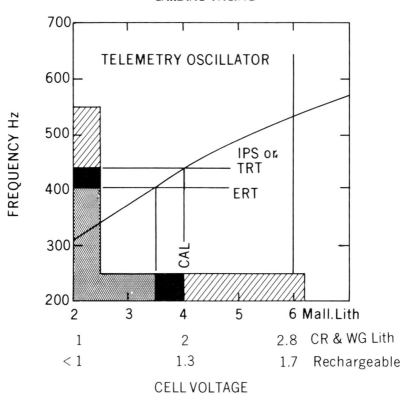

Fig. 23–3. Calibration of a pacemaker telemetry oscillator so that transmission of a particular frequency directly correlates with a particular voltage for a given implanted pacemaker power source. The calibration frequency and increased patient surveillance points are identical at 440 Hz. CAL = calibration point; IPS = increased patient surveillance point; TRT = total recharge required for a rechargeable system; ERT = elective replacement time; Mall. Lith = Mallory lithium pacemaker battery; CR & WG Lith = Catalyst Research or Wilson Greatbatch lithium-iodine cells; Rechargeable = rechargeable silver-mercury-silver-zinc pacemaker cell.

pacemaker power cell. Frequencies below A indicate a depleted or near-depleted power cell.

More sophisticated monitoring is required to determine impedances, timing intervals, and precise power source voltage. Figure 23–3 illustrates the calibration of a variety of voltages against the chosen range of telemetry frequencies. The diagnostic telemetry oscillator is trimmed during manufacture, so that it transmits at a frequency of over 500 cycles per second when the power source is adequate and at a frequency of 400 cycles per second or below when the power source requires replacement.

Power Source Voltage

Since the data are not carried by the stimulation rate of the pacemaker, the telemetric information pertaining to cell voltage is more comprehensive than previously possible. Figure 23–4 indicates the scale of a typical analog meter for direct determination of implanted pacemaker power source voltage. From Figure 23–3, it can now be understood that the implanted pacemaker, when activated magnetically, transmits a frequency that is a direct function of its power source voltage. The received frequency is converted back to voltage and displayed on the meter or a digital

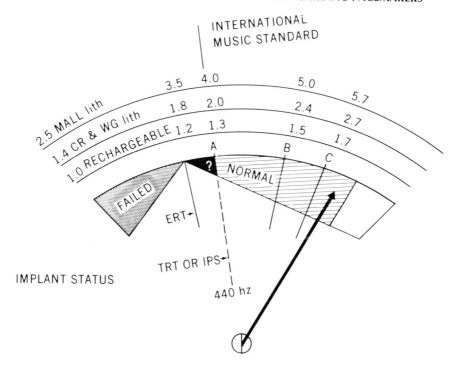

Fig. 23–4. Dial of an analog meter for direct determination of voltage of implanted pacemaker power cell or battery as determined by transmission of different frequencies as explained in Figure 23–3 (same abbreviations). For physicians and patients who prefer a self-monitoring technique, the precise voltage readouts can be deleted from the scale and the monitor used as a self-assessment device based on a red light, green light system. All frequencies above 440 Hz will activate a green light assuring the patient that function of the implanted pacemaker system is normal. Frequencies below 440 Hz will activate a yellow or red light indicating that the patient should contact professional follow-up more or less urgently, depending upon the color of the light.

readout. A frequency of 440 Hz would indicate 4 volts for a Mallory lithium battery (21 cells), 2 volts for a Catalyst Research or a Wilson Greatbatch cell, and 1.3 volts for a Mallory silver-mercury-silver-zinc rechargeable cell (Figs. 23–3, 23–4). In the third model, this frequency defines the need for total recharging.

Figure 23–5 shows voltage and rate telemetry data from a silver-mercury-silver-zinc rechargeable pacemaker used in a clinical program at the Pennsylvania State University. The telemetry system was initially developed for direct voltage monitoring of the rechargeable cell because the relatively large voltage fluctuations of 1.35 to 1.7 volts during recharging far exceeded the voltage changes with total cell discharge, i.e., the drop from 1.35 volts to 1.25 volts. In a voltage-sensitive rate monitoring system, each recharging of the pacemaker would have been associated with rate variability. Pacemakers of this type have functioned for over four years in patients without a single pacing or telemetry failure.

In the two lithium cells that have been used in clinical implantations of our telemetry system, 440 Hz is the point at which patient surveillance should be increased. When this frequency is reached, after several years of implantation in the usual case, biweekly monitoring is recommended.

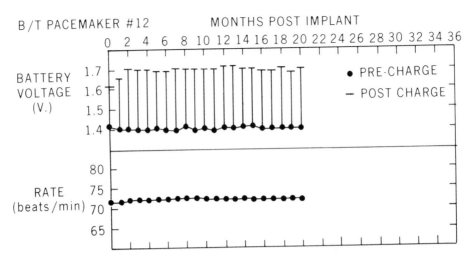

Fig. 23–5. Telemetry follow-up data from a patient with a Brownlee-Tyers, Penn State, silver-mercury-silver-zinc rechargeable pacemaker. Relatively large fluctuations in voltage with recharging are evident. Also evident is the lack of sensitivity of the pacing circuit in this device to battery voltage changes, a desirable feature for a rechargeable pacemaker.

It should be stressed that the intent of the inventors was to have a common end-of-life indicator frequency regardless of the power cell chosen for the implantable pacemaker. This feature would greatly simplify pacemaker follow-up, and an inexpensive standard that allows gross determination of normal or abnormal function, without the need for sophisticated monitoring equipment, is internationally available. Further, the time to replace the pacer is the most critical information required, regarding patient safety. It is feasible, however, to design a built-in pacemaker telemetry system and specific receiver of the type under discussion, to provide end-of-life indicators and dynamic data transmission, using a different range of frequencies. The design of interference-free transmission equipment for frequencies in the 1000 to 2000 Hz range is somewhat simplified, a potential advantage of a higher frequency system. For the individual unit, the critical factor is not the frequency range chosen but the matched calibration of a given implanted pacemaker and its external diagnostic analyzer.

Hermetic Integrity of Encapsulation

"Hermetic encapsulation" of pacemakers through the use of welded metallic enclosures has been as instrumental as the invention of the lithium cell in the development of long-life pacemakers. The massive number of early failures and recalls of epoxy-potted units, due principally to body fluid intrusion, is evidence enough that the delicate electronics used in pacemaker circuits require sophisticated protection from the caustic biologic environment.[4] Although there is little doubt that welded metallic hermetic pacemaker enclosures can withstand the implant environment for periods of up to five years, there is no real time *in vivo* data to substantiate the hermetic integrity of the encapsulation technology used, for the up to 20-year range currently being estimated by pacemaker manufacturers. At this phase of the lithium era, there are too few pacemakers implanted for periods over five years for any real assurance that hermetic encapsulation will not eventually present another weak link in the pacemaker system, just as the inadequacies of current electrodes are being exposed by the greater reliability of solid state lithium cells. There is no guarantee that the helium leak rate measured by manufacturers during construction of pacemakers can be maintained several years postimplant, and even if maintained there are still unknowns regarding the correlation of the water vapor penetration rate and the measured helium leak rate.[8] Metal and weld corrosion effects, and helium-to-water leak rate correlations are under serious investigation at several institutions.

As an added assurance of patient safety, it would be desirable to monitor the chronic long-term hermetic integrity of pacemakers noninvasively, using a method that allows elective replacement prior to pacemaker failure from gradual or premature fluid penetration of the hermetic enclosure. Even if current encapsulation technology proves to be adequate for 20-year electronic implants, occasional random weld or enclosure failures can be expected in any large commercial product series. Such random failures can potentially lead to unnecessary and costly recalls of all units in the related manufacturing series, the majority of which may well be inviolate and capable of years of normal function. Thus, chronic hermeticity monitoring has great potential for eliminating both morbidity and expensive replacement surgery for the majority of pacemaker patients. Constant checking of the internal relative humidity of the implanted pacemaker noninvasively is another feature of the telemetry diagnostic system.

Two hermeticity detection systems have been applied. The oldest and simplest was incorporated in a series of Mallory lithium battery-powered pacemakers. These units transmitted the usual range of frequencies indicative of power cell voltage and also stimulation rate by periodic modulation of the basic carrier frequency. The electronics and the cell were independently hermetically sealed within a third outer hermetic

package, the pacer case. The telemetry circuit was located between the inner and outer hermetic packages so that failure of the main outer seal would result in wetting and shorting of only the telemetry circuitry, leading to deviant or abnormal telemetry frequencies and thereby alerting the physician or follow-up center. Figure 23–6 illustrates voltage, pulse rate, and hermeticity monitoring data from one of the Mallory lithium battery-powered pacemakers. Continued hermeticity of the outer case seal is confirmed by the presence of the normal telemetry transmission frequencies at each monitoring session.

An alternative form of hermeticity detection has been developed. Sensors are available (for example, lithium chloride polyvinyl alcohol) which change their electrical conductivity when exposed to moisture. At a given humidity (we have chosen 65%) the high resistance or low conductivity of the humidity grid (in the range of several megohms at low humidities) acutely decreases. The sudden appearance of this low resistance component in the telemetry circuit produces a characteristic PacerGram (Fig. 23–7) and voltage changes.

A variety of methods of employing the humidity grids are under study. In future digital monitoring systems, LED readouts could indicate a dry, moist, or wet implant, or the relative humidity within the pacemaker capsule could be calibrated and externally monitored. Pacemakers are now assembled in a dry, inert gas environment, and internal humidities well below 10% are sought. An internal humidity detector set to indicate a warning when humidity reaches 65% would thus have no significant risk of false positive indication of impending moisture-related failure, as a significant defect of the hermetic capsule would be required for the internal humidity to rise from less than 10% to over 60%. On the other hand, it could be assumed that this would be a relatively effective early warning system, as the pacemaker circuitry might be expected to function for some time even in

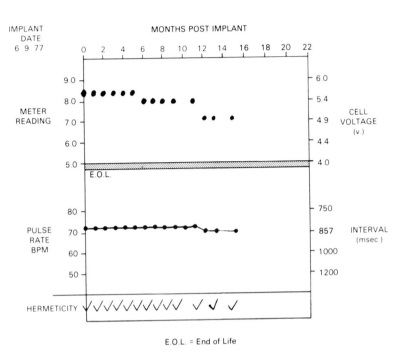

Fig. 23–6. Data from 15 months of transtelephonic telemetry follow-up of a Mallory lithium battery-powered pacemaker showing the multiple voltage plateaus of this complex cathode battery and the continued integrity of the hermetic seal.

PACERGRAM

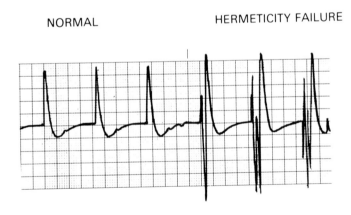

Fig. 23–7. Normal tracing compared with the tracing resulting from an internal humidity grid being exposed to greater than 65% relative humidity.

a relative humidity of 80 to 90%. With a coating of parylene or other barrier material over the internal components, except the humidity sensor, the pacemaker might be expected to continue to function for a year or more after 65% humidity is reached. It should be emphasized that a hermeticity monitor not only would protect those few patients in whom a hermetic seal failure occurred, but also would allow examination of all patients with an implant from any given manufacturing series. It would be possible to determine which units (the majority) are indeed dry and to exclude them from any moisture-related pacemaker recall requiring pacemaker explantation. If a significant number of units in a given series have hermeticity problems, it would still be prudent to increase the frequency of monitoring the whole series.

Electrode Stimulation Impedance

Electrode resistance/impedance parameters and internal lithium-iodine cell resistance phenomena are contained in the data transmitted from an implanted pacemaker that harbors our diagnostic telemetry system. According to the inventor of the lithium-iodine cell, power cell impedance is the most critical direct parameter to monitor, to establish the depletion mechanism and remaining energy of a lithium-iodine power cell.[9] Electrode impedance parameters play an important role in the rate of cell depletion.

The reasons for developing an improved method of pacemaker follow-up include the introduction of improved power source, encapsulation, circuit, and electrode technologies which for the first time give credence to the advertising claims that pacemakers of present design have potential implant lifetimes in the range of 3 to 20 years depending on the multiple variables discussed in the introduction. The critical factor controlling longevity is the energy requirement during pacing, and this de-

pends on a number of stimulus parameters (programmable in some pacemakers), electrode surface area and other factors. Stimulation impedance includes the resistance in the electrode wire carrying the stimulus from the pacemaker to the heart (relatively small, ranging from 5 to 120 ohms) and the resistance to the passage of the electrical pulse from the end of the electrode into the myocardial tissue (electrode-tissue interface impedance) which may vary from measurement to measurement.

Physicians are used to thinking of high resistance or impedance conditions as being detrimental. However, a large surface area electrode or a lead with rupture of its silicone or other insulating material sheath requires high pulse energy to provide a given threshold of myocardial current density. Thus, low resistance phenomena result in early battery depletion, whereas high resistance electrode designs with small surface areas are associated with much lower energy utilization during pacing and thus extended pacemaker battery or cell life.[10-12] The normal stimulation impedance for a large surface area electrode of 50 to 100 mm² approximates 300 ohms, whereas the normal impedance for a 5 to 8 mm² electrode is in the range of 1000 to 2000 ohms.[13] The Lewin-Parsonnet differential current density electrode can register impedances in the range of 3000 ohms under conditions that are optimal as far as pacing threshold and battery energy conservation are concerned.[13]

Regardless of the impedance of a particular electrode system, it should be evident that a drop in postimplant impedance indicates potential loss of the insulating sheath and development of excess energy drain. A sharp rise in impedance indicates potential fracture of the metallic conductive material of the lead.[14] With a stimulation impedance measured in the 1000 ohm range at the time of pacemaker lead implantation, acute and chronic variations consistent with normal function following implantation may potentially range from as little as 500 ohms, to as high as 3000 ohms, since limited clinical data are available on this subject. However, a decrease in stimulation impedance below 500 ohms will likely indicate a problem either with sealing of the electrode hub in the connector of the pacemaker or failure of the electrode lead insulation sheath. In contrast, an impedance rising acutely towards infinity after a long, relatively stable period will indicate fracture of the metallic coil or multistrand conductor. The availability of noninvasive telemetry monitoring of the impedance of chronically implanted pacemaker electrode systems should also help to expand our knowledge of the normal range of variability of stimulation impedance.

Power Cell Impedance

The noninvasive determination of the stimulation impedance and electrode continuity with the telemetry system is closely tied in with the noninvasive assessment of internal resistance change in the pacemaker power source. Even with frequent and early postimplant monitoring of rate to establish the baseline from which cell voltage decay must be measured, multiple factors complicate the usefulness of stimulation rate change as the primary pacemaker follow-up parameter. Cell voltage is dependent on both the power cell impedance and stimulation energy requirements.

With the older Mallory mercury-zinc batteries, there was little internal resistance at any time during the functional life of a cell. With a number of the lithium systems, especially the organic cells, low internal resistance is also the rule, but with the Wilson Greatbatch and Catalyst Research lithium halogen (lithium-iodine, lithium-bromine) power cells used in the majority of pacemakers, resistance within the power cell is initially in the range of a few hundred to a few thousand ohms and gradually rises during depletion of the cell energy, to a level, depending on cell design, of from

15,000 to 30,000 ohms.[9] Unlike voltage and therefore rate, which change minimally and very late in a solid state lithium cell as it is slowly discharged, impedance in the lithium halogen systems rises in a more or less time linear fashion from beginning to end-of-life, if the energy consumption rate is continuous. Thus the cell impedance defines the energy removed from the cell and the approximate capacity remaining (Fig. 23–8).

If the end-of-life impedance of a lithium system was 30,000 ohms and it could be determined that the impedance within the implanted cell was 29,000 ohms, end of pacemaker life would be imminent and prophylactic replacement would be indicated. This would be no more informative than the usual monitoring of rate change with the older mercury-zinc systems where a decreasing rate at the same time point would indicate the need for prophylactic replacement. However, a measured impedance of 15,000 ohms would indicate that about half the capacity had been removed from the power source. With a stimulation rate changed related system, the rate at this halfway point in the life of the pacemaker could be nearly identical with the rate at the time of implant, particularly with small surface area electrodes.

The PacerGram

Figure 23–9 illustrates the next step in the monitoring procedure after voltage determination, although it must be emphasized that all of the monitoring steps are performed simultaneously and only a few minutes of the patient's time are required. In Figure 23–9, an in-hospital electrocardiogram (ECG) that was obtained following pacemaker implantation is illustrated on the left. A Teletronics analyzer was used at the time of implantation to measure the intraoperative electrode impedance. At 1200 ohms it is somewhat higher than usually encountered with the Intermedics' lead, model number 465, with a surface area of 12

LITHIUM-IODINE POWER SOURCE END-OF-LIFE
MONITORING BY CELL IMPEDANCE

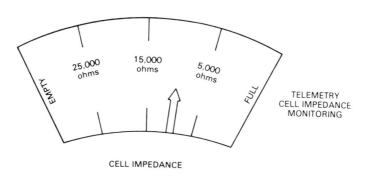

CELL IMPEDANCE

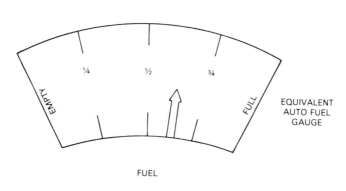

FUEL

Fig. 23–8. Comparison of telemetry monitoring of implanted lithium iodine power cell impedance (above) to a standard auto fuel gauge (below). With cell impedance monitoring, the follow-up physician can determine within 10%, the relative capacity remaining at the power source ¼, ½, and ¾ depletion points.

mm². The accuracy of this reading was verified by a direct method involving the measurement of average current drain during stimulation with a calibrated external pacemaker. A transtelephonic PacerGram is illustrated on the right side of Figure 23–9.

The PacerGram is obtained on ECG paper, and at first glance looks somewhat like an aberrant ECG. Comparison with the ECG to the left shows that this is an entirely different type of strip chart recording. The implanted telemetry system taps into the pacemaker circuitry and transmits dynamic functions of the pacemaker, including the output stimulus pulse energy, represented by the large upward deflection. The deflection is a measure of the brief increase in telemetry frequency required to transmit that data.

Activation of the sensing circuit at the end of the refractory period following the pacemaker stimulus is indicated by the small marker pulse just prior to return of the tracing to baseline. The size of the large positive deflection correlates with pulse width and stimulus current and thus with the energy delivered to the myocardium with each pacemaker stimulus. The refractory period is determined by counting the

DEMAND PACER WITH TELEMETRY (T) MONITORING —

Interlith model No. 223-04   S. No. 01000   Patient G.M.   Date 2/24/78
Pacer rate 72/minute   Pulse width 0.58 msec.
Stimulation impedance at time of implantation 1200 ohms
Intermedics TV lead Model No. 465, surface area 12 mm^2

EKG

John Sealy Hospital, Galveston, Texas

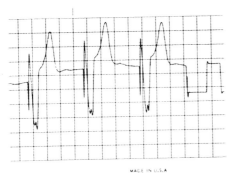

MADE IN U.S.A

TRANSTELEPHONIC PACERGRAM

Intermedics Inc., Freeport, Texas
T-stimulus current - 13 mm
T-meter reading 7.6 (cell voltage 2.7v)
T-pacing + sensing refractory interval
320 msec.
T-rate - 73/min.

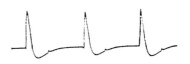

T-stimulation impedance 1100 ohms
T-cell impedance 2 Kohms

Fig. 23–9.   Implant data, a postimplant electrocardiogram, and a transtelephonic PacerGram transmitted approximately 100 miles the day following pacemaker implantation. T indicates transtelephonic transmission of telemetered data from the implanted pacemaker. The derivation of all the telemetered parameters including refractory interval is explained in the text.

spaces on the paper, (each small division is 40 msec as with the standard ECG running at a paper speed of 25/mm/sec). Thus, the 8 divisions from the beginning of the large spike to the end of the small spike equal 320 msec, the specified refractory period for this particular implanted unit. The pacemaker implanted in this patient is an Intermedics model 223–04, a standard InterLith with the addition of our telemetry transmitting circuit. The Intermedics Cyberlith, a multiprogrammable pacer also incorporates our telemetry circuitry, including a sense event marker as a small positive deflection of the PacerGram that corresponds to each sensed spontaneous beat. This feature confirms normal functioning of the demand circuitry and also allows for telemetry transmission of the normal spontaneous rate.

At the bottom right of Figure 23–9, T-stimulation impedance of 1100 ohms and T-cell impedance of 2000 ohms (2 kohms) are recorded. The stimulation impedance measured 1200 ohms at the time of implantation the previous day, affirming the accuracy of this feature of our system. As the power cell within the pacemaker is relatively new, depending on pacemaker shelf life and elapsed time since manufacture, the impedance of the power cell would also be expected to be low, and this is confirmed.

Nomogram

Figure 23–10 illustrates the derivation of the electrode stimulation impedance and power cell impedance from the telemetered stimulus energy (PacerGram, in Fig. 23–9) and telemetered power source voltage (analog meter, Fig. 23–4). Stimulus energy is plotted vertically and voltage is plotted horizontally. Calibration at the time of pacemaker manufacture allows postimplant derivation of cell impedance and electrode impedance from cell voltage and energy drain, employing the Figure 23–10 nomogram, by transecting the known points of pulse energy and cell voltage. Thus a meter reading of 7.7 (2.7 volts for a Catalyst Research 802 series cell) and a PacerGram

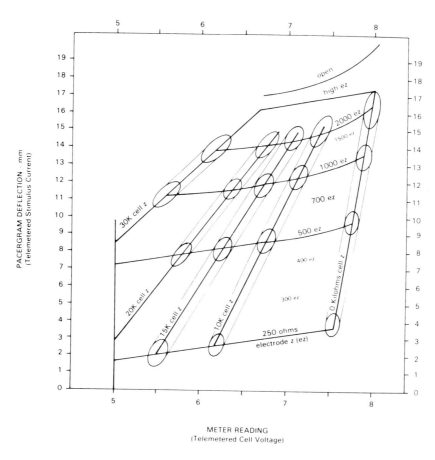

STANDARD DEVIATION ELLIPSES OF TELEMETRY DATA FOR INTERLITH TL MODEL
NO. 223-04s Serial Nos. 01000 - 01019

METER READING
(Telemetered Cell Voltage)

Fig. 23–10. Diagnostic chart for determination of stimulation impedance and implanted power cell or battery impedance. As several different cells with different voltage ranges have been used to power recent pacers, both parameters are in arbitrary units. Conversion tables are available for particular cells. Use of this Ohm's law nomogram to determine the impedances is explained in the text. A simplified method involving direct digital readout of all of the telemetered parameters is currently being developed. ez = electrode stimulation impedance; cell z = cell impedance; mm = millimeters.

deflection of 9.5 mm transect the point where the 500 ohm electrode impedance and zero ohm cell impedance lines cross. Similarly, a meter reading of 7.5 and a PacerGram deflection of 13 mm indicates an electrode stimulation impedance of 1000 ohms and power cell impedance of 2000 ohms.

The nomogram method of determining impedances from telemetered coordinate points may seem a little difficult but is no more complex than the acid-base nomograms formerly used in the clinical practice of medicine. Digital techniques now being developed will provide printout or display of the numerical values for voltage, rate, refractory interval, electrode impedance, cell impedance, and other parameters all virtually instantaneously with placement of the monitor probe over the site of the pacemaker implant. The frequency data may be recorded by a digital display analyzer in the physician's office or may be transmitted from the patient's home to the physician's office or to a centralized monitoring service.

Pacing Energy Capacity

The fuel gauge in an automobile and power source monitoring of a pacemaker have the same objective: to determine the status of the fuel supply so that it can be replaced prior to an emergency. Rate change monitoring can result in a nearly constant stimulation rate until just prior to loss of all pacing function. This is equivalent to an automobile fuel gauge that flashes a green light from the time the tank is full until it is 98% empty and begins to flash a red light only when the tank is 99% empty. With this type of fuel gauge one must continually stop the car and put a dip stick in the tank to determine the actual fuel level, a situation not entirely different from weekly or biweekly transtelephonic pacemaker rate change monitoring with conversion of the pacemaker to the fixed rate

mode. The equivalence of periodic cell impedance monitoring to a standard automobile fuel gauge is illustrated in Figure 23–8. Thus lithium halogen cell impedance monitoring allows the following physician not only to predict impending end of life but also to assess the relative pacing energy capacity remaining.

By knowing the energy consumption rate for the individual patient (PacerGram), telemetry follow-up allows almost total power source energy to be utilized prior to pacemaker replacement. Figure 23–11 illustrates a sample follow-up data form for a patient with a multiparameter programmable output pacer featuring our multiparameter noninvasive telemetry follow-up system. Direct assessment of pacemaker cell voltage, pacemaker power cell impedance, stimulation rate, stimulation impedance, electrode conductor integrity, electrode insulation integrity, sensing circuit refractory interval, and hermetic integrity are all possible. Although not indicated on the chart, the important parameters related to assessment of energy usage (PacerGram) and prediction of end of life are obtained as illustrated for the nonprogrammable demand pacer in Figure 23–9.

Clinical Trials

Multiparameter telemetry monitoring is no more difficult than commonly used transtelephonic ECG monitoring methods. In fact, the patient's telemetry monitoring equipment indicates when the magnet or telemetry probe is in the correct position over the pacemaker. The patient is actually assisted in activating the fixed rate mode for standard rate change monitoring as well as multiparameter telemetry monitoring. With some elderly patients, the precise positioning of the magnet to activate the fixed-rate mode for rate change monitoring is a problem that may extend the individual's monitoring time for as long as 10 or 15 minutes. The personnel involved in the

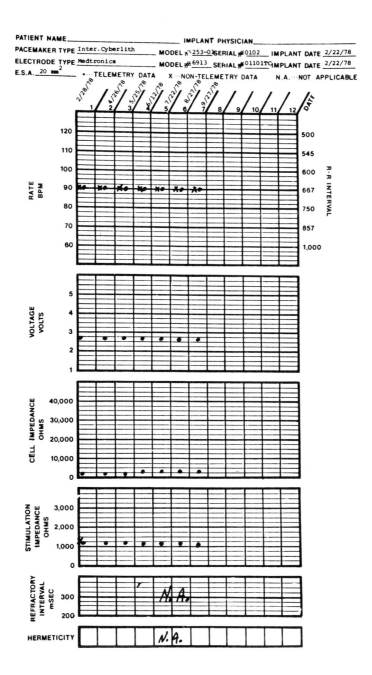

Fig. 23–11. Multiparameter telemetric follow-up data from a patient with an Intermedics Cyberlith multiparameter programmable pacer and a transthoracic 20 mm² surface area Medtronic electrode. This unit features a sense event marker rather than a refractory interval marker as illustrated in Figure 23–9. Initial models did not contain a relative humidity grid.

trials of this follow-up system are appreciative of the time saved during combined ECG and telemetry monitoring.

To date several hundred clinical telemetry implants have been performed. Pacemaker and lead functions are plotted regularly as illustrated in Figures 23–5, 23–6, and 23–11. After one to four years, normal voltage curves for the power cells used have been recorded. Seven to 10 months following implantation of the solid state lithium systems, power cell impedance has risen into the range of 3000 to 5000 ohms, while cell voltage and rate have dropped only fractionally from the values measured after manufacture. Electrode impedance has ranged from 300 to over 2000 ohms, depending on electrode surface area and implantation site. Stimulation impedances in most units have been stable after an initial rise during the first six weeks or so following implantation. In an occasional patient, stimulation impedances have shown fluctuations with time, probably on a physiologic basis. To date, since no lead in the test series has failed, no acute fall or rise in stimulation impedance, indicative of insulation or conductor failure, has been demonstrated.

The telemetry system is used for self-monitoring in a limited number of patients and for monitoring in the physician's office or clinic, including transtelephonic transmission of all of the multiparameter data. The refractory interval has been precisely monitored in all of the Intermedics 223–04 implanted units and has remained in the 315 to 320 millisecond range in all cases. In a few patients, it has been possible to demonstrate that early non-sensed premature ventricular contractions fell within the refractory period and were not indicative of abnormal slew rate or abnormal pacemaker function.[15]

Monitoring Packaged Pacemakers

The maximum transmission distance from a telemetry pacer to the external monitoring probe is approximately 2½ inches. Another application of the telemetry system is its activation through the shipping container. Multiparameter normal function of a pacemaker can thus be confirmed prior to its final distribution to a hospital or the operating field, without interfering with the container or sterile seal. The functions that can be telemetered through the sterile package include rate, cell voltage, refractory period, and hermeticity. Although a failed unit can be detected under these circumstances, the pacemaker is not loaded by an electrode and the heart, so that a relatively rundown battery would still show a relatively normal voltage and rate.

Verification of Telemetry Function

Accurate function of our telemetry system can be verified in a number of ways. The rate of the telemetry output energy waveform as displayed on a PacerGram can be checked against the rate on an ECG or digital chest probe (e.g., Instromedix Inc. Miniclinic). Telemetry electrode stimulation impedance can be checked against the intraoperative determination with one of a variety of analyzers available. Unless the new power cell has been damaged or shorted, its voltage and impedance fall within narrow ranges and can be verified by initial telemetry recordings. Similarly, the limits of normal refractory intervals of a given type of unit are generally well defined, and the refractory period as initially determined by the first telemetry transmission should fall within these limits.

Telemetry voltage transmissions are accurate to two decimal places. Standard deviations of impedance parameters are indicated by ellipses around the calibration points on Figure 23–10. When the telemetry system reads an electrode stimulation impedance of 1100 ohms, the true impedance of the implanted system may be only 1000 ohms. However, a 10 to 20% range in readout of cell and electrode stimulation impedance values is not of clinical significance. Reading a stimulation impedance of 1100 ohms when the true value is really 1000 ohms does not significantly affect power drain or longevity calculations and will not be mistaken for failure of either a conductor (impedance approaching infinity) or an insulation sheath or connector (a very low impedance). Similarly, internal power cell impedances of 1000, 2000 or 3000 ohms all indicate a relatively new cell.

The prime function of the telemetry system is to provide a method for noninvasively assessing the condition of the implanted pacemaker power cell, circuitry, lead, and hermetic enclosure. When malfunction is suspected, the telemetry system will usually allow the physician to assure himself and the patient that the pacemaker is performing its life-sustaining or life-improving function normally, or to determine the precise malfunction, so that appropriate treatment may be instituted without delay.

Perspective

Used in conjunction with a standard transtelephonic ECG system, our telemetry system provides an unprecedented advance in the technology of follow-up care for pacemaker patients. The general efficacy of applying a multiparameter monitoring system within an implanted pacemaker has been clinically proven. Several refinements and additions to the telemetry pacemaker follow-up system are currently being studied. To obtain follow-up data about the patient and the pacemaker with the current system, both a surface ECG probe and a telemetry PacerGram "radio" probe are required. The surface ECG is sensed with chest or wrist electrodes. Vital pacemaker data are obtained by applying a telemetry probe directly over the pacemaker implant site. The simplicity of this technology can be advanced by the addition of subcutane-

ous or noncardiac intravenous electrodes to monitor ECG data and/or the intracardiac electrogram. The signal detected from the implanted ECG sensing electrode is connected directly to the pacemaker telemetry transmitter. All comprehensive ECG and telemetry data can then be received with a single external monitoring probe, eliminating the need for separate ECG and telemetry probes and wrist bands. Advantages related to simplification of the patient's transtelephonic monitoring exercise are obvious. Automatic performance of most of the monitoring tasks minimizes the patient's difficulties. Elimination of the skin-ECG probe contact also eliminates many interference problems associated with skin potentials, as well as placement difficulties commonly encountered with patient ECG monitoring systems.

The number of specific physiologic and pacemaker parameters that can be monitored is limited only by the imagination of those implementing the system and, of equal import, the increased production costs related to calibrating and trimming the diagnostic transmission system. For example, calibration of an intrinsic sense event marker at the time of pacemaker manufacture allows chronic noninvasive evaluation of R-wave magnitude and assessment of its physiologic variations. There is little doubt that acquisition of comprehensive data, through study of calibrated electromagnetic "radio waves" transmitted directly through the pacemaker capsule to external reception equipment, is the optimal link for assessing the physiologic condition of the patient and the status of the implant.

It is somewhat ironic that recent technical advances enhancing the potential for improved pacemaker longevity also dictate the need for improved patient follow-up surveillance techniques. The new implant monitoring system incorporating the built-in independent surveillance transmitter circumvents the numerous deficiencies encountered with the simpler rate change systems historically used for power source surveillance. Widespread adoption of a standard reference tone (international music tone A suggested) for indicating impending implant dysfunction may eventually allow implementation of a true standard for implant surveillance, applicable to all pacemakers and to newer biologic implants for cardiac arrhythmia control.

REFERENCES

1. Tyers, G.F.O., and Brownlee, R.R.: Current status of pacemaker power sources. Ann. Thorac. Surg., 25:571, 1978.

2. Simmon, A. B., and Zloto, A.E.: Atrioventricular block; natural history after permanent ventricular pacing. Am. J. Cardiol., 41:500, 1978.

3. Bruce, R.G.: Cardiac pacemaker usage survey. Paine, Webber, Mitchell, Hutchins Inc. Status Report, pp. 1–14, 1978.

4. Tyers, G.F.O., and Brownlee, R.R.: The non-hermetically sealed pacemaker myth, or, Navy-Ribicoff 22,000—FDA-Weinberger O. J. Thorac. Cardiovasc. Surg., 71:253, 1976.

5. Tyers, G.F.O.: Monitoring programs for pacemaking. Cardiovascular Surgery, Amer. Coll. Surg. Postgrad. Course, pp. 17–20, 1978.

6. Cordis Corp.: Reported inadvertent reprogramming of Omni-Stanicor pacers with a permanent magnet. Cordis Technical Memorandum 24, Feb. 25, 1977.

7. Brownlee, R.R., et al.: Monitoring system for cardiac pacemakers. Trans. Am. Soc. Artif. Intern. Organs, 13:65, 1977.

8. DerMarderosian, A., and Gionet, V.: An experimental and theoretical analysis of the rate of water vapor penetration into nonhermetic enclosures. *In* Reliability Technology for Cardiac Pacemakers. National Bureau of Standards, Gaithersburg, Maryland, 1977.

9. Schneider, A.A., and Kraus, F.E.: End life characteristics of the lithium iodine cell. *In* Reliability Technology for Cardiac Pacemakers. National Bureau of Standards, Gaithersburg, Maryland, 1977.

10. Furman, S., Parker, B., and Escher, D.J.W.: Decreasing electrode size and increasing efficiency of cardiac stimulation. J. Surg. Res., 11:105, 1971.

11. Tyers, G.F.O., Torman, H.A., and Hughes, H.C. Jr.: Comparative studies of "state of the art" and presently used clinical cardiac pacemaker electrodes. J. Thorac. Cardiovasc. Surg., 67:849, 1974.

12. Fangman, T. R., and Michie, D. D.: Effects of an increase in operating load upon the energy output of implantable cardiac pacemakers. J. Cardiovasc. Surg., 12:286, 1971.

13. Tyers, G.F.O., et al.: Myocardial stimulation impedance—the effects of electrode, physiologic and stimulus variables. Ann. Thorac. Surg., 27:63, 1979.

14. Calvin, J.W.: Intraoperative pacemaker electrical testing. Ann Thorac. Surg., 26:165, 1978.

15. Furman, S., Hurzeler, P., and DeCaprio, V.: Cardiac pacing and pacemakers. III. Sensing the cardiac electrogram. Am. Heart J., 93:794, 1977.

Index

Page numbers in *italics* indicate illustrations; "t" indicates tabular matter.

369

Linder, transesophageal cardiac rhythm control by, 7
Lithium cell. *See* Battery(ies), lithium
Lithium iodine cell. *See* Battery(ies), lithium iodine
Lown, cardioversion and, 8
Ludwig, electrical current of heart and, 77

MACWILLIAM, on transthoracic rhythmic stimuli, 6
Magnet, location of, telemetric monitoring of, 352
Magnetic coupling, 329–331, *330*
Magnetic fields, low frequency, 334
Mahaim fibers, 77, *76*
"Map," ventricular, myocardial testing sites designated by, 260, *260, 261*
Marmorstein, electrostimulation by, 5, 7
Mauro, radiofrequency receiver of, 10
Mediastinoscopy, placement of electrode lead by, 169
Medtronic sutureless myocardial leads, 146, 160–162, *161, 162*
Medtronic Xyrel pacemakers, 252, *253*
Mercury-zinc battery, problems with, 45–46
Microwave fields, pacemakers and, 335
Minithoracotomy, anterior transaxillary implantation of myocardial leads by, 155, *155, 156*
Mobile transmitters, pacemakers and, 335–336
Mobitz type block. *See* Atrioventricular block, second degree
Monaca, interim external pacing by, 10
Morgagni-Adams-Stokes syndrome, electrostimulation in, 1, 7, 8–9
Muscle(s), activity of, demand pacemaker inhibition by, 302
 cardiac, electroresponsive quality of, 2–3
 chest wall, stimulation of, 236
 diaphragmatic, stimulation of, 236
 skeletal, stimulation of, 236
Myers, energy from body fluids and, 10
Myocardial infarction, acute, bifascicular block in, 113–114
 permanent pacing in, 94–95
 temporary pacing in, 113, 139, 139t
 with atrioventricular and bundle branch blocks, mortality rate in, 94, 95
 anterior, temporary pacing in, 140
 heart rate and pacing in, 218
Myocardial test electrode, in pacing site selection, 155, 160, 259–261, *158–159, 259, 260, 261*
Myocardium, anatomy of, 74
 cells of, 74
 nonstimulatable, 63
 perforation of, by electrode, 288–289, *289*
 ventricular electrogram displaying, 275
 testing sites of, electrophysiologic measurements of, 261–262
 ventricular "map" designating, 260, *260, 261*

NACLERIO, threshold tester probe of, 11
Nathan, pulse generator used by, 10, 145
Needle, percutaneous, insertion of, 192–193
Nerve stimulators, pulse-producing, demand pacemaker and, 333–334
Noble, "platform" bipolar lead of, 9
Noise sampling period, of demand pacemakers, 295, *295*
Nomogram, for determination of impedances, 363–364, *363*
Nuclear power for pulse generators, 46, *47*
Nurse(s), 14
 clinical care by, 319
 predischarge teaching by, 321–323
 reassurance of patient by, 321

role of, in pacemaker malfunction, 320
 postoperative, in permanent pacing, 318
 in temporary pacing, 312–313
 preoperative, in permanent pacing, 316–317
 in temporary pacing, 308–309
 primary objectives of, 318
 technical care by, 319
 wound care by, 319
Nursing management, of patient with pacemaker, 307–324
Nysten, direct galvanization of heart by, 3–4

OCCUPATIONAL ASPECTS of permanent pacing, 317
Ohm's law, 193–194, 327–328, *193*
 in calculation of lead impedance, 233, 249, 251
 stated in equivalent way, 328
Omni external pacemakers, 199
Oscilloscopic recorder, 265
Overdrive system, external, in atrial programmed pacing, 175, *174*
 in supraventricular tachycardia, 183–184
 in sinus nodal dysfunction, 134–135
 suppression of sinus node by, 115, *115*
Oversensing, causes of, 234–235, 298, 299
 characteristics of, 298
 diagnosis of, 235
 of false signals, magnet eliminating, 301, *300*
 management in, 235
 secondary to large T wave voltage, 299, *299*

PACEMAKER(S), 39–45. *See also* Asynchronous pacemakers; Demand pacemakers; Synchronous pacemakers
 artificial, development of, 7, 9–10
 as mainstay of cardiac therapy, 59
 atrial, compared, 129–130
 discharge rates of, 219
 external, 310
 programmed, 171, 172–175, *174*
 atrioventricular, bifocal, 43
 in restoration of synchrony, 198
 sequential, 92–93
 external, 310
 benefits of, explained to patient, 321
 bipolar, and unipolar, compared, 71, 68t
 definition of, 67–68
 capture abnormalities of, causes of, 287–291
 cardiac output and, 197–198
 categories of, 39, 30t
 clinical applications of, during cardiac surgery, 195–198
 complications with, 229–238
 diagnosis of, 229
 in children, 238
 unusual, 238
 constant current, theoretical behavior of, 194, *195*
 constant voltage, relationship of current output to lead impedance in, 249, *249*
 theoretical behavior of, 194, *195*
 contemporary, 29, *49, 53*
 using hermetically sealed hybrid, 51, *53*
 costs of, 56, 346
 coupled, functions of, 219
 cumulative survival summary for, 344t
 "current-limited," 249
 cycle of, alert period of, 284
 downward displacement of, 137, *137*
 electrical discharge of, 194, *194*
 energy capacity of, telemetric follow-up data form showing, 364, *365*